Cancer Diagnosis

Cancer Diagnosis
New Concepts
and Techniques

Editors

Richard J. Steckel, M.D.

Professor of Radiological Sciences and
Professor of Radiation Oncology
UCLA School of Medicine and
Director, UCLA Jonsson Comprehensive Cancer Center
Los Angeles, California

A. Robert Kagan, M.D.

Associate Clinical Professor of Radiation Oncology
UCLA School of Medicine and
Chief, Department of Radiotherapy
Southern California Permanente Medical Group
Los Angeles, California

GRUNE & STRATTON

A Subsidiary of Harcourt Brace Jovanovich, Publishers
New York   London
Paris   San Diego   San Francisco   São Paulo
Sydney   Tokyo   Toronto

LIBRARY OF CONGRESS
CATALOG CARD NO.: 82-80605

Steckel, Richard J. and A. Robert Kagan
Cancer diagnosis: new concepts and techniques

New York : Grune & Stratton

450 p.

8203   820201

Grune & Stratton, Inc.
111 Fifth Avenue
New York, New York 10003

Distributed in the United Kingdom by
Academic Press Inc. (London) Ltd.
24/28 Oval Road, London NW 1

Library of Congress Catalog Number 82-80605
International Standard Book Number 0-8089-1451-0
Printed in the United States of America

Contents

Preface

It is not unusual for new developments in diagnostic techniques to occur parallel to developments in therapy. Whether diagnostic improvements catalyze new treatment techniques, or the reverse, is probably immaterial; both diagnostic and therapeutic progress often occur within the same or similar time frame. In the over 100 diseases known as cancer, many advances in palliative and curative treatment would not have been possible without the advent of new techniques for diagnosis and staging. The combined application in Hodgkin's disease of ordinary radiologic procedures, lymphography, diagnostic laparotomy (in selected cases), and now CT and ultrasound exemplifies how the targeting of specific therapy for different stages of this disease has been facilitated by improvements in diagnostic techniques and their judicious application. By effecting earlier diagnosis of certain cancers, imaging techniques may also make curative approaches more feasible.

In considering recent improvements in imaging that have implications for cancer diagnosis, one must address not only conventional radiography and the newer techniques of CT and ultrasound but also direct visualization through endoscopy. Improved cytologic techniques and histopathologic approaches to the classification of tumors (e.g., with Hodgkin's and non-Hodgkin's lymphomas) are important advances that are continuing to evolve. Finally, the identification of serum and urine "tumor markers" has made it easier to monitor responses in certain patients, particularly for those tumors that secrete substantial amounts of a specific substance or substances into the circulation.

While progress in treating cancer depends heavily on developing more accurate methods for diagnosing and staging the disease, insufficient research emphasis has always been given to the development of new diagnostic techniques. Along with the national concern for rising costs of health technologies, however, there has recently been an increased interest in evaluating clinical diagnostic methods, particularly the expensive newer imaging techniques. It has nevertheless been observed that high-volume utilization of relatively inexpensive diagnostic tests and procedures, rather than overutilization of more expensive techniques such as computed tomography, has accounted for much of the rising costs of patient care.* Dr. Arnold Relman

*Moloney, T.W., and Rogers, D.E.: Medical Technology—A Different View of the Continuous Debate Over Cost. New England Journal of Medicine, Vol. 301 #26, pp. 1413–1419, December 27, 1979.

has remarked that, while we spent $12–$14 billion on laboratory tests last year in the United States, the total bill for diagnostic radiological procedures was $8 billion, and less than 10 percent of the latter was for CT scanning.* Even if we succeed in devising more effective restraints on the use of diagnostic tests, we must consider whether we currently possess the knowledge necessary to discriminate between the useful and the less useful diagnostic examinations that are now in use. Oncologists often use radiologic studies in an ineffectual and costly manner. This "blunderbuss" method must be replaced by a better planned and more reasoned approach. More careful selection of diagnostic procedures with an understanding of their limitations as well as their advantages, improved communications between radiologists and clinicians, and a better understanding by the diagnostic radiologist of therapeutic goals will decrease patient expense, doctor frustration, and the inefficient use of hospital beds. Is it usually wise, for example, to order bone scans, liver and brain scans, etc., in an asymptomatic patient with a localized cancer? While the research community and its funding sponsors continue to lavish support on therapeutic clinical trials (particularly for cancer, and often for advanced stages of disease), still relatively limited resources are being directed to research on the pretreatment side of the clinical management spectrum, including studies of new diagnostic techniques and staging strategies for cancer patients.

There is no doubt that expensive new treatment equipment such as clinical neutron therapy generators must be subject to careful study and evaluation; however, the imbalance between the support accorded clinical therapeutic trials as opposed to evaluation of new diagnostic techniques still remains unaddressed. Many clinical therapeutic trials contain impressive budgetary support for patient diagnostic tests on the apparent premise that it is better to gather large amounts of diagnostic information indiscriminately and to evaluate later which data will contribute to a study's conclusions. How important are protocol-prescribed examinations to find additional lesions in the patient who already has known metastatic disease? Overuse is also encouraged by gaping holes in our knowledge of the exact sensitivity and specificity of many diagnostic tests and procedures that are applied to cancer patients.

The unnecessary profusion of overlapping diagnostic studies in cancer research trials has also carried over into community practice, where diagnostic tests are sometimes ordered on the premise that ". . . they can do no harm and might teach us something useful." The current overuse (and misuse) of various diagnostic techniques, "large" and "small," can be attributed again to our ignorance of their sensitivity and specificity and their exact implications for clinical management. If ever there were a fertile area for intensive clinical investigation, it is today in the diagnostic realm. However, diagnostic or "pretreatment" investigations do not command the resources or the attention accorded therapeutic research: in our enthusiasm to "cure" cancer, we have neglected the need to define better *what* we are treating and to be able to evaluate accurately what has been accomplished therapeutically in the individual patient. *Cancer Diagnosis* is an attempt to collate information on some of the new diagnostic techniques and strategies that are being developed for cancer,

---

*Relman, Arnold S.: Technology Costs and Evaluation, New England Journal of Medicine, Vol. 301 #26, pp. 1444–1445, December 27, 1979.

including some methods that are still being evaluated and others that have recently entered clinical practice.

Richard J. Steckel, M.D.
A. Robert Kagan, M.D.

Contributors

Zoran L. Barbaric, M.D.

Associate Professor of Radiological Sciences, UCLA School of Medicine, Los Angeles, California

Marshall Bein, M.D.

Associate Clinical Professor of Radiological Sciences, UCLA School of Medicine, Los Angeles, California

George Berci, M.D.

Associate Clinical Professor, UCLA School of Medicine; Associate Director, Department of Surgery, Cedars-Sinai Medical Center, Los Angeles, California

Patricia A. Ganz, M.D.

Adjunct Assistant Professor of Medicine, UCLA School of Medicine—San Fernando Valley Program, Sepulveda VA Medical Center, Sepulveda, California

Richard H. Gold, M.D.

Professor of Radiological Sciences, UCLA School of Medicine, Los Angeles, California

Thomas P. Haynie, M.D.

Chief, Section of Nuclear Medicine, M.D. Anderson Hospital and Tumor Institute, The University of Texas System Cancer Center, Houston, Texas

A. Robert Kagan, M.D.

Associate Clinical Professor of Radiation Oncology, UCLA School of Medicine; Chief, Department of Radiotherapy, Southern California Permanente Medical Group, Los Angeles, California

Frederick S. Keller, M.D.

Assistant Professor, Department of Radiology, University of Oregon, Portland, Oregon

Stanley G. Korenman, M.D. — Professor, Department of Medicine, UCLA School of Medicine—San Fernando Valley Program, Sepulveda VA Medical Center, Sepulveda, California

Robert J. Lukes, M.D. — Professor, Department of Pathology, University of Southern California, Los Angeles, California

Anthony A. Mancuso, M.D. — Assistant Professor of Radiological Sciences, UCLA School of Medicine, Los Angeles, California

William Odell, M.D., Ph.D. — Chairman, Department of Medicine, University of Utah College of Medicine, Salt Lake City, Utah

John W. Parker, M.D. — Professor, Department of Pathology, University of Southern California, Los Angeles, California

Josef Rösch, M.D. — Professor, Department of Radiology, University of Oregon, Portland, Oregon

Richard J. Steckel, M.D. — Professor of Radiological Sciences, and of Radiation Oncology, UCLA School of Medicine; Director, UCLA Jonsson Comprehensive Cancer Center, Los Angeles, California

Clive R. Taylor, M.D., D.Phil. — Associate Professor of Pathology, University of Southern California, Los Angeles, California

Ada R. Wolfsen, M.D. — Associate Professor of Medicine, Harbor-UCLA Medical Center, Los Angeles, California

Chapter 1

Advances in the Classification of Lymphomas Using Histologic and Diagnostic Criteria

Clive R. Taylor, M.D., D.Phil.
Robert J. Lukes, M.D.
John W. Parker, M.D.

INTRODUCTION

The diagnosis and treatment of neoplasms of the lymphoreticular system is based upon assessment of the morphological characteristics of neoplastic cells seen in cytologic or histologic preparations. While it is true that the exact form that therapy may take, whether surgery, radiotherapy, chemotherapy, or some combination thereof, is to a degree governed by the extent of the disease (stage) at diagnosis, the staging data do not become relevant until a firm diagnosis is achieved.

In recent years immunologic marker techniques, borrowed from the rapidly advancing field of cellular immunology, have been adapted for the study of lymphoid neoplasms in man. At the present time such methods, if applied in isolation, cannot be said to have major diagnostic value. They have, however, served in the elucidation of new concepts, the reappraisal of nomenclature, and the reassessment of cytologic and histologic criteria. The present chapter describes the attempts that have been made to integrate knowledge derived from experimental immunology with the traditional morphologic standards upon which diagnosis of the lymphoid neoplasms depends. A number of new techniques, new in the sense that they first found application in the last ten years, will be described; their impact upon the diagnosis of lymphocytic neoplasms will be discussed.

MALIGNANT LYMPHOMAS: DEFINITION AND DIAGNOSIS

The first use of the term "malignant lymphoma" is generally attributed to Theodore Billroth (circa 1870), although prior to that time a number of related conditions had been described using diverse terminology. The honor of the first description of a primary neoplastic process of the lymphoreticular system is accorded to Thomas Hodgkin who, in 1832, delivered a paper upon the "Morbid Appearances of the Absorbent Glands and Spleen." Hodgkin described seven examples of a condition that he considered to be a primary disease of the absorbent glands: "This enlargement of the glands appeared to be a primitive affection of these bodies, rather than the result of an irritation propagated to them from some ulcerated surface or other inflammed texture." Hodgkin, with becoming modesty, made no attempt to claim priority for his description. Indeed he expressed the opinion that similar appearances must have been observed previously by others in the course of cadaveric inspection, citing the work of Marcello Malpighi (in De Viscerum Structura, 1666) among others.

It is imporant to recognize that Hodgkin's work was based upon interpretation of gross pathologic findings at autopsy, unaided by microscopic examination. Some 20 to 30 years later Samuel Wilks (1856, 1865) rediscovered and redescribed some of Hodgkin's original cases. Initially Wilks confused the condition with lardaceous disease (or amyloidosis - Wilks, 1856), but later he clearly recognized the distinct and separate nature of the process to which he affixed the eponymous title of "Hodgkin's disease:" "I will not say that the cases described by Hodgkin may not have certain affinities with the lardaceous disease, but there is sufficient peculiarity in them to warrant them standing alone, and without any support from any other affection" (Wilks, 1865). Wilks was convinced that Hodgkin's disease represented a distinct entity and was a form of "cancer:" "This disease of Hodgkin is clearly separable from lardaceous disease, from cancer and tubercule...It is as much a disease sui generis as any other and deserves a description of its own...It must take its place in the rank of malignant diseases, or amongst those affections which are characterised by the development of new growths in the system" (Wilks, 1865).

Histopathology: Art or Science?

At about this time a distinct advance in the area of the basic biological sciences was at last finding more widespread application with reference to the pathology of human diseases. Although the basic principles for construction of the light microscope were known to such men as Athanasius Kircher (1607-1680) and Atonj van Leeuwenhock (1632-1723), it was not until the middle of the 19th century that the microscope gained widespread use in the study of human disease. John Hughes Bennett introduced a course on microscopic pathology at the University of Edinburgh in the 1840's and described the use of the microscope for the study of blood diseases in a text "Leukocythaemia" published in 1854. Meanwhile Rudolf Virchow also identified and described leukemia and went on to apply the principles of microscopic examination to a wider area of pathology, giving a series of 28 lectures that culminated in the publication of "Cellular Pathologie" in 1858. If the gestation period of histopathology had been long, the appearance of Virchow's book can probably be considered to represent the moment of birth.

With the increasing use of the microscope for the study of blood and lymphatic diseases a number of more-or-less distinct new "entities" were described, albeit on the basis of imprecise criteria and obscure nomenclature. The use of the term "malignant lymphoma" as a generic name for these conditions dates from the beginning of this period.

Morphologic criteria were developed by successive generations of pathologists, based upon detailed microscopic examination of biopsy tissue, clinico-pathological correlations and associated autopsy findings. Upon these principles a number of entities were recognized and set apart from one another (e.g., Kundrat, 1893, lymphosarcoma; Sternberg, 1898, and Dorothy Reed, 1904, Hodgkin's disease; Brill, Baehr and Rosenthal, 1928, follicular lymphoblastoma; Roulet, 1930, reticulum cell sarcoma; and in more recent times Burkitt's lymphoma and Lennert's lymphoma).

Today, more than 100 years after initial use of the term "malignant lymphoma," diagnosis and differentiation of this group of conditions continues

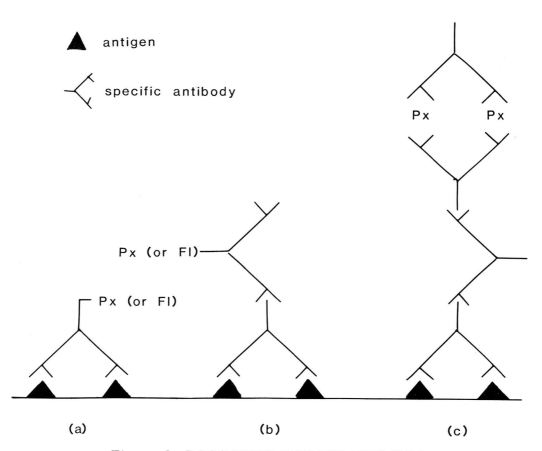

Figure 1. IMMUNOPEROXIDASE METHODS

(a) Direct conjugate

(b) Indirect conjugate

(c) PAP immunoperoxidase procedure

to rest upon histologic examination; although the criteria used in attaining a histologic diagnosis have been refined, the essential principles have not changed. Neoplastic cells are recognized, and the neoplasms named, according to the normal cell type that the neoplastic cell most closely resembles morphologically. Without independent means for validating the histologic identification of cells, the criteria for recognizing normal cells and their neoplatic derivatives remain to a large degree subjective. Therefore, it is perhaps not surprising that the diagnosis of these conditions is often hedged with uncertainty, even in the light of more than 100 years of experience.

The Advent of "Special Stains": Histochemistry and Immunohistologic Techniques

Pathologists have long recognized the subjective nature of their opinions and have sought methods of confirming their histologic judgments. Histochemical staining methods have proved helpful to the surgical pathologist in some aspects of tissue diagnosis, but have been of little value with reference to the lymphoreticular neoplasms, for cells of the lymphocytic series manifest few distinctive histochemical reactions; indeed the findings in most histochemical studies of the lymphomas might be said to fall into the unhelpful category of "weakly negative."

The introduction of the fluorescent labelled antibody method (Coons et al., 1941) was hailed by a few discerning pathologists as a potentially useful method for cell identification, independent of morphologic criteria. However, the application of immunofluorescence methods in surgical pathology was limited by the belief that such methods were restricted to the study of fresh frozen tissues (Sainte Marie, 1962). The poor morphologic resolution obtained in immunofluorescence preparations also served as an obstacle, precluding more general acceptance. The advent of enzyme-labelled antibodies (Fig. 1) offered a means of circumventing some of these difficulties, and with the application of the method to fixed paraffin-embedded tissues, the surgical pathologist's demands for excellent morphologic detail, coupled with specific cell identification, were at long last answered (Fig. 2).

Certain important limitations still apply. The possibility of denaturation or destruction of tissue antigens by the processes of fixation and embeddment is a problem, but the problem is not insurmountable. Similarly, the limited range of specific antisera presently available for the performance of immunohistologic studies seems to be a transient difficulty, for advances in the methods of preparing conventional antisera and the development of hybridoma systems to produce monoclonal antibodies hold imminent promise of providing a wide range of specific antisera for such studies (vide infra).

Immunohistologic methods, by virtue of their capability for identifying cells on the basis of infracellular structure (antigenicity), serve to link the disciplines of immunology and histology and promise thereby to transform histopathology from something of an art to more of a science.

In general terms, the minimum degree of fixation and processing that is compatible with the attainment of satisfactory histologic detail, should be employed. In practice, some compromise is usually necessary. If the preservation of antigenicity is at a premium, frozen sections (subject to brief fixation) are generally preferred, whereas if morphologic detail is most important there is still no substitute for adequate fixation followed by embedding in paraffin.

IMMUNOHISTOLOGIC METHODS: PRACTICAL AND THEORETICAL ASPECTS

If the preservation of antigenicity is the highest priority, then the method detailed in Table 3, based upon the recommendation of Tubbs (1979), may be used. Similar procedures have been advocated by Stein (1980), Warnke (1979), Janossy (1980), and others. Tissues processed in this way may be stained either by immunofluorescence methods or by immunoperoxidase methods, with results that are closely compatible in terms of sensitivity and specificity. An advantage of the immunofluorescence method is that it is usually more rapid. The principal advantage of the immunoperoxidase method is that morphologic resolution is somewhat better; in addition, permanent preparations are achieved and examination is possible by light microscopy without resort to the intricacies of fluorescence microscopy. If good morphologic detail is required, then one or another variation of the immunoperoxidase method applied to fixed paraffin sections is recommended (Table 3).

Immunoperoxidase Methods Applied to Paraffin Sections

Direct or indirect conjugate procedures may be employed for the demonstration of antigen in fixed, paraffin-embedded tissue. Alternatively, one may resort to the use of so-called nonlabelled methods, such as the enzyme bridge technique or the PAP technique (Taylor review, 1978), or to protein A or biotin-avidin linkage systems (Guedson et al., 1979). The direct and indirect procedures, together with the PAP method, are illustrated in the accompanying figure (Figure 1).

The direct conjugate procedure has the advantage of simplicity and rapid performance, but suffers from the potential disadvantage that partial denaturation of antibody may occur during the act of chemical conjugation. Residual unlabelled antibody may also remain in the conjugate preparation, thereby reducing the sensitivity of the method. A similar argument militates against the use of conjugated antibody in the direct method. In addition, the indirect method is more time-consuming but has the compensatory advantage of being more versatile than the direct method; one may substitute several different primary antibodies for the detection of different antigens using the same system.

The enzyme bridge method and the PAP method were both introduced to circumvent some of the problems involved in the chemical conjugation of enzyme with antibody (Taylor, 1978). The enzyme bridge method has no particular advantages over the PAP method; it is more cumbersome and perhaps

Table 1.

PRINCIPAL MARKERS FOR MONONUCLEAR CELLS OF MAN

First Generation (prior to 1974)	T	B	Monocytes
E rosette (sheep red cell)	+	–	–
Fc receptor (IgG)	–	+	+
C3 receptor	–	+	+
Surface Ig	–	+	–[1]
PHA response	+	–	–

Second Generation			
Fc receptors (IgG, IgA, IgM)	(+)[2]	+	+
C3 receptors (C3b, C3d, C4b)	(+)[2]	+	+
M rosette (mouse red cell)	–	+	–
T-cell antigens	$\overline{+}$[3]	–	–
B-cell allo-antigens (Ia-like)	$\pm$	+	+

―――――――――――――

The early "immune classifications" were stimulated by findings with "first generation markers." Second generation markers revealed several additional lymphocyte populations, a so-called null cell population (non-marking or "third population," lacking first generations markers), and subsets of T cells and B cells. Classifications incorporating second generation markers have yet to be devised (see Table 10).

[1]Monocytes may bear surface Ig by adsorption (Fc receptor or other mechanism.

[2]T cell subsets express Fc and C3 receptors in various combinations.

[3]At least 10 different T cell antigens have been identified using monoclonal antibodies (Reinherz et al., 1980); some are present only in certain T cell subsets.

less sensitive than the PAP method and will not be described further here. The PAP method involves the production of a stable immune complex of antibody to horseradish peroxidase and horseradish peroxidase antigen. The horseradish peroxidase-containing moiety then serves as the labelled reagent, as depicted in Figure 1. In the example shown, linkage of the PAP reagent (containing rabbit immunoglobulin) to the primary rabbit antiserum is done by means of a swine antiserum having specificity for rabbit immunoglobulin. Thus, attachment of the labelled moiety to the tissue section is immunological, avoiding the dangers inherent in chemical conjugations. It has been claimed that the PAP method is 100 to 1000 more sensitive than the conjugate procedures, at least in some systems. The procedure for the PAP method is detailed in Table 3.

Horseradish peroxidase is the most commonly used enzymatic label, principally because of its ready availability in pure form and the existence of a number of substrate systems yielding colored reaction products that are visible by light microscopy. A disadvantage of using horseradish peroxidase is that these same substrate systems show reactivity with various forms of endogenous peroxidase; this can led to confusion in the interpretation of staining patterns in tissue sections. If appreciable staining for endogenous peroxidase is anticipated or observed in pilot studies, and it is found to interfere with interpretation of specific labelling, then endogenous peroxidase activity may be blocked by prior treatment of the sections with a solution of hydrogen peroxide in methanol (Step 3, Table 3). This blocking procedure has been shown not to have adverse effects upon the antigenicity of tissue antigens, at least as exemplified by immunoglobulin and lysozyme (Burns et al., 1974). Step 4 in Table 3, advocating the addition of normal swine serum prior to the use of the primary antibody, is optional; it may be employed for reducing specific background staining attributable to nonspecific binding of the primary antiserum to charged components within the tissue sections.

The PAP procedure described here can be completed in five hours from the time that paraffin tissue sections are first deparaffinized for immunostaining, and 40 or more slides can be "batch stained" simultaneously. This time requirement has been considered by some to represent a serious disadvantge; however, with reasonable organization and strategy the method can be introduced into the routine laboratory without disruption of more routine staining procedures that are carried out concomitantly.

One disadvantage of existing immunohistologic techniques is that all of the antisera employed must first be shown to be specific, and must be titrated to optimal dilutions for use in immunostaining of tissue sections. This can be a tedious procedure for technologists not accustomed to the intricacies of checkerboard titrations. With the advent of immunostaining kits (DAKO, 22 N. Milpas, Santa Barbara, CA; Immulok, 1019 Mark Ave., Carpinteria, CA) containing pre-titrated compatible antisera, together with appropriate substrate systems, many of these difficulties have been resolved. In fact, with some "rapid kits" (Immulok) the entire staining procedure may be completed in two hours or less.

The patterns of staining that may be observed in "B cell-derived" neoplasms, including "plasma cell" neoplasms, are illustrated in Figures 2-6.

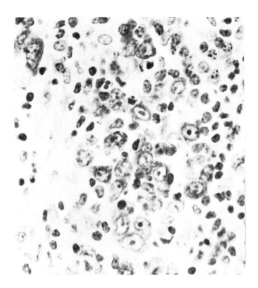

Figure 2. IMMUNOPEROXIDASE STAIN OF REACTIVE LYMPH NODE showing positive immunostaining (grey-black cytoplasm) in mature plasma cells and in B cell immunoblasts. The morphology of the immunoblasts is quite variable; these are the cells that once were regarded as forms of the reticulum cell or as histiocytic derivatives. Formalin paraffin section, counterstain hematoxylin x650.

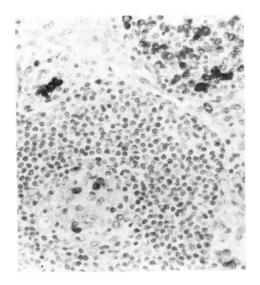

Figure 3. IMMUNOPEROXIDASE STAIN OF REACTIVE LYMPH NODE showing a small reactive center and part of a medullary cord packed with plasma cells. Section has been double stained for κ light chain (grey cytoplasm) and λ light chain (black cytoplasm) by a method described by Falini et al. (1981). B5 fixed section, counterstain hematoxylin, x250.

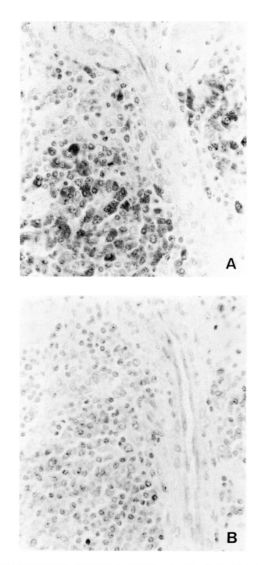

Figure 4. IMMUNOPEROXIDASE STAIN FOR A PLASMACYTOMA OF THE SKIN showing positive cytoplasmic staining for κ chain (a). There was no staining with anti-λ serum (b), again revealing the monoclonal nature of this B cell neoplasm. Bouin's fixed paraffin section, counterstain hematoxylin x400.

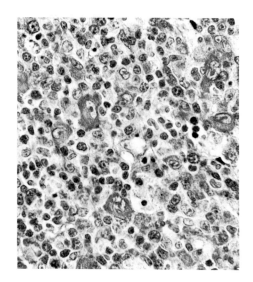

Figure 5. IMMUNOPEROXIDASE STAIN OF A B CELL IMMUNOBLASTIC
SARCOMA. Note that the neoplastic immunoblasts resemble the
reactive immunoblasts depicted in Figure 2. Stain was monoclonal
for $\lambda\gamma$. Formalin paraffin section, counterstain hematoxylin x400.

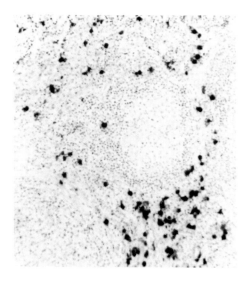

Figure 6. IMMUNOPEROXIDASE STAIN OF A LYMPH NODE showing scattered
muramidase (lysozyme) positive cells in the paracortex and sinuses.
Morphologically these cells were epithelioid histiocytes. Formalin
paraffin section, counterstain hematoxylin x250.

IMMUNOLOGY AND THE LYMPHOMAS - PRACTICAL ASPECTS

The division of the lymphoid system into at least two functional compartments, the B cell and T cell compartments, was of critical importance to the research immunologist but was of little practical value to the histopathologist, for T cells and B cells were found to be indistinguishable by morphologic criteria.

So-called "functional techniques" for identifying and distinguishing B cells, T cells and monocytes are listed in the accompanying table (Table 1). These techniques were designed for the study of cells in suspension, and they have been applied principally to the study of peripheral blood mononuclear cells or to suspensions obtained from fresh tissue biopsies. The requirement for suspensions of fresh viable cells precluded general use of these techniques by the surgical pathologist, because the need for such studies often becomes apparent only when the fixed paraffin section is examined (usually one or two days following the biopsy).

Details of these surface marker techniques have been given elsewhere, and they will be reiterated here only with reference to correlations of immunological methods with the more traditional morphologic criteria for the diagnosis of malignant lymphoma. A selected bibliography is included in Table 2.

Immunohistologic methods relate most to the surgical pathologist, for they offer at least the possibility of combining immunologic methods of cell identification directly with the morphologic parameters upon which tissue diagnosis is presently based. Two basic immunohistologic methods exist, using either fluorescein or enzyme labelling. They are strictly analogous in principle. Much of the debate considering the relative merits of these two techniques has focused upon attempts to prove that one method is superior to the other. The debate seems somewhat sterile, for the methods are similar and should be considered complementary to one another, each with its peculiar advantages and limitations.

Coons and colleagues (Coons et al., 1941) were perhaps the first to demonstrate clearly the potentialities of the immunofluorescence method. Antibody against the antigen in question is either labelled directly with fluorescein ("direct method"), or alternatively it is applied to the section in a natural unlabelled state and is then localized using a second "labelled" antibody directed against the first antibody (fluorescein-labelled, "indirect technique") (Figure 1, A & B). Until recently, it was assumed that fluorescein-labelled antibody methods could not be applied to fixed paraffin-embedded sections (Sainte Marie, 1963); it was believed that cryostat sections, or specially processed sections, were required for tissue antigen localization using immunofluorescence. However, with the discovery that immunoperoxidase methods are applicable to the demonstration of many antigens in fixed paraffin-embedded tissues, it has become evident that immunofluorescence techniques can also be applied successfully to paraffin sections.

The act of fixation and the subsequent processing and embeddment in paraffin does, nevertheless, have deleterious effects upon some tissue antigens.

Table 2. LYMPHOCYTE MARKER STUDIES OF THE NON-HODGKIN LYMPHOMAS[1]

Reference	Marker Employed/ Number of Cases	Comments
Payne et al, 1977	E, SIg, Fc, C3 cytoplasmic Ig on 28 non-Hodgkin lymphomas (24 reactive node controls)	Tissue cells -- 24 B-cell, 2 histiocytic, 2 unclassified, 0 T-cell. Elevated T-cells in follicular lymphoma
Bloomfield, 1979	Review	B- and T-cell markers in ALL and lymphomas; survival better in B-cell group than null
Michlmayr et al, 1976 Huber et al, 1976	E (neuraminidase), Fc (agg. Ig), C3, SIg on 170 lympho-proliferative diseases	Includes CLL, B-cell type; Hodgkin's disease, normal B- and T-cell proportions; non-Hodgkin, mostly B-cell type. Sometimes involved peripheral blood
Davey et al, 1976	E, SIg, cyto-chemistry on 28 non-Hodgkin lymphomas (24 normal controls)	15/28 B-cell (various types); Diffuse histiocytic, 1/7 T-cell. Diffuse PDL, 3/4 T-cell. Peripheral blood involved in 4/12 tested
Habeshaw et al, 1979	157 non-HD lymphomas	Divisible into B, T and "null" groups; correlation with morphology
Berard et al, 1978	Review, and new cases of non-Hodgkin lymphoma	11/17 histiocytic lymphomas of B-cell type; 1 T-cell, 1 histiocytic, other "null" cell
Stein et al, 1978	179 lymphomas	Tested lyophilized tissue for Ig content, Kiel classification utilized
Catovsky et al, 1978	Lymphomas/ leukemias	Surface markers including mouse red cell rosettes
Frizzera et al, 1978	70 non-Hodgkin lymphomas	Morphology (Lukes/Collins) as a predictor of surface marking
Greaves, 1978	Review	Surface markers in relation to lymphoproliferative disease and lymphocyte differentiation
Lukes et al, 1981	Review and Report of 790 cases	Surface markers and immunohistology in relation to Lukes/Collins scheme

[1]Selected from Tables 3.1 and 3.2 of Taylor, 1980a, to include large comprehensive studies and reviews.

Table 3. IMMUNOHISTOLOGIC STAINING
(PAP—PEROXIDASE-ANTI-PEROXIDASE METHOD)

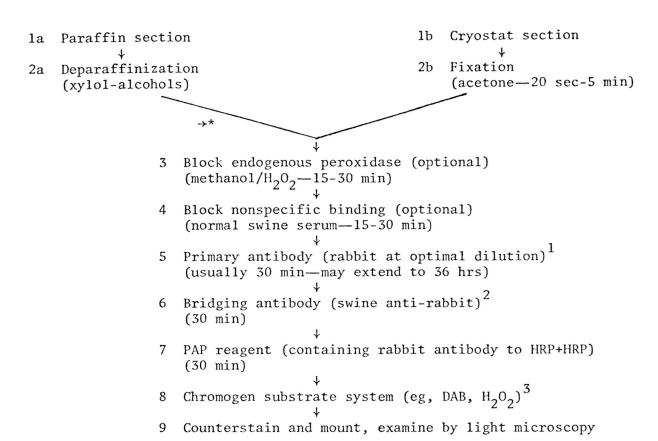

1a Paraffin section   1b Cryostat section

2a Deparaffinization   2b Fixation
    (xylol-alcohols)   (acetone—20 sec-5 min)

→*

3 Block endogenous peroxidase (optional)
   (methanol/H_2O_2—15-30 min)

4 Block nonspecific binding (optional)
   (normal swine serum—15-30 min)

5 Primary antibody (rabbit at optimal dilution)[1]
   (usually 30 min—may extend to 36 hrs)

6 Bridging antibody (swine anti-rabbit)[2]
   (30 min)

7 PAP reagent (containing rabbit antibody to HRP+HRP)
   (30 min)

8 Chromogen substrate system (eg, DAB, H_2O_2)[3]

9 Counterstain and mount, examine by light microscopy

---

[1]In direct conjugate procedure, FITC or HRP conjugated primary antibody would be used at this point, proceeding directly to mounting in glycerol for FITC, or to addition of chromogen/substrate for HRP conjugate. If the biotin-avidin system is used, the biotinylated primary antibody would be used at this point followed by the avidin-peroxidase conjugate (Guedson et al, 1979).

[2]In indirect conjugate procedure, substitute the FITC or HRP conjugate at this stage and proceed as in (1) above.

[3]DAB=diaminobenzidine; other chromogens given in text.

→*Removal of mercury pigments, if present, may be effected at this point.

FITC=fluorescein isothiocyanate; HRP=horseradish peroxidase.

The principal applications of the method in hematopathology are given in Table 4.

IMMUNOLOGY AND THE LYMPHOMAS: CHANGING CONCEPTS

The Reticulum Cell Epoch

When histology alone was the final arbiter of diagnosis, the nomenclature and classification of lymphoreticular neoplasms were based upon the apparent resemblance of the neoplastic cells to one or another of the cell types normally present in the lymph nodes, spleen, or bone marrow. Normal cell types, in turn, were recognized and distinguished on the basis of morphologic judgments alone. The judgments dispensed by different pathologists were often at variance with one another, giving rise to serious confusion and argument.

For a considerable period the reticulum cell-stem theory of Maximow held sway; numerous classifications were developed to reflect, in neoplasms, the supposed derivations and interrelations of the corresponding normal cells (Table 5). However, the term "reticulum cell" was applied loosely, signifying all things to all people; correspondingly, the designation "reticulum cell sarcoma" was not used uniformly, and in different classifications the same words might or might not have signified the same lesions (Table 5). Nevertheless, the underlying concepts remained relatively simple, namely that a large primitive-appearing stem cell ("reticulum cell" or reticulum cell variant) existed within the lymphoreticular tissues and served as the progenitor of the lymphocyte and plasma cell. The same cell, according to various doctrines, antedated the monocyte, histiocyte, granulocyte, megakaryocyte, and/or the fibrocyte.

Willis saw the problem too clearly: "Nowhere in pathology has a chaos of names so clouded clear concepts as in the subject of lymphoid neoplasms" (Willis, 1948). Unfortunately, Willis' solution was to devise his own personal classification (Table 5), and thus he fell into the trap that had ensnared many of his colleagues.

The idea that the reticulum cell serves as a "mother lode" for all the cellular elements of the lymphoreticular tissues saw its final flowering in the work of Custer and his associates. Based on the premise that the majority of the lymphoreticular cells were derived from a common progenitor cell and were thus related by lineage, Custer concluded that the corresponding lymphomas must also be of common lineage and must, therefore, be related to one another (Custer, 1953). It followed that one lymphoma might merge into another, and composite forms might be encountered. This "fluid lymphoma" concept proved too much for many histopathologists; taken to its logical conclusion, if different morphological forms of lymphoma could "transmute" at will the value of histologic classifications for predicting prognosis might be severely diminished.

Table 4. APPLICATIONS OF IMMUNOHISTOLOGIC METHODS IN HEMATOPATHOLOGY

Immunoglobulin
   1. Distinction of reactive B-cell proliferations from B-cell neoplasia
      a. Myeloma—benign monoclonal gammopathy—reactive plasmacytosis
      b. Plasmacytoid lymphocytic lymphoma/plasmacytoma—chronic reactive lymphadenitis
      c. Follicular center cell lymphoma (some cases)—reactive follicular hyperplasia
      d. B-cell immunoblastic sarcoma—reactive immunoblastic proliferations
   2. Subclassification of lymphomas
      a. Recognition of B-cell tumors by Ig content
      b. Subclassification of B-cell tumors
   3. Recognition of anaplastic tumor as B-cell in origin according to content of monoclonal Ig (distinction of B-IBS[a] from carcinoma, melanoma, etc)
   4. Recognition of morphologically unusual tumors as B-cell in origin, eg, "signet ring cell" lymphoma

J Chain
   Recognition of B-cell nature of normal or neoplastic cells

Lysozyme
   1. Histiocytic marker in reactive and neoplastic proliferations
   2. Marker of primary granule formation in myeloid maturation
   3. Distinction of granulocytic sarcoma from other "anaplastic" tumors
   4. Rapid identification of numbers of granulocytes in marrow (marrow granulocyte reserve)

α-1-antitrypsin
   Aid to recognition of reactive and neoplastic histiocytes

Lactoferrin
   1. Marker of secondary granule formation in myeloid maturation
   2. Aid to assessment of mature granulocytes in marrow

Hemoglobin A and F
   1. Distinction of erythroid precursors from lymphoid cells
   2. Rapid and specific identification of marrow erythroid reserve, from stage of hemoglobin synthesis
   3. Assessment of extent of HBF production in marrow in hemolytic diseases

Additional Antigens
   Other antigen systems of potential interest include anti-terminal transferase,[b] anti-free light chains, anti-B cell (Ia-like) antigens, anti-human T cell antigens, anti-tumor associated antigens of various types (eg, common ALL antigen), anti-factor VIII.[c]

RESEARCH
   Powerful investigative tool; widely applicable

TEACHING
   Morphologic and functional correlations

---

[a]B-IBS = immunoblastic sarcoma, B cell type
[b]C. Halverson. University of Southern California, personal communication
[c]M. Nadji. University of Miami, personal communication

16

Table 5

Robb-Smith 1938	Gall & Mallory 1942	Jackson & Parker 1947	Custer & Bernhard 1948	Willis 1948
Reticulosis (systematized hyperplasia)	Malignant lymphomas	Malignant lymphomas	Malignant lymphomas	
(a) Follicular reticulosis	Follicular lymphoma	Giant follicle lymphoma	Follicular lymphoma	Follicular lymphoma
(b) Sinus reticulosis				
(c) Medullary reticulosis (incudes Hodgkin's disease	Hodgkin's lymphoma	Hodgkin's disease paragranuloma granuloma	Hodgkin's disease paragranuloma granuloma	Hodgkin's disease
Reticulosarcomas (malignant)	Hodgkin's sarcoma	sarcoma	sarcoma	
(a) Undifferentiated Syncytial	Stem cell lymphoma (reticulum cell sarcoma)	Reticulum cell sarcoma	Reticulum cell sarcoma	Reticulum cell sarcoma
(b) Differentiated to histioid cells Dictyosyncytial Dictyocytic				
(c) Differentiated to haemic cells Lymphoblastic Lymphosarcoma Plasmacytoma Monocytoma Myelocytoma Erythroblastoma	Lymphoblastic lymphoma Lymphocytic lymphoma Plasmatocytic lymphoma	Lymphoblastoma Lymphosarcoma Lymphocytoma	Lymphosarcoma	Lymphosarcoma $\pm$ leukemia
(d) Mixed haemic & histoid polymorphic				
(e) Differentiated to sinus lining cells				
(f) Differentiated to haemic, histioid & sinus lining				

Drawn from Robb-Smith and Taylor, 1981.

17

The Histiocyte Dynasty

Against this background the need for a more strictly-defined system of nomenclature was widely felt; a proposal along these lines by Rappaport and colleagues (1956) thus fell on fertile ground. Rappaport put forward the basic idea that the large cell neoplasms were histiocyte-derived, and the small cell neoplasms lymphocyte-derived. Neoplasms consisting of a mixture of large and small cells were designated simply as mixed histiocytic-lymphocytic lymphomas. All three of these principal categories could occur in nodular or diffuse forms. Some 10 years later a modified version of this classification appeared in an AFIP Fascicle (Table 6) and was accepted by pathologists and clinicians alike - by pathologists for its simplicity and ease of application, by clinicians for its value in predicting prognosis and determining therapy. However, by 1966, during the heyday of the Rappaport scheme, the seeds of its destruction could already be found to be sprouting by those who knew where to look.

The Immunologic Era

Knowing where to look was the crux of the problem. Histopathologists, in attempting to unravel the mysteries of the lymphoreticular neoplasms, had for almost a century not looked much beyond the microscopic appearances of cells. The first signs that the discoveries of experimental immunologists were beginning to impinge upon the collective consciousness of histopathologists are to be found in the report of the International Symposium on Lymphology held in Zurich, Switzerland on July 19-23, 1966. Under the banner of "Classification of Malignant Lymphomas (the European Concept)" Karl Lennert noted that "...at present we have no exact knowledge of that progressive hyperplasia of the basophilic stem cells, the immunoblasts of Dameshek (1963) and the phytohaemagglutinin cells of tissue cultures." Lennert went on to state that "in Europe most of the authors do not separate stem cell lymphoma from reticulosarcoma. The large basophilic cells must be considered accordingly as the neoplastic cells of the reticulary tissues....We should take into consideration the possibility that lymphogenous stem cells may be present as a malignant neoplasm, which therefore should be called immunoblastic sarcoma."

The early in vitro studies of lymphocyte transformation and the development of surface marker methods applicable to the study of lymphoid cells in man (Table 1), served as the stimuli for formulating these new concepts. Subsequently the widespread application of these laboratory methods confirmed the initial impressions recorded above, and thereby insured that future lymphoma classifications must take cognizance of:

(1) the radical morphologic changes occurring in the process of lymphocyte transformation; and

(2) the division of lymphocytes into two or more functional categories (B cells, T cells, and possibly other functional cell types).

Table 6. CLASSIFICATION OF NON-HODGKIN LYMPHOMAS[1]

Traditional Terminology	Rappaport	Lukes/Collins	Lennert (Kiel)
NODULAR (FOLLICULAR)	Lymphocytic W.D.		[Centrocytic-cleaved]
	Lymphocytic P.D.	[Small cleaved]	
		[Small noncleaved]	
Follicular lymphoma	Mixed		[Centroblastic-noncleaved]
	Histiocytic	[Large cleaved] [Large noncleaved]	
DIFFUSE	Lymphocytic W.D.	Small lymphocytic (B or T)	Lymphocytic
Lympho-sarcoma*	Lymphocytic P.D.	Plasmacytic lymphocytic	Lymphoplasmacytoid
	Mixed	[Small cleaved]	[Centrocytic]
		[Large cleaved]	
- - - - - - - - - -	- - - - - - - - - -	- - - - - - - - - -	- - - - - - - - - -
Reticulum cell sarcoma	Histiocytic	[Large noncleaved]	[Centroblastic]
		Immunoblastic sarcoma (B or T cell)	Immunoblastic sarcoma (B or T cell)
		Histiocytic	
Burkitt's lymphoma	Undifferentiated	[Small noncleaved]	Burkitt
			Lymphoblastic
		Convoluted (T)	Convoluted (T)

[1]Shows approximate correspondence of cytologic types—precise matching is not feasible (from Taylor, 1980b.

- - - interrupted line separates good histology from bad in the Kiel classification, and may be extended across the other classifications, the principal exception being that convoluted lymphoma makes up part of the lympho-sarcoma and lymphocytic P.D. groups.*

☐ Boxed entries in the Lukes/Collins and Kiel classifications designate follicular center cell tumors.

An Epidemic of Immune-Based Classifications

Following the 1966 Zurich meeting, there was a seven-year interval during which new immunological knowledge slowly diffused to those pathologists concerned with the classification and nomenclature of lymphoid neoplasms in man. This was followed by a period of exponential growth, during which many new classifications of lymphomas were published as pathologists attempted to integrate their newfound knowledge of immunology with traditional histologic classifications. Soon the problem was not so much a lack of immune-based classifications of the lymphomas, but a surfeit (Table 7).

After considerable controversy, the classifications proposed by Lennert and by Lukes and Collins (Table 6) emerged as front runners. Neither of these schemes has attained universal acceptance; the Lennert classification is used extensively in Europe, while the Lukes/Collins classification has gradually supplanted the Rappaport scheme in the United States. While assignment of cases within the Lennert and Lukes/Collins classifications is dependent upon morphologic criteria, both systems lend themselves to correlations with immunologic and immunohistologic methods.

Lukes and his colleagues at the University of Southern California recently reported findings using immunologic surface marker studies in the histopathologic diagnosis of 790 cases of non-Hodgkin lymphomas (Lukes et al., 1981) (Table 8). The majority of lymphomas were of the B cell type, and among these the follicular center cell lymphomas were most common. T cell lymphomas occurred less frequently. Lymphomas and leukemias made up of unmarked cells were even less common. Of 790 cases, only two appear to be truly of histiocytic origin, whereas 160 cases might have been categorized as histiocytic lymphomas using the Rappaport system. Clearly, the histiocytic lymphoma category of Rappaport conceals lymphomas of several distinct cell types that may be distinguished by immunologic criteria, or by judicious application of fine morphologic distinctions incorporated within the Lukes/Collins classification. Histiocytic lymphoma of Rappaport encompasses the following cytologic types of Lukes and Collins: large cleaved follicular center cell lymphoma, large non-cleaved follicular center cell lymphoma, immunoblastic sarcoma of the B cell type, immunoblastic sarcoma of the T cell type, and true histiocytic lymphoma (Table 6).

Thus the adoption of immune-based classification systems has permitted recognition of cytologic types that were not recognized in pre-existing classification schemes. It must be remembered that the simple fact that such distinctions can be made is not in-and-of-itself sufficient cause for making them, or for discarding the older classification systems. Clinical relevance must be demonstrated.

"A difference is only a difference if it makes a difference."

Recently, evidence has been forthcoming supporting the clinical relevance of at least some of the categories in the Lukes/Collins and Lennert systems (Table 2). In the lymphoblastic lymphoma/leukemia category (including acute lymphocyte leukemia), non-marking or "null cell" cases fare better than

Table 7. AN EPIDEMIC OF LYMPHOMA CLASSIFICATIONS

Bennet et al	1974
Chelloul	1974
Diebold	1974
Dorfman	1974
Hamilton-Fairly & Freeman	1974
Lennert et al	1974
Lukes & Collins	1974
Mathe & Belpomme	1974
Tubiana & LeBourgeois	1974
Beard	1975
Burg & Braun-Falco	1975
Schnitzer	1975
Bryon et al	1976
Mathe, Rappaport (WHO)	1976
Jaffe et al	1977

_____

(from Taylor, 1980b)

Table 8. IMMUNOLOGICAL-HISTOPATHOLOGICAL CORRELATIONS IN LYMPHOMAS:
FREQUENCY OF OCCURRENCE OF DIFFERENT TYPES[1]

Cytologic Type by Lukes/Collins	Immunological Type[2]	
	B Cell %	T Cell %
Small lymphocytic	11	3
Plasmacytoid lymphocytic	7	0
Follicular center cell	49	0
Immunoblastic sarcoma	4	4
Convoluted lymphocytic	0	9
Cerebriform lymphocyte	0	3
Lymphoepithelioid cell	0	1
Total	71	20

In addition, 6% of cases were designated as 'U' cell, a term used for a primitive cell type, lacking morphologic or functional markers. Less than 0.5% of cases were true 'histiocytic' cases.

[1] Based on 790 cases of non-Hodgkin lymphoma (modified from Lukes et al, 1981).

[2] Designation as B or T was based on morphology, supported by surface markers in the majority of cases; in a minority of cases morphologic B-cell or T-cell lymphomas failed to mark convincingly for technical or other reasons (eg, apparently 20% of follicular center cell lymphomas showed low or absent markers).

those in which E rosettes (T cells) or surface immunoglobulin (B cells) can be demonstrated. However, this cannot be regarded as a generalization for all the lymphomas, and the determination of immunologic markers without reference to cytologic type is of no value. Clearly much remains to be done in assessing the clinical significance of even the conventional "first generation" markers, let alone the second generation immunologic markers (Table 10) for which even less clinical data are available.

Finally, a cooperative venture sponsored by the National Cancer Institute has examined the reproducibility of several of the recently-proposed classifications, including those of Lennert and of Lukes and Collins. The findings have yet to be reported in the medical literature, but have been described verbally at a number of meetings. Twelve pathologists participating in this study were unable to reach complete accord upon a universally acceptable classification system; they were unable to agree that any one of the classification schemes examined was significantly better than any of the others. In a spirit of compromise the participating pathologists settled upon a "formulation," or a recommendation of an "International Panel of Experts" (Table 9). This formulation serves as a crude framework into which the other classifications may be fitted, and it has the merit of arranging lymphomas into low grade, intermediate grade, and high grade malignancies with obvious clinical relevance. However, it seems likely that this proposal is destined to serve only as an interim measure, for not all pathologists (even among the "Panel of Experts") are currently using it. Even more important is the fact that the new formulation takes no cognizance of the impact that immunology has had on basic understanding of the biology of these neoplasms; instead it falls back upon the traditional premise of clinicopathologic correlation, and it includes immunological parameters only to the extent that they are part of some of the immune-based classifications used in parallel with the formulation.

IMMUNOLOGY WAITS FOR NO MAN

Reference to studies describing immunologic and histopathologic correlations in the lymphomas (Table 2) reveals that the classifications of Lennert and of Lukes and Collins are generally predictive of the immunological findings, albeit imperfectly and to a variable degree. This holds true as long as the immunologic parameters are restricted to those listed in Table 1 as "first generation" tests. However, the march forward of immunology continues, and additional cellular markers have been described that appear now to warrant the distinction of new subclasses of lymphocytes within the basic B and T cell categories. For example, certain conventional antisera and some monoclonal hybridoma antisera are now able to discriminate between several subsets of T lymphocytes: subsets in a developmental sense, and subsets in a functional sense. There is preliminary evidence that some of these subset phenotypes may also be expressed by neoplastic lymphocytes. If these findings are reproducible, then new immune-based classifications may be devised to incorporate this information. At the present time, classifications using these new discriminators have been confined primarily to the acute lymphocytic leukemias (Table 10), distinguishing five or six categories where only three existed previously. Extension of these parameters to the subclassification of

Table 9. A WORKING FORMULATION OF NON-HODGKIN'S LYMPHOMA FOR CLINICAL USAGE: RECOMMENDATIONS OF AN EXPERT INTERNATIONAL PANEL[1]

LOW GRADE	LUKES-COLLINS
A. ML small lymphocyte (CLL plasmacytoid)	Small lymphocyte (B or T cell) Plasmacytoid lymphocytic (B cell)
B. ML follicular Predominantly small cleaved cell (diffuse areas, sclerosis)	Small cleaved FCC, follciular (B cell)
C. ML follicular Mixed small cleaved and large cleaved	Small cleaved FCC, follicular (B cell)

INTERMEDIATE GRADE

D. ML follicular Predominantly large cell (diffuse areas, sclerosis)	Large cleaved FCC, follicular (B cell) Large noncleaved FCC, follicular (B cell)
E. ML diffuse Small cleaved cell ($\pm$ sclerosis)	Diffuse small cleaved FCC (B cell) with sclerosis
F. ML diffuse Mixed small and large cell ($\pm$ epithelioid cell component)	Lymphoepithelioid cell (T cell)
G. ML diffuse, large cell Cleaved cell Noncleaved cell (sclerosis)	Large cleaved FCC, diffuse (B cell) Large noncleaved FCC, diffuse (B cell)

HIGH GRADE

H. ML large cell immunoblastic Plasmacytoid Clear cell Polymorphous (Japanese Pleomorphic type)	Immunoblastic sarcoma B cell type T cell type
I. ML lymphoblastic Convoluted cell Nonconvoluted cell	Convoluted T cell
J. ML small noncleaved cell Burkitt's Follicular areas	Small noncleaved FCC, diffuse (B cell) Burkitt's Variant (B cell)
K. Miscellaneous Composite Mycosis Fungoides Histiocytic Extramedullary plasmacytoma Unclassifiable Other	Cerebriform T cell Histiocytic (genuine)

[1]From material distributed at the Tutorial on Neoplastic Hematopathology, Pasadena, California, February 1980. Director, Dr. H. Rappaport.

Table 10. ACUTE LYMPHOCYTIC LEUKEMIA: SUBCLASSIFICATION BY
FIRST AND SECOND GENERATION MARKERS (Table 1)

(adapted from Catovsky et al, 1979, and Kersey et al, 1979)

First Generation   Second Generation

T-cell ---------- E rosette +   T-cell ---------- E+ TAg+ SIg-
                  SIg -
                                            ---------- E+ TAg+ C3+ SIg-

                                     Pre-T ---------- E- TAg+ SIg-

                                            ---------- E- TAg+ ALL+ SIg-

Null cell ------- E- SIg-   Non-T, non-B ---- E- SIg- ALL+

                                                 ---- E- SIg- ALL- TAg-?

                                     Pre-B ---------- E- SIg- Cytop Ig+
                                                       ALL+ Ia+

B-cell ---------- SIg+   B-cell ---------- E- SIg+ Ia+

    ALL=common ALL antigen

    TAg= thymocyte antigen [by conventional antisera; subdivision by the
monoclonal antibody defined T cell subsets of Reinherz et al (1980) not as
yet established.]

    Ia=Ia-like antigen

all lymphomas would involve the creation of whole new categories of lymphomas, and the process of correlating clinical findings with immunologic and histopathologic parameters (attempted so recently for the Lennert and Lukes/Collins classifications) would begin anew. It is essential that immunologists, pathologists and clinicians now reach some accommodation or agreement, in an attempt to assimilate the wealth of new knowledge in an orderly fashion. The creation of an interdisciplinary "panel of experts" to develop a generally acceptable system might serve as valuable prophylaxis against a new epidemic of immune-based classifications that will otherwise soon descend upon us.

Let us select our "experts" with care, however, for even in a matter as simple as this one can only hope that the older definitions will be superseded by more helpful and clinically useful criteria.

> An expert is a person who tells you a simple thing
> in a confused way, in such a fashion as to make you
> think the confusion is your own fault.

> (W.D. Castle; Harvard Medical Bulletin, 1955)

REFERENCES

Berard, C.W., Jaffe, E.S., Braylan, R.C., Mann, R.B., Nanba, K. Immunologic markers of non-Hodgkin's lymphomas. In: Lymphoid Neoplasias I. Classification, Categorization, Natural History, Proceedings of the CNRS International Colloquium held in Paris, France, June 22-24, 1977. Vol. 64, Swiss League Against Cancer. Mathe, G., Seligmann, M., Tubiana, M., eds. Berlin, Springer-Verlag, Recent Results in Cancer Research, 1978, pp. 138-145.

Bloomfield, C.D. Gajl-Peczalska, K.J., Frizzera, G., Kersey, J.H., Goldman, A.I. Clinical utility of lymphocyte surface markers combined with the Lukes-Collins histologic classification in adult lymphoma. N. Engl. J. Med. 301:512-518, 1979.

Brill, N.E., Baehr, G., Rosenthal, N. Generalized giant lymph follicle hyperplasia of lymph nodes and spleen. A hitherto undescribed type. J.A.M.A. 84:668, 1925.

Burns, J., Hambridge, M., Taylor, C.R. Intracellular immunoglobulins. A comparative study on three standard tissue processing methods using horseradish peroxidase and fluorochrome conjugates. J. Clin. Pathol. 27:548-557, 1974.

Catovsky, D., Cherchi, M., Galton, D.A., Hoffbrand, A.V., Ganeshaguru, K. Cell differentiation in B- and T-lymphoproliferative disorders. In: Cold Spring Harbor Conference on Cell Proliferation, Vol. 5 (Book B). Cold Spring Harbor, 1978, pp. 811-822.

Catovsky, D., Pittman, S., O'Brien, M., Cherchi, M., Costello, C., Foa, R., Pearce, E., Hoffbrand, A.V., Janossy, G., Ganeshaguru, K., Greaves, M.F. Multiparameter studies in lymphoid leukemias. Am. J. Clin. Pathol. 72 (Suppl 4):736-745, 1979.

Coons, A.H., Creech, H.J., Jones, R.N. Immunological properties of an antibody containing a fluorescent group. Proc. Soc. Exp. Biol. 47:200-202, 1941.

Custer, R.P. Borderlands dim in malignant disease of the blood forming organs. Radiology 61:764-770, 1953.

Davey, F.R., Goldberg, J., Stockman, J., Gottlieb, A.J. Immunologic and cytochemical cell markers in non-Hodgkin's lymphomas. Lab. Invest. 35:430-438, 1976.

Frizzera, G., Gajl-Peczalska, K., Bloomfield, C.D., Kersey, J.H. Predictability of immunologic phenotype of malignant lymphomas by conventional morphology. A blind study of 70 cases (abstract). Lab Invest 38:345, 1978.

Greaves, M. Cell surface structures, differentiation and malignancy in the haematopoietic system. Symp. Soc. Exp. Biol. 32:429-442, 1978.

Guedson, J.L., Ternynck, T., Avrameas, J. The use of avidin-biotin interaction in immunoenzymatic techniques. J. Histochem. Cytochem. 27:1131-1139, 1979.

Habeshaw, J.A., Catley, P.F., Stansfield, A.G., Brearley, R.L. Surface phenotyping, histology and the nature of non-Hodgkin's lymphoma in 157 patients. Br. J. Cancer 40:11-34, 1979.

Hodgkin, T. On some morbid appearance of the absorbent glands and spleen. Trans. Med. Chir. Soc. London 17:658, 1832.

Huber, H., Michlmayr, G., Huber, C., Falkensammer, M. Immunological characterization of lymphoproliferative disorders by membrane markers. Clin. Wochenschr. 54:699-708, 1976.

Kersey, J.H., LeBien, T.W., Hurwitz, R., Nesbit, M.E., Gajl-Peczalska, K.J., Hammond, D., Miller, D.R., Coccia, P.F., Leikin, S. Childhood leukemia-lymphoma. Heterogeneity of phenotypes and prognoses. Am. J. Clin. Pathol. 72 (Suppl 4):746-752, 1979.

Kundrat. Uber Lympho-Sarkomatosis. Wien. klin. Wschr. 6:211, 1893.

Lennert, K. Classification of malignant lymphomas (European concept). In: Progress in Lymphology, Ruttimann, A., ed. Verlag, Stuttgart, 1967, pp. 103-109.

Lennert, K., Stein, H., Kaiserling, E. Cytological and functional criteria for the classification of malignant lymphomata. Br. J. Cancer 31 (Suppl 2):29-43, 1975.

Lukes, R.J., Collins, R.D. New approaches to the classification of the lymphomata. Br. J. Cancer 31 (Suppl 2):1-28, 1975.

Lukes, R.J., Taylor, C.R., Parker, J.W. Immunological surface marker studies in the histopathological diagnosis of non-Hodgkin lymphomas based on multiparameter studies of 790 cases. In: Advances in Malignant Lymphoma: Etiology, Immunology, Pathology, and Treatment. Proceedings of the Third Annual Bristol-Myers Symposium in Cancer Research, held at Stanford University, November 20-21, 1980. (in press, 1981).

Michlmayr, G., Pathouli, C., Falkensammer, M., Huber, C., Huber, H., Braunsteiner, H. (Rosette tests in lymphoproliferative diseases.) Schweiz. Med. Wochenschr. 106:794-799, 1976.

Payne, S.V., Smith, J.L., Jones, D.B., Wright, D.H. Lymphocyte markers in non-Hodgkin's lymphomas. Br. J. Cancer 36:57-64, 1977.

Rappaport, H., Winter, H.J., Hicks, E.B. Follicular lymphoma: a reevaluation of its position in the scheme of malignant lymphoma, based on a survey of 253 cases. Cancer 9:792-821, 1956.

Rappaport, H. Tumors of the hematopoietic system. In: Atlas of Tumor Pathology, fascicle 8, section 3. Washington, D.C.: Armed Forces Institute of Pathology, 1966.

Reed, D.M.   On the pathological changes in Hodgkin's disease, with especial reference to its relation to tuberculosis.   Johns Hopkins Hosp. Rep. 10: 133-196, 1902.

Reinherz, E.L., Moretta, L., Roper, M., Breard, J.M., Mingori, M.G., Cooper, M.D., Schlossman, S.F.   Human T lymphocyte subpopulations defined by Fc receptors and monoclonal antibodies.   J. Exp. Med. 151:969, 1980.

Robb-Smith, A.H.T., Taylor, C.R.   The Lymph Node Biopsy.   Harvey Miller Publishers, Marryat Road, Wimbledon, London, and Oxford University Press, 1981.

Roulet, F.   Das primare Retothelsarkom der Lymphoknoten.   Virchows Arch. Path. Anat.   277:15, 1930.

Sainte-Marie, G.   A paraffin embedding technique for studies employing immunofluorescence.   J. Histochem. Cytochem.   10:250, 1962.

Stein, H., Papadimitriou, C.S., Bouman, H., Lennert, K., Fuchs, J. Demonstration of immunoglobulin production by tumor cells in non-Hodgkin's and Hodgkin's malignant lymphomas and its significance for their classification. In: Lymphoid Neoplasias I.   Classification, Categorization, Natural History, Proceedings of the CNRS International Colloquium held in Paris, France, June 22-24, 1977.   Vol. 64, Swiss League Against Cancer.   Mathe, G., Seligmann, M., Tubiana, M., eds.   Berlin: Springer-Verlag, Recent Results in Cancer Research, 1978, pp. 158-175.

Sternberg, C.   Euber eine eigenartige unter dem Bilde der Pseudoleukamie verlaufende Tuberkulose des lymphatischen Apparates.   Z. f. Heilk.   19:21-90, 1898.

Taylor, C.R.   Immunoperoxidase techniques: theoretical and practical aspects. Arch. Pathol. Lab. Med.   102:113-121, 1978.

Taylor, C.R.   Hodgkin's Disease and the Lymphomas, Vol. 4.   Annual Research Reviews, D.F. Horrobin, series editor.   Montreal: Eden Press; and Edinburgh/London: Churchill Livingstone, 1980a.

Taylor, C.R.   Changing concepts in the classification of lymphoma.   In: Malignant Lymphoproliferative Diseases.   van den Tweel, J.G., Taylor, C.R., Bosman, F.T. (eds.).   Leiden University Press, Leiden, 1980b, pp. 175-184.

Wilks, S.   Cases of lardaceous disease and some allied affections, with remarks.   Guy's Hosp. Rep. 17 (Series II, Vol. 2):103-132, 1856.

Wilks, Sir S.   Cases of enlargement of the lymphatic glands and spleen (or, Hodgkin's disease), with remarks.   Guy's Hosp. Rep.   11:56, 1865.

Willis, R.A.   Pathology of Tumours.   Butterworths, London, 1948.

Chapter 2

The Clinical Value of Steroid Receptors in Cancer

Patricia A. Ganz, M.D.
Stanley G. Korenman, M.D.

Introduction

The clinical observation of hormone-dependent growth in breast cancer led to laboratory investigations which have brought about major advances in the classification, treatment, and basic biology of this neoplasm. In this review we focus on the use of steroid receptors for predicting response to endocrine therapy using breast cancer as a model, and extend the analysis to other neoplasms.

Therapeutic hormonal manipulations in breast cancer include ablative therapy (castration, adrenalectomy, hypophysectomy, anti-hormones) or additive therapy (estrogens, androgens, progestogens, glucocorticoids). Historically, the specific treatment was selected empirically in relation to the hormonal milieu in which the tumor became clinically recognized (e.g., castration was performed in premenopausal women whose tumors develped in an estrogen-rich milieu; conversely, estrogens were given to postmenopausal women whose tumors arose in an estrogen-poor milieu). An objective measurable response to therapy was observed in about 30% of patients so treated, regardless of the particular manipulation that was chosen. Patients with an earlier therapeutic response were expected to have a high incidence of remissions upon receiving subsequent endocrine therapy. However, prior to the clinical use of the estrogen receptor assay, there was no rational basis for selecting therapy and many patients with metastatic breast cancer in fact received ineffective endocrine-directed therapy. With the development of very effective combination chemotherapy regimens (objective response rates of 70-80%) during the past decade, it became essential to predict which tumors specifically were apt to be hormone responsive.

Until recently, there was little understanding of the biologic mechanism by which hormones affect the growth of tumors. The current model of steroid hormone action asserts that cells whose growth and metabolism are influenced by these hormones must contain specific high-affinity receptors in the cytoplasm. The steroid hormones are lipid soluble and easily diffuse across the cell membrane. After the steroid binds to its specific cytoplasmic receptor, the steroid-receptor complex is translocated to the nucleus where it binds to chromatin acceptor sites. Resulting alterations in transcription produce the specific changes in protein synthesis which lead to the altered cellular function characteristic of the hormone effect. Cells which lack a sufficient concentration of specific receptor will not respond on exposure to the hormone. On the other hand, while the presence of the cytoplasmic steroid receptor is necessary for hormone response, it is not sufficient to ensure a biological response because of the many sub sequent steps required after binding.

During the past decade, improvements have been made in the measurement of a variety of steroid receptors in vitro, and this area of basic

32

research has made a major impact on the management of patients. Steroid receptors for estrogens, androgens, progesterone and glucocorticoids can now be measured in every tissue of the body, and in neoplasms. Their role in clinical medicine is the subject of this review.

Historical Development

In 1959, it was observed that radioactively labeled estrogen injected into animals, localized in the normal target tissues.[1,2] Jensen and Jacobson reported selective, prolonged uptake of unmetabolized tritiated estradiol in estrogen targets implying tight binding of the steroid in the cell. It was soon shown that binding moieties were present in the cytoplasm and the nucleus of target tissues and that both may be measured by their uptake of radioactive hormone in vitro.[3] Breast cancer patients undergoing endocrine ablative surgery were subjected to a similar experiment, and the patients who had an objective clinical response were noted to have concentrated larger quantities of the labeled estrogen within their tumors.[4] In experimental mammary carcinomas it was shown that excised tumors also concentrated more hormone if they were hormone-responsive.[5] These results suggested that it might be possible to analyze human tumor specimens and predict subsequent hormone responsiveness.

During the 1970's, techniques were developed to quantify estrogen receptor (ER) in human breast cancer.[6] It was shown that non-neoplastic breast tissue had minimal amounts of estrogen receptor, and that circulating levels of estradiol did not interfere with the assay.[6]

The clinical response of patients to endocrine therapy was correlated with the receptor assay results.[7,8] This information was shared and reviewed in 1974 at a National Institutes of Health workshop[9] which concluded that receptor assays were indeed valuable in predicting the results of endocrine therapy in breast cancer. A second NIH workshop on estrogen receptors in breast cancer was recently convened.[10,11] The original findings correlating endocrine responsiveness and receptor content have now been confirmed and extended.

Because progesterone receptor (PR) concentration was known to be dependent on estrogen stimulation, McGuide developed the PR assay[12] to augment the predictive value of the ER assay; this theoretically assesses the entire pathway of estrogen action.

Technical Aspects of Steroid Receptor Assays

Since steroid receptors are thermolabile, the tumor must be processed immediately by the pathologist and kept cold while being transported to the laboratory and during all subsequent manipulations. A piece of tissue adjacent to the tumor should be identified by the pathologist for microscopic examination and correlation with the tissue being sent for receptor analysis. All tissue should be kept deep frozen in dry ice for transportation.

There are two established methods for steroid receptor quantitation, the charcoal assay and the sucrose density gradient assay. In the charcoal method, the specimen is pulverized and homogenized while frozen, and then subjected to ultracentrifugation in order to obtain the cytosol receptors. Aliquots of cytosol are incubated with varying concentrations of hormone in competition with radio-labeled hormone. Bound and free hormone are separated by activated charcoal and a Scatchard plot constructed to calculate the number of receptor sites and their affinity. In the sucrose density gradient method, cytosol is incubated with an excess of radioactive estrogen and subjected to ultracentrifugation in a gradient of sucrose. The number of counts in the receptor peak determines receptor concentration.

These assays which measure unoccupied cytosol receptors (at 0° C) may be sufficient for evaluation of breast neoplasms. Additional receptor assays which may become clinically useful are nuclear receptor assays and exchange assays which measure the occupied and free receptor in the nucleus or cytoplasm. For example, in prostate cancer measurement of occupied as well as unoccupied cytoplasmic and nuclear receptors may be necessary for studying receptor quantity and physiology, and for clinical utility.[13]

It is essential that the ER assay for breast cancer be performed accurately and reliably because of its now-established clinical and therapeutic implications. Key technical problems remaining include: 1) the difficulty in developing transportable standard specimens; 2) the current lack of quality control arrangements between laboratories; 3) the need for laboratory precision in performance of the assay; and 4) the need for careful follow-up analysis of assay results. Receptor assays which are more complex (e.g., exchange assays) will require even greater technical expertise for performance in the clinical laboratory.

Distribution of Steroid Receptors in Tumors

Steroid receptors are present in a variety of hormonal target tissues and neoplasms. However, they are also present in some tissues which are not considered to be endocrine responsive (e.g., colonic mucosa: see Tables I and II). Androgen receptor has been described in breast, prostate and colon cancers. Glucocorticoid receptor has also been reported in a number of tumors, particularly in breast and lymphoid neoplasms, but since fibroblasts and other tissue elements contain glucocorticoid receptors it is uncertain which cells actually harbor the receptor.

Because of the wide distribution of steroid receptors in normal tissues, it is important to define the normal range of receptor content in the adjacent (non-neoplastic) tissue so that the source of receptor in a given specimen may be identified. In prostate and endometrial carcinomas the high concentration of receptors in surrounding tissues raises questions about the cellular source of receptors reported for the neoplasms. The role of steroid receptors in tumors derived from tissues that are not ordinarily regarded as hormonal targets is unknown.

Steroid Receptors in Breast Cancer

The normal non-lactating breast is dependent on the multiple and synergistic actions of estrogens, progestins, prolactin, and cortisol for its

TABLE I

Normal Tissues Reported to Contain Estrogen Receptors

Classical Targets	Other
Endometrium	Kidney
Myometrium	Prostate
Oviduct	Adrenal
Vagina	Pancreas
Fallopian Tube	Colon
Cervix	Spinal Cord
Brain	Eosinophils
- hypothalamus	Heart
- pituitary	Skin
Liver	
Placenta	
Leydig Cell	
Ovarian Cells	

TABLE II

Steroid Receptors in Diverse Malignancies

Tumor Type	Receptor			
	ER+	PR+	AR+	Glucocorticoid+
Colon [91,95-98]	19/67	9/31	7/24	20/25
Gallbladder [95]	2/3			
Pancreas [95,98]	2/6			
Liver [95,96]	2/4			
Squamous Cell Ca. [95]	2/2			
Rectal [95]	1/2			
Sarcomas [93,95,98]	9/18			
Carcinoid [94]	2/2			
Thyroid [96,98]	2/8			
Lung [95,96,98]	0/9			
Stomach [95,98]	1/7			

growth. Estrogens stimulate ductal proliferation. Progesterone (in addition to prolactin) is required for the complete functional development of the alveolar lobules and the secretion of milk. Progesterone can also suppress lactation by end organ inhibition during pregnancy in spite of high levels of prolactin. Lactation proceeds in the post-partum period after a fall in maternal progesterone levels. Many investigators have studied the relationship between animal as well as human breast tumors and the mammotropic hormones. Prolactin, glucocorticoid, and androgen receptors have all been demonstrated in human breast cancer, in addition to the well-studied ER and PR.[14,15]

1. ER and response to endocrine therapy

Whenever correlations have been made between tumor ER status and the response to endocrine therapy, 50-60% of estrogen receptor positive (ER+) tumors have shown objective responses. The results were comparable in a variety of countries using diverse receptor assays and therapeutic modalities. When objective responses to endocrine or ablative therapy in patients independent of their ER status were correlated retrospectively with tumor ER content, a common pattern of anti-tumor response was seen[9] (Table III). Whereas patients with ER+ tumors had a 55-60% response rate, patients with estrogen receptor negative (ER-) tumors had an 8% response rate independent of the kind of therapy or the metastatic site (soft tissue, bone, viscera). These results have been confirmed repeatedly.[11]

There is a quantitative relationship between ER concentration in the tumor and the likelihood of a subsequent endocrine response[16] (Table IV). Primary tumors which contain > 100 fmoles/mg tissue have an 80% probability of showing an objective response, while tumors with lower levels of ER are less responsive as a group. For this reason, clinicians should now insist on obtaining the results of a quantitative ER assay.

Why do 40% of patients with ER+ tumors (overall) and 20% of tumors with a high receptor concentration fail endocrine therapy? One possible explanation is that different metastatic sites may vary in their ER concentration. The most likely explanation, however, is that even tumor cells possessing ER do not necessarily depend on the ER complex for their continued growth and division. It is reassuring, however, that tumors which contain a high level of ER or which possess both ER and PR have almost an 80% response rate[17] (Table V).

2. Distribution of ER with regard to menopausal status and stage of disease

Seventy percent of primary breast cancers contain estrogen receptors[18], with a wide range of concentrations from 3 to greater than 1000 fmol/mg of protein (a femtomole is 10^{-15} moles); the highest levels occur in postmenopausal women. Some groups report a lower overall incidence of receptor positivity in premenopausal patients.[19,20]

The presence of ER in the primary tumor is independent of the axillary node status at presentation.[21-23] Since nodal status is traditionally accepted as the most significant prognostic factor, the independent relationship between

TABLE III

ER Status and Response to Endocrine Therapy[1]

Therapy	ER+	ER−	ER+
Adrenalectomy	32/66	4/33	3/8
Castration	25/33	4/53	0/2
Hypophysectomy	2/8	0/8	−
Total	59/107=59%	8/94=8%	3/10=30%
Androgen	12/26	2/24	0/1
Estrogen	37/57	5/58	0/2
Glucocorticoid	2/2	−	−
Total	51/85=60%	7/82=8%	0/3=0%
Antiestrogens	8/20	5/27	−
Other	2/3	0/5	−
Total	10/23=43%	5/32=16%	

[1]Adapted from Reference 9.

TABLE IV

ER Level and Clinical Response to Therapy[1]

	Objective Response	
	Primary Biopsy	Metastatic Biopsy
ER fm/mg		
0-3	1/6 (17%)	4/47 (8%)
3-100	17/38 (45%)	26/67 (40%)
>100	5/6 (83%)	22/36 (61%)

*Fmoles/mg cytosol protein

[1]Adapted from Reference 16.

39

TABLE V

Objective Response to Endocrine Therapy when ER and PR
Concentration are Known[1]

Receptor Content	Response Rate
ER-, PR-	9/63 = 14%
ER-, PR+	3/6
ER+, PR-	20/71 = 28%
ER+, PR+	67/91 = 74%

[1]Adapted from Reference 17.

ER concentration and status of the axillary nodes is an important finding and adds a new prognostic variable. As one might expect, there is no correlation between the size of the primary tumor and ER status.[20,22]

There have been no reports describing the relationship of PR to axillary node involvement or to primary tumor size. However, PR has been related to ER in a large number of tumor biopsies[16] (Table VI). PR is uncommon in ER-tumors. This tends to support the hypothesis that PR is under the control of ER in breast cancer, in a manner similar to that described in other estrogen responsive target tissues. The incidence of PR positivity is independent of menopausal status.

An analysis has not been made of PR concentration and endocrine responsiveness. There is essentially no correlation between ER concentration and PR concentration because the estrogenic state of the woman may influence the receptor concentration in her tumor.* Increasing concentrations of endogenous estrogen favor translocation of ER to the nucleus, as well as PR synthesis.

3. Steroid receptors in the primary vs. metastatic tumor

Primary tumors are more often ER+ than metastases.[9] However, the predictive value of the ER assay is independent of whether the measurement is made in a primary tumor or in a metastasis.[9] The degree of concordance of the ER concentration in metastases with the primary tumor may be an important consideration when receptor data is not available from the primary tumor. Most studies which have examined this question have compared multiple biopsies of metastatic tumors, with only a few samples actually comparing the primary with the metastasis in an individual patient.[24-26] There is a 95% concordance in receptor content in synchronous metastases. In asynchronous metastases without any intervening therapy, there is usually no apparent change in ER status; however, there is some suggestion that the longer the interval between biopsies the more likely a change in ER status (almost always from ER+ to ER-).[25]

Intervening chemotherapy or hormonal therapy may lead to a change in receptor content of the tumor. This may be a clinical problem in a patient who has received adjuvant chemotherapy and then relapsed. Allegra et al.[24] reported a marked decrease in ER content after hormonal therapy. In patients with intervening chemotherapy between biopsies, the median ER content was similar overall in the pre- and post-therapy biopsies; however in a few patients there was a slight increase in ER concentration, or ERtumors converted to ER+.

4. The value of assays of additional steroid receptors in predicting response to endocrine therapy

The measurement of PR in breast cancer may increase the predictive value of the ER assay.[27] Results from McGuire's laboratory suggest that the presence of both ER and PR in a tumor increases the likelihood of hormone response to about 80%; however, some tumors which are ER+ but lacking in

---

*Korenman, unpublished data

TABLE VI

ER and PR Distribution in 1366 Biopsies[1]

	Distribution (%)	
	Premenopausal	Postmenopausal
ER-, PR-	30	19
ER-, PR+	9	3
ER+, PR-	12	23
ER+, PR+	49	55

[1]Adapted from Reference 16.

PR still demonstrate endocrine responsiveness (Table V). Bloom et al.[28] recently presented similar results. Since 80% of tumor with >100 fmoles/mg protein of ER are known to respond to endocrine therapy, the PR assay may have greater prognostic value in those tumors with low and intermediate values of ER.

Allegra et al.[15] measured progesterone, androgen and glucocorticoid receptors, in addition to ER, in 85 patients with metastatic breast cancer. They reported that the presence of PR increased the predictive value of ER only in a group of patients with no prior therapy. Concentration of ER appeared to have the most important influence on response rate.

Prolactin receptors have been demonstrated in mammary cell membranes of animal breast tumors[29], human breast cancer cell lines[30], and in tissue from human breast tumors[14]. There have been technical difficulties in the assay and clinical correlations are not yet available.

Recently McGuire et al.[27,31], in studies of nuclear ER in tissue culture and in samples from human breast cancers, documented both occupied and unoccupied nuclear ER, but not enough data were available to correlate this information with responses to therapy. When translocation of the ER complex to the nucleus was assessed in a small number of patients as a measurement of an intact hormone response, the ability to translocate correlated strongly with objective endocrine response.[32]

5. ER as an independent prognostic variable in breast cancer.

In 1977, Knight et al.[33] suggested that ER was an independent prognostic factor for early recurrence in breast cancer. Their recently updated results on survival in 281 patients after mastectomy demonstrates a significantly improved survival in those patients with ER+ primary tumors. Improved survival was independent of tumor size, axillary node status, age, or menopausal status. This patient group received no adjuvant hormonal or cytotoxic therapy.[16] When node positive patients were analyzed separately, survival was strikingly worse in the ER- group of patients. At two years, overall survival for the ER+ patients was 90% compared to 70% for the ER- group, and at three years the survivals were 80% and 55%, respectively. Several other groups have confirmed Knight's original report.[34-37] These data indicate that receptor status should now be used as a stratifying variable in clinical trials for breast cancer treatment.

6. ER as a reflection of tumor differentiation

Several groups have suggested a relationship between histologic differentiaton of breast neoplasms and ER concentration. In a recent study of 140 primary breast cancers[38], there was indeed a tendency for the concentration of ER to correlate positively with the degree of differentiation of the tumor. Tumors were evaluated for their histologic classification, degree of differentiation, epithelial cellularity, lymphoid reaction, calcification and necrosis. Carcinomas without a specifically classifiable histologic type were divided into low, average or high grade according to the degree of tubule formation, cellular pleomorphism, and number of mito-tic figures. Because of the subjectivity and tediousness of this kind of pathologic evaluation, ER may prove to be an easier and more accurate measurement of tumor differentiation.

The relationship between growth rate and ER status has been examined by two investigative groups using the thymidine labeling index. Meyer et al.[39] found that tumors with the highest labeling index were ER-, and these tumors also tended to occur in the younger patients. A small number of specimens were also graded for histologic differentiation, and there was a positive association between older age, better differentiated tumors, ER positivity and low thymidine labeling index. This was confirmed by Silvestrini et al.[40] who did thymidine labeling in explants incubated in tissue culture in 199 patients and correlated the results with ER assays. The lowest labeling indices occurred in the postmenopausal ER+ cases and the highest indices in the ER- premenopausal patients, but ER remained a much better indicator of responsiveness to endocrine therapy.

7. ER and response to chemotherapy

Since ER- tumors were thought to be more poorly differentiated and had a more aggressive natural history, there was interest in examining the relationship between ER status and response to cytotoxic chemotherapy.[41] This question has been examined retrospectively by many groups.[17,41-49] Most studies show no significant difference in response rate between ER+ and ER- tumors; however, in some reports there has been a more favorable response rate in the ER+ tumors, while the reverse was noted in a widely quoted paper.[41]

8. Conclusion

Measurement of cytosol ER is of established value in improving the clinician's ability to select appropriate therapy for metastatic breast cancer. ER- tumor are often poorly differentiated, have a higher proliferative rate, and recur earlier than ER+ tumors, leading to poorer survival. Clinical observations regarding metastatic breast cancer tend to correlate with estrogen receptor analyses (e.g., postmenopausal women have more indolent cancers which tend to be endocrine responsive; their tumors are more often ER+ and also have higher quantitative levels of ER). ER does not seem to be predictive of response to chemotherapy but does seem to be an independent prognostic variable for survival. Assessment of PR in the same sample may increase the predictive value of ER.

Steroid Receptors in Other Tumors

1. Prostate Cancer

Cancer of the prostate is the third most common cancer in men, increasing in prevalence with advancing age. The pathogenesis of this malignancy is uncertain, but there has been considerable study of its rela-tionship to the changing hormonal milieu of aging men. Normal, hyperplastic and neoplastic prostate contains androgen receptors (AR), ER, PR, and glucocorticoid receptors. Prostatic cancer is known to be androgen dependent, and in 60% of patients responds to androgen withdrawal or estrogen administration.[50] Because of the demonstrated clinical usefulness of the ER assay in breast cancer, investigators have pursued androgen receptor (AR) in prostate cancer.

Until recently, specific high affinity AR have been difficult to measure because of the rapid metabolism of the natural intracellular androgen (5αdihydrotestosterone) and its tight binding to sex hormone-binding globulin. A synthetic androgenmethyltrienolone (R1881), which is now being used, does not have these problems. Since methyltrienolone has been shown to bind PR as well as AR, PR binding must be blocked by the addition of triamcinolone or a progestin.

The presence of AR in benign as well as malignant prostatic tissue complicates the interpretation of receptor analysis on prostatic biopsy material. The usual steroid receptor assay does not allow for separation of various tissue elements. Most of these problems can be circumvented by assaying metastatic sites; however, accessible metastases are infrequently available in this tumor.

Procurement of adequate amounts of tissue is also a problem because the diagnosis of prostate cancer is often made by needle biopsy or trans urethral resection, rather than by the prostatectomy.[51] Needle biopsies contain only about 50 mg of tissue, and the specimens from transurethral resection are small and are often partially denatured by the cautery. Biopsies of metastases are also small (95% of the time from bone). Since steroid receptor analysis usually requires 200-300 mg of tissue, these sources are usually inadequate. However, they have been employed by some groups by using multiple biopsies and single point assessments.[52-54] As stated, histologic examination of prostate samples also usually reveals a mixture of normal and neoplastic tissue, and this must be kept in mind when evaluating the results of receptor assays.

Recently Shain et al.[13] found that the mean AR concentration of carcinomatous prostate specimens was similar overall to that of non-carcinomatous prostates. However, when carcinomatous and non-carcinomatous areas from the same prostate were compared, the AR concentration of the carcinoma was consistently lower. They raised serious questions about the prognostic value of prostatic AR determinations. Some groups have turned to immunofluorescent staining of tissue sections to help define and locate steroid receptors in prostatic cancer because of the technical problems described.[55] To date, the presence of ER, PR, and glucocorticoid receptor in normal and neoplastic prostate has not been shown to have clinical significance.[53,56,57]

While several groups have examined AR in human prostatic carcinoma[13,52,53,54,58,59], only a small number of patients have been studied in each report and only a few studies have actually correlated steroid receptor levels with endocrine response[52-54] (Table VII). Only the investigative series involving previously untreated patients are discussed here, since receptor content has been reported to change after endocrine therapy in breast cancer and several reports demonstrate a fall in AR content after

TABLE VII

Androgen Receptors and Response to Endocrine Therapy
in Prostate Cancer

Reference	Tissue Source	Number of Patients	Response to Hormone Rx	
			AR+ Tumors	AR-Tumors
Ekman[52]	Prostate	23	15/18 (80%)	1/5 (20%)
Young[53]	Prostate	9	6/9 (60%)	-
deVoogt[54]	Prostate	19	10/12 (83%)	6/7 (85%)
Totals		52	31/38 (82%)	7/13 (54%)

endocrine therapy in prostate cancer. Ekman et al.[52] detected AR in 20 out of 25 prostate tumors. In 23 patients who could be evaluated, 15 out of 18 AR+ patients had a response to endocrine therapy. Unfortunately, it is uncertain to what extent the measurements actually reflected AR concentrations within tumor, since the specimens varied from 10-80% pure cancer on histologic examination. In a small series, Young et al.[53] showed that AR was present in all patients without prior hormonal therapy, and that response to endocrine therapy seemed best in patients with the lowest AR levels. In de Voogt's series[54] the distribution of AR concentrations was similar to Ekman's group (above), but their reported response rate for endocrine therapy in the AR- group was no different from the AR+ group.

While a response to endocrine therapy is seen in 60% of patients with advanced prostate cancer[50], the therapeutic alternatives with chemotherapy are limited. A number of cytotoxic antineoplastic agents (e.g., Adriamycin and cis-platinum) show activity in prostate cancer[60], but many patients with this malignancy are elderly with systemic medical problems such as cardiac and renal failure which preclude their use. Bone marrow reserve diminishes with age, and malignant infiltration of the marrow also leads to decreased tolerance for myelosuppressive therapy. These factors make chemotherapy less attractive as an alternative to endocrine therapy in the initial treatment of metastatic prostate cancer. Younger patients with prostate cancer tend to have more biologically aggressive and hormonally unresponsive tumors. Because of their better general health, this group can better tolerate the side effects of chemotherapy; if absence of steroid receptors can be demonstrated to predict a failure of endocrine response, these patients may benefit from earlier chemotherapy.

In conclusion, there is currently no established clinical role for the measurement of steroid receptors in prostate cancer. Technical improvements are necessary before meaningful clinical studies can be done. The measurement of steroid receptors in metastatic sites may prove to be more useful than in the primary tumor.[61,62]

2. Endometrial Cancer

Estrogenic hormones cause proliferation of the endometrial epithelium, and progesterone converts the proliferative endometrium to a mature secretory epithelium. Prolonged unopposed estrogen effect will produce hyperplasia of the endometrium. There is a large body of epidemiologic evidence linking exposure to unopposed estrogens and the development of endometrial hyperplasia and (eventually) endometrial cancer.[63] Naturally occurring examples include women with Stein-Leventhal syndrome (anovulatory menstrual cycles) and obese postmenopausal women (increased peripheral conversion of precursors to estrogen); exogenous intake of estrogens also leads to an increased risk of endometrial cancer.[64] Therefore the investigation of ER in endometrial carcinoma seemed appropriate.

The human endometrium has been relatively easy to sample and to evaluate for steroid receptor analysis. The levels of ER and PR in endometrium are influenced by circulating hormone levels: estrogen stimulates production of ER and PR; progesterone inhibits production of both ER and PR. In addition,

Gurpide and Tseng[65] have demonstrated that progesterone and progestagens increase the activity of estradiol-17β dehydrogenase which in turn inactivates estradiol in the tissue by accelerating its conversion to estrone, a much weaker estrogen. This factor contributes to the anti-estrogen effect of progesterone, in addition to its inhibition of ER synthesis.

The normal endometrium shows periodic fluctuations in receptor content which are highly dependent on prior hormonal exposure.[66-70] In the premenopausal woman the ER peak occurs just before the estradiol peak in the late follicular phase of the menstrual cycle, which is then associated with a decrease in ER (figure). The endometrial PR is lowest at the beginning and end of the menstrual cycle, and is maximum at mid-cycle. In hypoestrogenic postmenopausal patients, endometrial ER is significantly lower than the lowest values recorded in premenopausal women, and PR cannot be detected. In the presence of estrogen effect ER may be found, as is PR in some specimens.[66] In endometrial hyperplasia, most investigators have described a slight decrease in PR content compared to normal proliferative endometrium; however, one group[67] found the highest cytosol levels of PR in hyperplastic endometrium. In general, a high PR level is usually associated with a low ER level in premenopausal women. In postmenopausal women PR is lower or may be undetectable.

The role of steroid receptor measurements in the management of endo-metrial cancer is not yet known. While several receptors can be measured easily, the possible therapeutic importance and prognostic significance of the receptor determinations are as yet uncertain. Endometrial biopsy specimens may contain focal carcinoma admixed with hyperplastic and normal endometrium. When the tissue specimen is prepared for receptor analysis there may be a substantial contribution of receptors from non-malignant tissue. This problem can be avoided if the tissue comes from a hysterectomy specimen where a piece of "pure" tumor can be obtained.

The majority of endometrial carcinomas contain both ER and PR. Two series relate the presence of both receptors with the most well-differentiated lesions.[67,71] Several reports demonstrate a direct correlation between the quantitative level of PR and tumor differentiation (with the highest PR values in the most well-differentiated lesions and in normal endometrium)[66,67,72], while a reverse correlation is noted for ER levels.[66,73]

Since progestins are a commonly-used therapy for metastatic endometrial carcinoma, PR concentration might prove more significant than ER in predicting endocrine response. This concept is supported by recent reports[66,73] suggesting that PR rich tumors may be more likely to respond than PR poor tumors. Some of the PR rich tumors which responded were poorly differentiated and would not normally have been thought to be endocrine responsive.

When reviewing the results of studies which correlate tissue receptor content and responses to endocrine therapy, it is critical to know whether the patient is receiving hormone therapy at the time of sampling. Several groups have demonstrated a significant fall in endometrial carcinoma PR with progestin therapy.[66,67] In theory, PR can be replenished by giving estrogen, and some authors have suggested that periodic administration of estrogen should be used to prolong the clinical response to progestin therapy.[67]

The role of steroid receptors in the clinical management of endometrial carcinoma remains uncertain at this time. As in breast cancer, only one-third of patients with metastatic endometrial carcinoma will respond to endocrine therapy[74], so that a biological parameter which can predict the likelihood of response would be very helpful. There is currently no highly effective cytotoxic therapy for endometrial cancer.[74,75] If and when there is sufficient improvement in the response rate to cytotoxic chemotherapy, steroid receptor measurements may assume a more important role in identifying patients who are endocrine responsive. At the present time, measurement of ER and PR in endometrial carcinoma cannot be recommended, except for investigative purposes.

3. Lymphoid Neoplasms

Because of the therapeutic effectiveness of glucocorticoids in lymphoid neoplasms (acute lymphoblastic leukemia, chronic lymphocytic leukemia, and the lymphomas), several groups have examined these tumors for glucocorticoid receptors.[76-78] Modulation of the glucocorticoid receptor is quite complex, and many variables affect its quantity and its measurement.[77] This may account for reported discrepancies between the results of several groups. The glucocorticoid receptor sites are similar in normal and in neoplastic cells.[77]

In evaluating patients with acute lymphoblastic leukemia, Lippman et al.[78] found that patients with the highest glucocorticoid receptor concentrations had null cell acute lymphoblastic leukemia, and they experienced the longest remission durations (see also, Chapter 1). Patients with T lymphoblasts had fewer receptor sites and shorter remission durations. It is doubtful that the prognosis of individual patients was being dictated by the concentration of glucocorticoid receptor sites; however, the presence of receptors may be a biologic marker of differentiation.

In a review of the prognostic value of steroid receptor determinations in leukemia, Duval and Homo[77] suggest that the simple measurement of glucocorticoid binding sites may not be sufficient to predict the response to therapy in this disease. Since not all lymphoid tumors which contain glucocorticoid receptors respond clinically to glucocorticoid therapy, they feel that the situation may be comparable to that of ER+ breast tumors in which only 60% of the receptor positive tumors respond.

Glucocorticoids can of course have serious side effects when given over prolonged periods of time, so that biochemical discriminants such as receptors which could predict hormone responsiveness would be very useful. At the present time there is not enough correlative data to recommend the measurement of receptors in these tumors.

4. Miscellaneous Neoplasms

a. Gynecologic neoplasms

All tissues of the female genitourinary tract are targets for estrogens. Except for the endometrium, the measurement of steroid receptors in these tissues has been carried out in a limited fashion[79], and the clinical significance of receptor content is still uncertain. Squamous tumors of the vulva, vagina, and cervix are not strongly influenced by steroids, and they contain only low levels of ER.[80,81] Adenocarcinomas of the vagina, cervix, and fallopian tubes have not been adequately studied, but they do occasionally show high ER or PR titers.[79] High ER and PR levels have also been found in some ovarian adenocarcinomas, but there are insufficient data correlating receptor content and response to endocrine therapy.[82] While there may be a potential application for endocrine therapy in these tumors, it is more likely that steroid receptor measurements will be used as an indicator of physiologic differentiation which in turn might predict their biologic behavior.[79]

b. Malignant melanoma

For many years there have been scattered (and conflicting) reports about the relationship between estrogens, pregnancy and melanoma.[83,84] Several groups have measured ER in melanoma[85,87], and there have been clinical trials of both estrogens and anti-estrogens in this malignancy with some surprising objective response rates.[88,89] However, some of the reported responses occurred in ER- tumors, and it is possible that the presence of steroid receptors in some melanoma cases reflects their presence in normal melanocytes.

c. Renal cell carcinoma

Interest in the hormonal treatment of renal cell cancer is derived from an animal model of this tumor. In the Syrian hamster only the male (or castrate female) is sensitive to the induction of renal cancer after prolonged administration of estrogens. Induction of the tumor can be blocked by the simultaneous administration of testosterone or progesterone. When these tumors are transplanted or become metastatic, a variety of endocrine therapies have been shown to affect their growth.[82] Sex hormones might conceivably influence the development of renal cell carcinoma in humans, as suggested by: 1) a low incidence of this tumor in children before puberty; 2) a predominance of males with this tumor (3:1); and 3) isolated reports of tumor regression with endocrine therapies (see below).

The therapeutic modalities for metastatic renal cell carcinoma are currently limited. Progestational agents are frequently given because of their minimal morbidity and occasional therapeutic benefit. An objective response rate of between 0% and 30% has been reported. There have been only a few studies of steroid receptors.[90,91] In an analysis of 27 patients, Concolino et al.[90] found that 59% of tumors were positive for ER and 59% for PR; 37% were positive and 19% negative for both ER and PR. Correlation of the results of progestin therapy and the presence of receptors in this report is complicated by the fact that only a few of the patients had measurable disease and most were treated in an adjuvant setting. In this particular tumor much more information is still needed on the occurrence of steroid receptors, and correlations with endocrine therapy must rely on objective (measurable) tumor responses.

d. Other tumors

Steroid receptors have been measured in a wide variety of tumors, from colon cancer to sarcomas[92-98] (Table II). The clinical and biologic implications of these findings are uncertain. In some instances they may indicate that trials of endocrine therapies in these tumors are warranted, or they may be a reflection of the neoplastic state and an epiphenomenon of no utility.

How steroid receptors might be used clinically

ER measurement has led to a more rational basis for determining therapy in advanced metastatic breast cancer. The role of steroid receptor measurement in other tumors is not as clearly defined, but the use of ER in breast cancer has formed the model upon which current investigations are based.

ER concentration should be determined in primary breast cancers, since tissue may not be available subsequently for this purpose. The information obtained may be essential for predicting the efficacy of hormone therapy should metastases occur. Whenever possible, a portion of the biopsy material should be rapidly frozen and kept frozen until a pathological diagnosis is made, so that the remaining specimen can be sent if indicated for receptor analysis. In some of these patients there may be no residual tumor in the mastectomy specimen or a breast-conserving approach may be chosen, so that information on the receptor status of the primary will be unavailable if not determined at biopsy.

Since ER seems to be an independent variable in breast cancer[16,33], it should be added to the traditional stratification variables when examining the natural history of breast cancer and the results of treatment interventions. It seems likely that ER status will soon play a more significant role in the adjuvant therapy of breast cancer. There are trials in progress evaluating the addition of the anti-estrogen tamoxifen to the adjuvant chemotherapy of ER+ patients with the hope of additional therapeutic benefit. While this is entirely speculative, it is possible that the absence of receptor may predict a higher risk group of axillary node negative patients who could benefit from adjuvant chemotherapy.

How does ER play a role in the management of metastatic breast cancer? Many patients presenting with metastatic breast cancer today may not have had receptor analysis performed on their primary cancer. In these patients an effort should be made to biopsy a metastatic site for receptor concentration. Receptor analyses have been performed on cells from pleural fluid[99], but samples are usually obtained from soft tissue and skin, and occasionally from visceral sites. If no tissue can be obtained, then one must select endocrine therapy on clinical grounds, as was traditionally done prior to ER analysis. If the ER status of the primary tumor is known, the therapy can be directed by these results; however, if there has been a long interval since biopsy of the tumor, then consideration should be given to rebiopsy if tumor tissue is easily accessible.

Since the therapeutic alternatives to endocrine therapy in disseminated prostatic and endometrial carcinoma are limited and there is less urgency for a predictive test for hormone response, the technical problems of steroid receptor measurements in these tumors make it unlikely that widespread clinical use will occur in the near future. More extensive data on the relationship of receptors to therapy must be obtained and there must be more standardization of sampling techniques and methods of measurement.

What is the clinical role of steroid receptors in other tumors? Steroid receptors have been found in a wide range of normal and neoplastic tissues (Tables I, II). Kiang and Kennedy[98] suggest that ER analysis should be performed with metastatic adenocarcinomas of unknown origin in female patients, since this conceivably may give a clue to the origin of the tumor. They report several cases in which the presence of ER in the tumor led to successful endocrine therapy that would not otherwise have been tried.

Summary on the Use of Steroid Receptors

Modern endocrinology has identified a mechanism by which most hormones interact with their target tissues to effect a specific hormonal action. Steroids bind to specific high affinity receptors in the cytosol and nucleus of the cell to initiate their actions. Receptor measurement by radioligand assays began a revolution in the understanding of hormone action in both normal and neoplastic tissues. In some tumors, such as breast cancer, the results are relatively straightforward. Since the non-neoplastic adjacent tissue is free of significant quantities of receptor[6], one can feel confident that the measured cytosol receptor concentrations are due to the neoplastic tissue. By contrast, normal as well as hyperplastic prostate and endometrium are rich in various steroid receptors, so that measured cytosol receptors in tumor specimens may be derived from several sources.

In order to evaluate the validity of reports of steroid receptors in cancer, one should consider several technical issues:

1. Is the tissue viable; has it been handled in the cold and properly prepared for analysis?

2. Is the tissue that is processed composed of pure tumor, and is there histologic confirmation of cancer?

3. Is care taken to insure that one is not measuring binding to serum proteins present in the tissue specimen?

4. Has it been demonstrated unequivocally that binding is to a receptor, by use of: a) competition curves; b) serum binder saturation; c) affinity and molecular weight data?

5. How sensitive is the receptor assay? Are quantitative results reported?

6. Have the circulating hormone levels been taken into consideration?

Predictions for the future

Analysis of steroid receptors in normal and neoplastic tissues can be anticipated to play a growing role in fundamental and clinical investigation. More sensitive assays are becoming available. Isolation and purification of receptors will permit quantitative assessments of receptor concentration independent of their ability to bind radioactive steroid. The roles of occupied and unoccupied nuclear and cytoplasmic receptors will be clarified and assessments of translocatability of the hormone-receptor complex will be developed. While immunofluorescence assessments of receptor content and histologic localization employing antibody to the steroid hormone have not been very useful, similar studies employing antibody to the receptor itself have a much greater potential.

Development of receptor panels for tumors may in the future provide additional useful information about the expected responses to endocrine therapies. Newer information about the regulation of receptor concentration and an enhanced ability to grow various tumor cells in culture may make it possible to develop therapeutic approaches based on an ability to induce receptors. Finally, new therapeutic agents focused on the presence of receptors in the tumor are being developed and may eventually lead to more selective chemotherapy based on the specific biological properties of the tumor.

References

1. Glacock, R.F., Hoekstra, W.G.: Selective accumulation of tritium-labelled hexeoestrol by the reproductive organs of immature female goats and sheep. Biochem. J. 72:673-682, 1959.

2. Jensen, E.V., Jacobson, H.I.: Fate of steroid estrogens in target tissues. in Pincus, G., Vollmer, E.P. (eds.) Biological activities of Steroids in relation to cancer. New York, Academic Press, 1969, pp. 161-178.

3. Jensen, E.V., Jacobson, H.I.: Basic guides to the mechanism of estrogen action. Rec Progr Hormone Res 18:387-414, 1962.

4. Folca, P.J., Glascock, R.F., Irvine, W.T.: Studies with tritium-labelled hexoesterol in advanced breast cancer. Lancet ii:796-802, 1961.

5. Jensen, E.V., DeSombre, E.R., Jungblut, P.W.: Estrogen receptors in hormone-responsive tissues and tumors. in Wissler, R.W., Dao, T.C., Wood Jr., S. (eds.) Chicago, U. of Chicago Press, 1967, pp. 15-30.

6. Korenman, S.G., Dukes, B.A.: Specific estrogen binding by the cytoplasm of human breast carcinoma. J. Clin. Endo. Metab. 30:639-645, 1970.

7. Jensen, E.V., Block, G.E., Smith, S. et al.: Estrogen receptors and breast cancer response to adrenalectomy. Nat. Cancer Inst. Monograph 34:55-70, 1971.

8. Savlov, E.D., Wittliff, J.L., Hilf, R. et al.: Correlations between certain biochemical properties of breast cancer and response to therapy: A preliminary report. Cancer 33:303-309, 1974.

9. McGuire, W.L., Carbone, P.P., Vollmer, E.P., eds.: Estrogen receptors in human breast cancer. New York, Raven Press, 1975.

10. DeSombre, E.R.: Steroid receptors in breast cancer. NEJM 301:1011-1012, 1979.

11. Steroid receptors in breast cancer, an NIH Consensus Development Conference, June 27-29, 1979. Cancer 46:2759-2963, 1980.

12. McGuide, W.L, Horowitz, K.B., Pearson, O.H. et al.: Current status of estrogen and progesterone receptors in breast cancer. Cancer 39:2934-2947, 1977.

13. Shain, S.A., Boesel, R.W., Lamm, D.L. et al.: Cytoplasmic and nuclear androgen receptor content of normal and neoplastic human prostates and lymph node metastases of human prostatic adenocarcinoma. J. Clin. End. Metab. 50:704-711, 1980.

14. Di Carlo, R., Muccioli, G.: Prolactin receptor in human mammary carcinoma. Tumori 65:695-702, 1979.

15. Allegra, J.C., Lippman, M.E., Thompson, E.B. et al.: Relationship between the progesterone, androgen, and glucocorticoid receptor and response rate to endocrine therapy in metastatic breast cancer. Can. Res. 39:1973-1979, 1979.

16. Osborne, C.K., Yochmowitz, M.G., Knight, W.A. et al.: The value of estrogen and progesterone receptors in the treatment of breast cancer. Cancer 46:2884-2888, 1980.

17. McGuire, W.L.: Hormone receptors: their role in predicting prognosis and response to endocrine therapy. Sem. Onc. 5:428-433, 1978.

18. McGuire, W.L.: Current status of estrogen receptors in human breast cancer. Cancer 36:638-644, 1975.

19. Jensen, E.V., Polley, T.Z., Smith, S. et al.: Prediction of hormone dependency in breast cancer. in McGuire, W.L., Carbone, P.O., Vollmer, E.P. (eds.): Estrogen Receptors in Human Breast Cancer, New York, Raven Press, 1975, pp. 37-56.

20. Hahnel, R., Vivan, A.B.: Biochemical and clinical experience with the estimation of estrogen receptors in human breast carcinoma. in McGuire, W.L., Carbone, P.P., Vollmer, E.P. (eds.): Estrogen receptors in Human Breast Cancer, New York, Raven Press, 1975, pp. 205-235.

21. McGuire, W.L., Pearson, O.H., Segaloff, A.: Predicting hormone responsiveness in human breast cancer. in McGuire, W.L., Carbone, P.P., Vollmer, E.P. (eds.): Estrogen Receptors in Human Breast Cancer, New York, Raven Press, 1975, pp. 17-36.

22. Heuson, J.C., Leclercq, G., Longeval, E. et al.: Estrogen receptors: prognostic significance in breast cancer. in McGuire, W.L., Carbone, P.P., Vollmer, E.P. (eds.): Estrogen Receptors in Human Breast Cancer, New York, Raven Press, 1975, pp. 57-72.

23. Maass, H., Engel, B., Nowakowski, H. et al.: Estrogen receptors in human breast cancer and clinical correlations. in McGuire, W.L., Carbone, P.P., Vollmer, E.P. (eds.): Estrogen Receptors in Human Breast Cancer, New York, Raven Press, 1975, pp. 175-191.

24. Allegra, J.C., Barlock, A., Huff K. et al.: Changes in multiple or sequential estrogen receptor determinations in breast cancer. Cancer 45:792-794, 1980.

25. Rosen, P.P., Menendez-Botet, C.J., Urban, J.A. et al.: Estrogen recetpro protein in multiple tumor specimens from individual patients with breast cancer. Cancer 39:2194-2200, 1977.

26. Kiang, D.T., Kennedy, B.J.: Factors affecting estrogen receptors in breast cancer. Cancer 0:1571-1576, 1977.

27. McGuire, W.L., Horowitz, K.B., Zava, D.T. et al.: Hormones in breast cancer: Update 1978. Metabolism 27:487-501, 1978.

28. Bloom, N.D., Tobin, E.H., Schreibman, B. et al.: The role of progesterone receptors in the management of advanced breast cancer. Cancer 45:2992-2997, 1980.

29. Kledzik, G.S., Bradley, C.J., Marshall, S. et al.: Effects of high doses of estrogen on prolactin binding activity and growth of carcinogen-induced mammary cancers in rats. Can. Res. 36:3265-3268, 1978.

30. Shiu, R.P.C.: Prolactin receptors in human breast cancer cells in long-term tissue culture. Can. Res. 39:4381-4386, 1979.

31. Horowitz, K.B., McGuire, W.L.: Estrogen control of progesterone receptor in human breast cancer. J. Biol. Chem. 253:2223-2228, 1978.

32. Macfarlane, J.K., Fleiszer, D., Fazekas, A.G.: Studies on estrogen receptors and regression in human breast cancer. Cancer 45:2998-3003, 1980.

33. Knight, W.A., Livingston, R.B., Gregory, E.J., et al.: Estrogen receptor as an independent prognostic factor for early recurrence in breast cancer. Can. Res. 37:4669-4671, 1977.

34. Maynard, P.V., Blamey, R.W., Elston, C.W. et al.: Estrogen receptor assay in primary breast cancer and early recurrence of the disease. Can. Res. 38:4292-4295, 1978.

35. Rich, M.A., Furmanski, P., Brooks, S.C.: Prognostic value of estrogen receptor determinations in patients with breast cancer. Can. Res. 38:4296-4298, 1978.

36. Blamey, R.W., Bishop, H.M., Blake, J.R.S. et al.: Relationship between primary breast rumor receptor status and patient survival. Cancer 46:2765-2769, 1980.

37. Furmanski, P., Saunders, P.E., Brooks, S.C., et al.: The prognostic value of estrogen receptor determinations in patients with primary breast cancer: An update. Cancer: 46:2794-2796, 1980.

38. Parl, F.F., Wagner, R.K.: The histopathological evaluation of human breast cancer in correlation with estrogen receptor values. Cancer 46:362-367, 1980.

39. Meyer, J.S., Rao, B.R., Stevens, S.C. et al.: Low incidence of estrogen receptor in breast carcinomas with rapid rates of cellular replication. Cancer 40:2290-2298, 1977.

40. Silvestrini, R., Dardone, M.G., DeFronzo, G.: Relationship between proliferative activity and estrogen receptors in breast cancer. Cancer 44:665-670, 1979.

41. Lippman, M.E., Allegra, J.C., Thompson, E.B., et al.: The relation between estrogen receptors and response rate of cytotoxic chemotherapy in metastatic breast cancer. NEJM 298:1223-1228, 1978.

42. Kiang, D.T., Frenning, D.H., Goldman, A.I., et al.: Estrogen receptors and responses to chemotherapy and hormonal therapy in advanced breast cancer. NEJM 299:1330-1334, 1978.

43. Hilf, R., Feldstein, M.L., Savlov, E.D. et al.: The lack of relationship between estrogen receptor status and response to chemotherapy. Cancer 46:2797-2800, 1980.

44. Jonat, W., Maass, H., Stolzenbach, G. et al.: Estrogen receptor status and response to polychemotherapy in advanced breast cancer. Cancer 46:2809-2813, 1980.

45. Kiang, D.T., Frenning, D.H, Gay, J., et al.: Estrogen receptor status and response to chemotherapy in advanced breast cancer. Cancer 46:2814-2817, 1980.

46. Lippman, M.L., Allegra, J.C.: Quantitative estrogen receptor analyses: the response to endocrine and cytotoxic chemotherapy in human breast cancer and the disease-free interval. Cancer 46:2829-2834, 1980.

47. Rosenbaum, C., Marsland, T.A., Stolbach, L.L. et al.: Estrogen receptor status and response to chemotherapy in advanced breast cancer. The Tufts-Shattuck-Pondville experience. Cancer 46:2919-2921, 1980.

48. Rubens, R.D., Hayward, J.C.: Estrogen receptors and response to endocrine and cytotoxic chemotherapy in advanced breast cancer. Cancer 46:2922-2927, 1980.

49. Samal, B.A., Brooks, S.C., Cummings, G. et al.: Estrogen receptors and responsiveness of advanced breast cancer to chemotherapy. Cancer 46:2925-2927, 1980.

50. Walsh, P.C.: Physiologic basis for hormonal therapy in carcinoma of the prostate. Urol. Clin. N.A. 2:125-140, 1975.

51. Catalona, W.J., Scott, W.W.: Carcinoma of the prostate: a review. J. of Urology 119:1-8, 1978.

52. Ekman, P., Snochowski, M., Zetterberg, A. et al.: Steroid receptor content in human prostatic carcinoma and response to endocrine therapy. Cancer 44:1173-1181, 1979.

53. Young, J.D., Sidh, S.M., Bashirelahi, N.: The role of estrogen, androgen, and progestogen receptors in the management of carcinoma of the prostate. Trans. Am. Assoc. of Genito-Urinary Surgeons 71:23-25, 1979.

54. De Voogt, H.J., Dingjan, P.: Steroid receptors in human prostatic cancer. Urol. Res. 6:151-158, 1978.

55. Pertschuk, L.P., Zava, D.T., Gaetjans, E. et al.: Histochemistry of steroid receptors in prostatic diseases. Ann. Clin. Lab. Sci. 9:225-229, 1979.

56. Murphy, J.B., Emmott, R.C., Hicks, L.L. et al.: Estrogen receptors in the human prostate, seminal vesicle, epididymis, testis, and genital skin: a marker for estrogen-responsive tissues? J. Clin. End. Metab. 50:938-48, 1980.

57. Bashirelahi, N., Kneussl, E.S., Vassil, T.C. et al.: Measurement and characterization of estrogen receptors in the human prostate. Prog. Clin. Biol. Res. 33:65-84, 1979.

58. Mobbs, B.G., Johnson, I.E., Connolly, J.G.: Protamine sulfate precipitation of androgen receptors of human benign and malignant prostatic tumors. Prog. Clin. Biol. Res. 33:13-32, 1979.

59. Olsson, C.A., DeVere White, R., Goldstein, I. et al.: A preliminary report on the measurement of cytosolic and nuclear prostatic tissue steroid receptors. Prog. Clin. Biol. Res. 33:209-221, 1979.

60. Torti, F.M., Carter, S.K.: The chemotherapy of prostatic adenocarcinoma. Ann. Int. Med. 92:681-689, 1980.

61. Ekman, P., Snochowski, M., Dahlberg, E. et al.: Steroid receptors in metastatic carcinoma of the human prostate. Eur. J. Cancer 15:257-62, 1979.

62. Kliman, B., Prout, G.R., MacLaugline, R.A.: Characterization of androgen receptor in human prostatic tissues and demonstration of decreased androgen receptor content in metastatic prostate cancer. Surgical Forum 30:550-1, 1979.

63. MacMahon, B.: Risk factors for endometrial cancer. Gynecol. Oncol. 2:122-9, 1974.

64. Mack, T.M.: Exogenous oestrogens and endometrial carcinoma: studies, criticisms, and current status. in Brush, M.G., King, R.J.B., Taylor, R.W. (eds.) Endometrial Cancer, London, Bailliere Tindall, 1978, pp. 17-28.

65. Gurpide, E., Tseng, L.: Potentially useful tests for responsiveness of endometrial cancer to progestogen therapy. in Brush, M.G., King, R.J.B., Taylor, R.W. (eds.) Endometrial Cancer, London, Bailliere Tindall, 1978, pp. 252-257.

66. Martin, P.M., Rolland, P.H., Gammerre, M. et al.: Estradiol and progesterone receptors in normal and neoplastic endometrium. Int. J. Cancer 23:321-329, 1979.

67. Janne, O., Kauppila, A., Kontula, K. et al.: Female sex steroid receptors in normal, hyperplastic and carcinomatous endometrium. Int. J. Cancer 24:545-54, 1979.

68. Bayard, F., Damilano, S., Robel, R. et al.: Cytoplasmic and nuclear estradiol and progesterone receptors in human endometrium. J. Clin. End. Met. 46:635-648, 1978.

69. Tsibris, J.C.M., Cazenave, C.R., Cantor, B. et al.: Distribution of cytoplasmic estrogen and progesterone receptors in human endometrium. Am. J. Obst. Gynec. 132:449-54, 1978.

70. Prodi, G., De Giovanni, C., Galli, M.C. et al.: 17B-estradiol, 5 α-dihydrotestosterone, progesterone, and cortisol receptors in normal and neoplastic human endometrium. Tumori, 65:241-253, 1979.

71. McCarty, K.S., Barton, T.K., Fetter, B.F. et al.: Correlation of estrogen and progesterone receptors with histologic differentiation in endometrial adenocarcinoma. Am. J. Pathol. 96:171-83, 1979.

72. Ehrlich, C.E., Cleary, R.E., Young, P.C.M.: The use of progesterone receptors in the management of recurrent endometrial cancer. in Brush, M.G., King, R.J.B., Taylor, R.W. (eds.) Endometrial Cancer, London, Baillière Tindall, 1978, pp. 258-264.

73. Pollow, K., Schmidt-Gollwitzer, M., Pollow, B.: Oestradiol-binding proteins in normal human endometrium during the menstrual cycle and in endometrial carcinoma dependent on the degree of tumor differentiation. in Brush, M.G., King, R.J.B, Taylor, R.W. (eds.) Endometrial Cancer, London, Baillière Tindall, 1978, pp. 265-274.

74. Berman, M.L., Ballon, S.C.: Treatment of endometrial cancer. Can. Treat. Rev. 6:165-175, 1979.

75. Kauppila, A., Jänne, O., Kujansuu, E. et al.: Treatment of advanced endometrial adenocarcinoma with a combined cytotoxic therapy. Cancer 46:2162-2167, 1980.

76. Crabtree, G.R., Smith, K.A., Munck, A.: Glucocorticoid receptors and sensitivity of isolated human leukemia and lymphoma cells. Can. Res. 38:4268-4272, 1978.

77. Duval, A., Homo, F.: Prognostic value of steroid receptor determination in leukemia. Can. Res. 38:4263-4267, 1978.

78. Lippman, M.E., Yabro, G.K., Levinthal, B.G.: Clinical implications of glucocorticoid receptors in human leukemia. Can. Res. 38:4251-4256, 1978.

79. Hoffman, P.G., Siiteri, P.K.: Sex steroid receptors in gynecologic cancer. Obst. Gyn. 55:648-652, 1980.

80. Hähnel, R., Martin, J.D., Masters, A.M. et al.: Estrogen receptors and blood hormone levels in cervical carcinoma and other gynecological tumors. Gyn. Onc. 8:226-233, 1979.

81. Johansson, R., Grönroos, M., Kouvonen, I. et al.: Oestrogen receptors in dysplastic and malignant vulval tissue. Acta Obstet. Gynecol. Scand. 58:213-214, 1979.

82. Friedman, M.A., Hoffman, P.G., Jones, H.W.: The clinical value of hormone receptor assays in malignant disease. Can. Treat. Reviews 5:185-194, 1978.

83. Shaw, H.M., Milton, G.W., Farago, G. et al.:   Endocrine influences on survival from malignant melanoma. Cancer 42:669-677, 1978.

84. Shiu, M.H., Schottenfeld, D., Maclean, B. et al.:   Adverse effect of pregnancy on melanoma. Cancer 37:181-187, 1976.

85. Fisher, R.I., Neifeld, J.P., Lippman, M.E.:   Oestrogen receptors in human malignant melanoma. Lancet ii:337-338, 1976.

86. McCarthy, K.S., Wortman, J., Stowers, S. et al.:   Sex steroid receptor analysis in human melanoma. Cancer 46:1463-1470, 1980.

87. Creagan, E.T., Ingle, J.N., Woods, J.E. et al.:   Estrogen receptors in patients with malignant melanoma. Cancer 46:1785-1786, 1980.

88. Fisher, R.I., Young, R.C., Lippman, M.E.:   Diethylstilbesterol therapy of surgically nonresectable malignant melanoma. Proc. Am. Soc. Clin. Oncol. 19:339, 1978.

89. Nesbit, R.A., Woods, R.L., Tattersal, M.H.N. et al.:   Tamoxifen in malignant melanoma. NEJM 301:1241-1242, 1979.

90. Concolino, G., Di Silverio, F., Marocchi, A. et al.:   Renal cancer steroid receptors: biochemical   basis   for   endocrine   therapy.   Eur.   Urol. 5:319-322, 1979.

91. Giulani, L., Pescatore, D., Giberti, C. et al.:   Usefulness and limitation of estrogen receptor protein (ERP) assay in human renal cell carcinomas. Eur. Urol. 4:342-347, 1978.

92. McClendon, J.E., Appleby, D., Claudon, D.B. et al.:   Colonic neoplasms: tissue estrogen receptor and carcinoembryonic antigen.   Arch. Surg. 112:240-241, 1977.

93. Lee, Y.T.N., Markland, F.S.:   Steroid receptors in sarcomatous lesions. J. Surg. Onc. 11:305-311, 1979.

94. Keshgegian, A.A., Wheeler, J.E.:   Estrogen receptor protein in malignant carcinoid tumor. Cancer 45:293-296, 1980.

95. Stedman, K.E., Moore, G.E., Morgan, R.T.:   Estrogen receptor proteins in diverse human tumors. Arch. Surg. 115:244-248, 1980.

96. Molteni, A., Bahu, R.M., Battifora, H.A. et al.:   Estradiol receptor assays in normal and neoplastic tissues. Ann. Clin. Lab. Sci. 9:103-108, 1979.

97. Alford, T.C., Do, H.M., Geelhoed, G.W. et al.:   Steroid hormone receptors in human colon cancers. Cancer 43:980-84, 1979.

98. Kiang, D.T., Kennedy, B.J.:   Estrogen receptor assay in the differential diagnosis of adenocarcinomas. JAMA 238:32-34, 1977.

99. McCarthy, K.S., Wortman, J., Moore, J.O. et al.: Malignant effusions in
    recurrent breast cancer. Cancer 45:1609-1614, 1980.

Chapter 3

Advances in the Use
of Peptide Hormones as Tumor Markers

Ada Wolfsen, M.D.
William Odell, M.D., Ph.D.

Introduction

Systemic symptoms from the production of humoral substances by tumors may be the first clue to the presence of a cancer. These systemic symptoms often wax and wane with the course of the disease. It was felt initially that the ectopic production of hormones by cancers was relatively uncommon. While the symptomatic expression of hormone production by tumors is unusual, in the past five years our understanding of the pathogenesis of these humoral syndromes has improved strikingly. Odell and Wolfsen have postulated[1-3] that in fact all carcinomas elaborate proteins "ectopically": tumors associated with clinically apparent syndromes are associated with bioactive forms of these proteins; those cancers not associated with clinically apparent syndromes elaborate biologically inactive or weakly active proteins, including protein hormone precursors. In this article, we review the information on which this hypothesis has been developed. We have selected as examples several of the syndromes of greatest interest, including those we have studied personally.

The hormones or hormonal precursors that have been found to be elaborated by cancers are listed in Table I. Note that, with the single exception of the prostaglandins, these hormones are protein or peptide in nature; steroid hormones or thyronines do not appear to be synthesized ectopically by nonendocrine cancers. Thus, the currently understood ectopic humoral syndromes are produced by the elaboration of a protein or a peptide by the cancer.

Chorionic Gonadotropin

Chorionic gonadotropin (CG) is a glycoprotein hormone composed of two protein chains, alpha and beta. The alpha chain is quite similar in amino acid sequence to the alpha chains of related human pituitary glycoprotein hormones, thyrotropin (TSH), luteinizing hormone (LH) and follicle stimulating hormone (FSH)[4-7]. These alpha chains themselves possess no biological activity and are indistinguishable by radioimmunoassays. The beta chain of CG, while similar in the first 117 amino terminal residues to LH, possesses in addition a carbohydrate-rich 30 amino acid tail at the carboxyl terminus. The beta chains of these glycoprotein hormones also possess no biological activity. The intact, biologically active protein hormones are composed of alpha and beta peptide chains which are not joined together covalently, but by charge-charge interactions.

Until about 1960, production of gonadotropin resembling human placental chorionic gonadotropin was recognized only in association with neoplasms derived from the placental cytotrophoblast, or with teratomas containing such

64

TABLE I

HORMONES REPORTED TO BE SECRETED BY CANCERS

ProACTH and ACTH

Lipotropin

Chorionic gonadotropin (CG)

alpha peptide chain of CG

beta peptide chain of CG

Vasopressin

Somatomedins

Hypoglycemic producing factors

Parathyroid hormone

Osteoclast activating factor

Prostaglandins

Erythropoietin

Hypophosphatemia producing factor

Calcitonin

Growth Hormone

Prolactin

Gastrin

Secretin

Glucagon

Corticotropin Releasing Hormone

Growth Hormone Releasing Hormone

Somatostatin

Chorionic somatotropin

Neurophysins

cells. In the years 1949 to 1968, isolated case reports of patients with various cancers and evidence of increased gonadotropin production appeared, but the assays available at that time could not distinguish LH from CG. The reported neoplasms included malignant melanoma[9], carcinoma of the lung[10-12], renal carcinoma[13], undifferentiated carcinoma[14], and breast carcinoma[15]. Braunstein et al.[16], using an assay with enhanced ability to distinguish CG from LH[17], found that between 6 and 13 percent of patients with a variety of carcinomas had increased blood CG concentrations. The greatest frequency of detectable CG was in gastrointestinal neoplasms: 167/363, or 18%.

A study of 532 patients with biopsy proven carcinoma of the lung, gastrointestinal tract, pancreatic islet cells or carcinoid, revealed elevations of CG and free CG-β in many tumor-bearing individuals as determined by a highly-specific assay in 41% of men with lung cancer, 28% of men with gastrointestinal cancer, and 6% of men with islet cell carcinoma, in women, CG and CG-β were elevated in 16% with lung cancer, 34% with gastrointestinal cancer, 50% with carcinoid and 19% with islet cell carcinoma.[18] None of 579 control subjects or men with carcinoid tumors had elevated levels of CG or CG-β.

Studies from our laboratory showed that extracts of a wide variety of carcinomas contained CG-like material, as determined by the CG-β radioimmunoassay and gonadotropin radioreceptor assay[19]. Surprisingly, using the same methods to extract normal human tissues obtained at autopsy from patients without cancers, we found that all normal human tissues contained CG[19,20]. This material was indistinguishable from placental CG as determined by CG-β radioimmunoassay and LH-CG radioreceptor assay. However, it was distinguishable from placental CG by its reaction with concanavalin (Con A). Placental CG is carbohydrate rich and binds to Con A via its carbohydrate units. By contast, normal tissue CG was found to exhibit little or no Con A binding and is probably carbohydrate free[19,20].

As opposed to CG extracted from normal tissues, the Con A binding properties of CG extracted from carcinomas was found to be variable, ranging from less than 5% binding (equivalent to that of normal tissue CG) to 93% (equivalent to hCG) (Table II)[21]. Previous investigators had reported that desialation of placental CG greatly decreases its biological potency in in vivo bioassays by increasing its metabolic clearance rate (shortening its half time of disappearance)[22,23]. This may explain the low concentrations of hCG reported in the blood of normal subjects (<20 pg/ml)[24], despite the apparent production of hCG by pituitary[25] and other normal human tissues[19,20].

CG detected by specific CG-β assay is a useful tumor marker for diagnosis and for monitoring response to therapy in patients with trophoblastic neoplasms[26,27]. Measurement of plasma and cerebrospinal fluid CG has been useful for detection and for monitoring the response to therapy of cerebral metastases of trophoblastic tumors[28]. The use of CG as a tumor marker has also facilitated the diagnosis and treatment of testicular germ cell neoplasms[29]. Approximately 75% of non-seminomatous testicular tumors are associated with elevated CG levels in blood. CG is produced by syncytiotrophoblastic giant cells of germ cell tumors and the

TABLE II

CON A BINDING OF CG EXTRACTED FROM VARIOUS HUMAN TISSUES

	% Bound $\pm$ SEM	Range
Normal tissues (10)	6.1 $\pm$ 1.6	0.0 - 14.6
Normal placenta (4)	92.5 $\pm$ 0.9	90.1 - 94.0
Carcinomas (9)	31.2 $\pm$ 9.1	4.0 - 86.0
Cancer serum (8)	54.7 $\pm$ 11.9	3.1 - 92.5
Pregnancy serum (3)	100	---

Modified from Yoshimoto, Wolfsen and Odell (21).

syncytiotrophoblastic cells of choriocarcinoma. Measurement of serum CG has been useful in the diagnostic classification of these tumors, in staging germ cell tumors, and in predicting the effects of therapeutic intervention. Following complete surgical removal of testicular tumors, a CG disappearance rate from blood which has a slower half-time than 20 hours has been shown to be predictive of occult nodal or distant metastases with a greater accuracy than the lymphangiogram. Serum CG concentrations have also been shown to predict remission or recurrence in response to chemotherapy in patients with advanced disease.

In patients with trophoblastic and germinal tumors, injected ^{131}I-labeled goat immunoglobulin G antibody to CG has been shown to localize in primary and metastatic tumors, and thus permit tumor localization by external gamma ray scintigraphy[30]. CG therefore has a potential for tumor imaging and localization, as well as for diagnosis and tumor surveillance following therapy.

In tumors that do not harbor trophoblastic cells, the determination of serum CG/CG-β may have limited use in screening for early cancer detection. Of 9 subjects who developed pancreatic carcinoma and 8 who developed gastric carcinoma while being followed in the Framinghan Heart Study, one patient with pancreatic carcinoma had a marked elevation of CG in the blood 2 months before clinical diagnosis and borderline elevation 26 months before diagnosis. Four of 34 postmenopausal control women also had borderline CG elevations in at least one of several blood samples [31]. Thus low sensitivity and specificity prevent the use of serum CG as a cancer screening test using current methodology.

Urinary CG measurements may be more useful for cancer screening. A greater percentage of patients with nontrophoblastic malignancies have increased CG immunoreactivity in urine than in serum. Of 70 patients studied with a wide variety of malignancies, 44.3% had elevated urinary excretion of CG and its β subunit while only 17.1% had elevated concentrations in serum obtained simultaneously[32]. Both male and female control subjects including patients with nonmalignant diseases were used to calculate normal ranges in the population.

Free Alpha Chain of CG

In addition to the synthesis and elaboration of a CG-like material, carcinomas also elaborate the free alpha subunit. The alpha subunit of CG is indistinguishable from that of TSH and LH. Studies from our laboratory [33,34] have shown that the normal human pituitary stimulated by thyrotropin releasing hormone (TRH) or gonadtropin releasing hormone (GnRH), releases respectively thyrotropin (TSH) or luteinizing hormone (LH) and abundant free alpha chain. The alpha subunit associated with TSH and LH is indistinguishable from the alpha chain of CG. The purpose (if any) of the secretion of excess alpha chain is uncertain, but it may insure maximum combination of the secreted beta chains with alpha chains to form intact, biologically active hormone. Normal alpha chain concentrations are higher in postmenopausal women than in premenopausal women or men. Rosen and Weintraub[35] first reported a patient with a carcinoma that produced free alpha chain. Kahn et al[36] reported elevated free alpha chain concentrations in the blood in 59% of patients with pancreatic islet cell carcinomas, but in no patients with benign islet cell tumors.   One-third of patients with malignant gastrinomas have elevated alpha subunit when compared to patients with benign gastrinomas or benign gastrointestinal diseases[37].   Further studies from our laboratory[3,38] revealed that blood concentrations of free alpha chain are increased in patients with a variety of different carcinomas more frequently than intact CG: 30% of men with untreated carcinoma of the lung, 20% of men with untreated gastric carcinoma, and 20% of women with untreated colon carcinoma had elevated free alpha chain concentrations in the blood. Furthermore, when we extracted a wide variety of carcinomas as well as normal human tissues, immunoreactive free alpha chain was detectable in over 95% of tissue extracts.

Braunstein et al.[39] found no correlation between alpha subunit concentrations and either the initial tumor burden or the occurrence of tumor progression or regression in patients with various malignancies. On the other hand, in a study of fifty-five patients with metastatic melanoma elevated alpha subunit concentrations prior to therapy were associated with reduced survival in premenopausal women[40]. Pretreatment alpha chain levels were significantly lower in premenopausal patients who responded to chemoimmunotherapy, compared to those who failed to respond.

The alpha subunit may be more valuable for tumor diagnosis when used in combination with other peptide hormones. Prospective studies in our laboratory combining determinations of alpha subunit, ACTH, LPH (see below) and calcitonin revealed an elevated plasma concentration of one or more peptides in 77% of 74 lung cancer patients at the time of diagnosis; none of the 26 patients who were evaluated for abnormal chest x-rays and found subsequently to have benign diseases had plasma peptide elevations[41]. Blackman et al.[18] reported elevated levels of alpha subunit in 11% of men with lung cancer, 32% of men with gastrointestinal cancer, 50% of men with carcinoid, and 61% of men with islet cell cancer. However, when combined with determinations of CG and CG-β concentration in blood, either alpha chain or CG-β levels were elevated in 45% of men with lung cancer, 48% of men with gastrointestinal cancer, 50% of men with carcinoid and 61% of men with islet cell cancer. For women, alpha subunit alone was elevated in 16% with lung cancer, 18% with gastrointestinal cancer, 13% with carcinoid, and 38% with islet cell cancer. Either alpha subunit or CG-β levels were elevated in 29% of women with lung cancer, 41% of women with gastrointestinal cancer, 50% of women with carcinoid, and 43% of women with islet cell carcinoma. While combined determinations of alpha subunit and CG/CG-β may be useful as markers for certain nontrophblastic malignancies, their clinical utility remains to be established in prospective studies.

Adrenocorticotrophin(ACTH)

The first ectopic hormonal syndrome to be reported was the association of Cushing's syndrome with oat cell carcinoma of the bronchus in 1928[42]. In the 1960's Liddle et al.[43] published extensive studies of this syndrome using in vivo bioassays to quantify ACTH. These investigators showed that in patients with cancer and Cushing's syndrome, the primary tumor as well as its metastases contained large amounts of biologically active ACTH. This particular ectopic hormonal syndrome shows a striking association with certain types of neoplasms. Approximately 80% of reported cases have been associated with six types of cancer: 50% with carcinomas of the lung (usually small cell or "oat cell" type), 10% with carcinoma of the pancreas, 10% with thymus carcinomas, 5% with neoplasms derived from neural crest tissues*, 5% with medullary carcinomas of the thyroid, and 2% with bronchial adenomas or carcinoids. The remaining patients cover many types of carcinoma. The association of tumors with clinically-apparent hypercortisolism is rare; for instance, only 2.8% of patients with oat cell carcinoma have elevated plasma cortisol levels which fail to suppress with 8 mg daily of dexamethasone[44].

However, studies performed by Ratcliffe et al.[45], Bloomfield et al.[46], Gewirtz and Yalow[47] and Wolfsen and Odell[3,48] have revealed that extracts of all carcinomas of the lung, regardless of histologic type, contain an ACTH-like material by radioimmunoassay. Further studies from our laboratory have revealed that extracts of all carcinomas of the colon, stomach, esophagus and pancreas contain the same immunoreactive ACTH, but generally in lower concentrations than lung carcinomas. This ACTH material is different from the biologically active ACTH secreted by the pituitary, in that it has a higher molecular weight, and has little biological activity in the in vitro dispersed adrenal cell bioassay (100 to 300-fold less potent than $hACTH_{1-39}$) and little activity in the radioreceptor assay for ACTH. This high molecular weight ACTH may be converted to biologically active ACTH by incubation with trypsin[47,48,49]. It might be noted that high molecular weight forms of ACTH that are purified from sheep pituitary block the action of bioactive $ACTH_{1-39}$ on adrenal cells from fetal sheep in vitro[50].

Investigations of ACTH biosynthesis in mouse pituitary tumor cell cultures by Eipper and Mains[51,52] have revealed that the first messenger RNA product possessing ACTH immunoreactivity is a glycoprotein with a molecular weight of 31,000. This is converted sequentially to 23,000 MW, then to a 13,000 MW precursor, and finally to the familiar 4500 MW biologically active form of ACTH. Presumably the immunoreactive, non-biologically active ACTH which has been shown by our studies to be extractable from all carcinomas is one of the precursor forms of ACTH ("ProACTH").

Based on our observations of ACTH immunoreactivity in all tumor extracts, we performed a blind prospective study to evaluate the potential of ProACTH measurements for the diagnosis of lung cancer. One hundred patients admitted to the medical service of Harbor-UCLA Medical Center with an abnormal chest x-ray had plasma ACTH determined on admission by radioimmunoassay. Any patient with clinical or laboratory evidence suggestive of ectopic ACTH syndrome (hypokalemia, elevated blood glucose) was excluded from study. Fifty-three of 74 patients (72%) subsequently shown to have lung cancer had elevated immunoreactive ACTH.† Like the ACTH extracted directly from carcinomas, the immunoreactive material exhibited little activity in our ACTH radioreceptor assay[3,48]. All 26 patients subsequently shown to have benign diseases had normal immunoreactive ACTH concentrations. ACTH was also quantified in patients with chronic obstructive pulmonary disease

---

*pheochromocytomas, neuroblastomas, ganglioneuromas, paragangliomas.
†For these studies, lightly heparinized plasma was obtained in an ice bath at the bedside. All samples were kept on ice until centrifuged at 4°C within 30 minutes. Aliquots were thawed only once for assay.

(COPD) and in patients with tuberculosis or other granulatomous diseases. Twenty of 111 patients with COPD had elevated ACTH levels, and after $2\frac{1}{2}$ years' follow-up 5 of these have been shown to have early lung carcinomas. Of 31 patients hospitalized for granulatomous lung diseases, 3 had elevated ACTH levels initially, but all were normal on subsequent sampling during convalescence. These data suggest that whereas all carcinomas may synthesize and secrete immunoreactive ACTH, those carcinomas associated with the clinically recognizable ectopic ACTH syndrome convert biologically inactive ProACTH to biologically active ACTH. These neoplasms possess the specific enzymes which are required to metabolize ProACTH to ACTH.

Other investigations have supported these concepts. Yalow reported that two-thirds of 36 patients whose tumors were considered resectable had elevated plasma ACTH levels[53]. Follow-up plasma ACTH levels within 3 months following surgical resection were lower than the preoperative concentrations in 20 of 25 patients. After administering 2 mg dexamethasone to patients with bronchogenic carcinoma, nonmalignant lung diseases and to normals, mean immunoreactive ACTH remained significantly higher in patients with cancer as compared to normals or patients with noncancerous lung diseases[54]. The percentage of cancer patients with elevated plasma ACTH (20%) did not change significantly after dexamethasone administration.

In two other reported studies involving patients with oat cell carcinoma and elevated ACTH concentrations prior to radiation or chemotherapy, reported ACTH determinations were useful for monitoring responses to therapy. Elevated plasma ACTH values were observed to decrease in patients who responded to therapy, and in some patients they increased again several weeks before tumor progression was demonstrated clinically[55,56]. However, clinical progression of disease was not heralded by an increase of ACTH in all patients, and plasma ACTH levels did not correlate with initial tumor stage.

A study of the usefulness of cerebrospinal fluid ACTH for detecting brain metastases in patients with small cell bronchogenic carcinomas revealed significantly higher ACTH concentrations in 14 patients with central nervous system metastases than in 8 patients without evidence of metastases[57]. Eleven of the 13 patients with brain metastases had CSF ACTH concentrations greater than the highest level observed in patients without metastases.

The clinical usefulness of ACTH measurements in blood and other biological fluids is still being investigated actively. In the future we look forward to the development of radioimmunoassays specific for the high molecular weight ACTH that represents the major species in tumor extracts and blood of cancer patients.

Lipotropin (LPH)

The ectopic production of melanocyte-stimulating hormone (MSH) by cancers in man has been described as a concomitant of ectopic ACTH production[58-60]. However, Bloomfield and Scott[61] and our own laboratory[62] have confirmed that βMSH as such is not secreted by the pituitaries of normal people or patients with endocrine diseases associated with hyperpigmentation

(Addison's disease, Cushing's disease, Nelson's syndrome). We believe βMSH is an artifact of the extraction-purification technique that was used originally to prepare it. Li et al.[63] originally purified and characterized the protein βlipotropin (LPH) from sheep pituitaries. Human βLPH contains within its structure the entire amino acid sequence of βMSH. We have shown that LPH circulates in the blood of normal individuals and is elevated in the blood of patients with Addison's disease, Cushing's disease and Nelson's syndrome[62]. Although βMSH may be produced by cancers that are associated with the ectopic ACTH syndrome[64], we believe that most of the immunoactivity that was previously identified in MSH radioimmunoassays was in reality lipotropin. It is not known whether the blood LPH that has been quantified in "MSH" bioassays is implicated in pigmentation, but it is certain that it is considerably less potent than alpha or beta MSH and it seems about equal to ACTH. Mains et al.[65] have shown that the same precursor molecule that gives rise to ACTH also gives rise to βlipotropin. Accordingly, as part of our study of ectopic hormone production by tumors, we have evaluated cancer patients for ectopic lipotropin production[66]. The story is reminiscent of that already described for CG and ACTH. All extracts from 79 carcinomas originating in the lung, colon, stomach, esophagus or breast contained LPH in concentrations greater than the blood. Sixty-one of 79 tumor extracts contained LPH in amounts greater than those observed in extracts of normal tissues.

Plasma LPH was quantified in a prospective study of 107 patients with a specific abnormality on chest radiographs admitted to the medical service at Harbor-UCLA Medical Center. Thirty-one of 33 patients subsequently diagnosed as having a benign disease had plasma LPH concentrations within the 95% confidence limits of a normal population, whereas 28 patients out of 80 (36%) subsequently diagnosed as having a malignant lung tumor had elevated LPH values. Twenty-two of 23 patients admitted with granulomatous lung diseases had normal LPH concentrations, as did 87 of 100 patients admitted with obstructive pulmonary disease. During a two-year follow-up, 3 of the 13 COPD patients with elevated LPH levels and 4 of the 87 patients with normal levels have been diagnosed as having lung carcinomas. In extracts of the carcinomas as well as in the plasma, LPH levels correlated well with ProACTH levels.

Corticotropin Releasing Hormone (CRH)

Cushing's syndrome has also been reported to occur in association with bronchial carcinoids[1,2,67]. This association is often attributed to ACTH production by the carcinoid tumor. However, approximately half the patients with carcinoids and "ectopic ACTH syndrome" show suppression of plasma cortisol concentrations with high-dose dexamethasone treatment and/or a response to metyrapone[68-72]. In some bronchial carcinoids, ACTH levels in the tumor have been shown to be very high[68-70]. There are three possible explanations: 1) the tumors' secretion of ACTH may be inhibited by glucocorticoids directly; 2) since hypothalamic production of CRH and the action of CRH on the pituitary have both been shown to be inhibited by glucocorticoids, these tumors may be responsive to CRH secreted by the normal hypothalamus; or 3) the tumors themselves may elaborate CRH as well as ACTH. The latter possibility gains support from Upton and Amatruda[73] who reported the presence of a CRH-like material in extracts of tumors from two patients who responded to metyrapone; the tumors were a pancreatic carcinoma and a small cell lung carcinoma. Yamamoto et al.[74] reported CRH activity in 7 out of 12 tumors associated with the ectopic ACTH syndrome. It appears likely that neoplasms associated with the "ectopic ACTH syndrome" and which suppress their ACTH production in response to dexamethasone elaborate a CRH-like material.

Calcitonin

Calcitonin is normally secreted by the parafollicular cells of the thyroid and is an excellent marker for tumors developing from these cells (e.g., medullary carcinomas). Calcitonin is also produced ectopically by a variety of other carcinomas. Even when plasma concentrations of immunoreactive calcitonin are greatly elevated, no symptoms appear to be caused by this substance in humans. Although single case reports appeared earlier, the first two series of cancer patients who were evaluated for hypercalcitonemia were reported by Coombs et al.[75] and by Hillyard et al.[76]. These workers found immunoreactive calcitonin in extracts of breast carcinomas, and they also reported that about 60 percent of patients with carcinomas of the lung and the breast had elevated plasma values. In studies from our laboratory Schwartz et al.[77] have investigated 240 patients who were admitted for diagnostic evaluation. In 123 patients subsequently shown to have carcinoma, 40 had highly elevated plasma calcitonin levels ($>$150 pg/ml; normal is $<$100 pg/ml). Those with elevated plasma calcitonins included 19 out of 49 patients (38%) with breast cancer and 6 out of 14 (42%) with pancreatic carcinoma. None was hypercalcemic. Noncancerous conditions such as acute hemorrhage, hypotension, renal failure, pancreatitis and pregnancy may also be associated with increased serum calcitonin levels. While for some of the ectopic hormonal syndromes already discussed synthesis by the tumor seems to be well established, this is not true for calcitonin. Silva et al.[78] demonstrated by selective thyroidal catheterization in a normocalcemic patient with hypercalcitonemia and cancer, that the normal thyroid was the source of calcitonin, and not the extrathyroidal neoplasm. In this patient, at least, it appears that the tumor might have elaborated a substance that stimulated thyroidal calcitonin production.

Radioimmunoassay of urine calcitonin identifies a greater percentage of cancer patients with elevated calcitonin values. Becker et al. reported that 76% of normocalcemic patients with bronchogenic carcinoma had urinary calcitonin levels which were abnormally elevated (versus 46% of the patients who had elevated serum calcitonin levels)[79]. When both serum and urine were assayed using an antiserum that recognized the carboxyl terminus as well as one that recognized the midportion of the calcitonin molecule, 90% of 41 cancer patients were found to have an abnormal value. Increased serum and urine calcitonin levels were observed in all cell types of lung cancer including epidermoid, adenocarcinoma, small cell and large cell carcinomas.

Studies of patients with all histologic types of lung cancer revealed that serum calcitonin concentrations paralleled the changes in clinical status[80,81]: serum calcitonin levels decreased when patients responded to therapy and increased with relapses. In patients with small cell carcinoma in remission, rising serum calcitonin levels preceded clinical evidence of relapse by up to 5 months[80,55]. Because not all patients with disease progression had elevated serum calcitonin, however, treatment decisions cannot be based on changes in peptide concentrations alone. No relation was found between the initial serum calcitonin concentrations and clinical stage of disease[81].

Parathyroid Hormone

The first suggestion that cancers might produce parathyroid hormone (PTH) was made by Albright in 1941[82]. In discussing a patient with cancer and hypercalcemia in whom the serum phosphorus was low, he commented that bony dissolution by metastases was not a likely cause since this would have resulted in an elevated serum phosphorus as well as an elevated calcium. He suggested that the tumor might be producing a parathyroid hormone-like material. Subsequently, Tashjian et al.[83], Berson and Yalow[84], and Sherwood et al.[85] found immunoreactive PTH in extracts from a variety of carcinomas. These data suggested that some cancers might indeed elaborate a PTH-like material. However, Buchle et al.[86] presented solid evidence of a carcinoma producing PTH when they reported a patient with renal carcinoma and hypercalcemia. Significant arterial-venous differences for PTH existed across the kidney containing the neoplasm, and following tumor resection the hypercalcemia disappeared. However, the debate continued about how frequently ectopic production of parathyroid hormone might be the cause of tumor-associated hypercalcemia. In a 1971 case record[87] the patient had a squamous cell carcinoma, hypercalcemia, and hypophosphatemia, but undetectable PTH levels in the plasma. In 1973 Powell et al.[88] carefully evaluated 11 cancer patients with hypercalcemia and hypophosphatemia who did not have bony metastases. In nine, treatment of the tumor either by surgical ablation or chemotherapy restored the serum calcium to normal. Parathyroid hormone levels were quantified using several radioimmunoassays that were selected to react with intact parathyroid hormone as well as with parathyroid hormone fragments. No parathyroid hormone was detected in either the blood or tumor extracts by these investigators, and they postulated that a substance other than parathyroid hormone was being elaborated by these tumors and was the cause of the hypercalcemia.

In 1972 Brereton et al.[89], Robertson et al.[90] and Ito et al. [91] each described single patients who had a renal carcinoma associated with hypercalcemia and who had prostaglandins extracted from their tumor[89] or elevated prostaglandins in their blood[90], or whose hypercalcemia responded to indomethacin treatment[91]. Seyberth et al.[92] evaluated 29 patients with solid tumors, 14 of whom were hypercalcemic. Twelve of the 14 hypercalcemic patients had marked increases in urinary prostaglandin metabolite excretion; whereas 7 our of the 15 patients with normal blood calciums had elevated prostaglandin excretion levels, the elevations were slight or moderate. Six patients with hypercalcemia were treated with aspirin or indomethacin, resulting in a fall in urinary prostaglandin metabolite excretion and a variable decrease (not to normal levels in all) in blood calcium. With these data as background, one might conclude that prostaglandin elaboration is a common cause of hypercalcemia in cancer, but the story is more complex. Tashjian noted in an editorial[93] that many investigators had found the majority of cancer patients did not respond to indomethacin therapy, suggesting that prostaglandin production may not be the predominant cause for their hypercalcemia. Secondly, it was suggested that the metabolism of parathyroid hormone differs in parathyroid adenomas from that in carcinomas elsewhere in the body. Benson et al.[94] reported that the carboxyl terminal fragment of parathyroid hormone (which is measured in many parathyroid hormone radioimmunoassays) is formed intracellularly by parathyroid tissue, but not (or to much lesser extent) by carcinomas producing parathyroid hormone. Although the carboxyl terminal fragment is also formed in peripheral tissues following secretion of hormone by a carcinoma, the formation of carboxyl terminal fragment is significantly less than that occurring in a parathyroid adenoma. Measurements of parathyroid hormone using an assay which reacts with the carboxyl terminus result in higher values in hyperparathyroidism than in cancer. Whereas hypercalcemia would be expected to suppress normal parathyroid gland secretion to undetectable levels, Benson et al.[95] using a radio-immunoassay directed primarily against the carboxyl terminus reported that 103 of 108 cancer patients (95%) with hypercalcemia had detectable plasma parathyroid hormone concentrations. Our experience is similar using an immunoassay directed against the middle and carboxyl terminal ends of parathyroid hormone. In a study of 62 cancer patients we observed that 86% had detectable plasma parathyroid hormone concentrations which were considerably lower for a given serum calcium than those which are observed in hyperparathyroidism. In a more recent study of normocalcemic patients with untreated lung cancer, elevated levels of immunoreactive parathyroid hormone were observed in 14 of 52 patients (27%) with oat cell carcinoma, 12 of 37 patients (32%) with squamous cell carcinoma, and 3 of 18 patients (12.5%) with large cell carcinoma[55].

An important clinical observation is that ordinary hyperparathyroidism and cancer not infrequently coexist in the same patient. Drezner and Lebovits[96] determined renal excretion of cyclic AMP (CAMP) in a study of 15 cancer patients with hypercalcemia. Six of these patients had elevated CAMP excretion, and all six subsequently had surgically proved hyperparathyroidism. Nine had CAMP excretion indistinguishable from normals and presumably had cancer-mediated hypercalcemia. The differential diagnosis may sometimes be difficult, since urinary CAMP excretion may be elevated in some lung cancer patients who have normal serum calciums and normal serum parathyroid hormone levels[97].

Vasopressin

The syndrome of hyponatremia, renal sodium loss, hypervolemia and inappropriately high urine osmolality associated with lung cancer (the Schwartz-Barter Syndrome), was initially attributed to sustained inappropriate antidiuretic hormone secretion (SIADH) by the tumor[98]. Subsequently, Amatruda et al.[99] and Bower and Mason[100] extracted the tumors of two patients with this syndrome and demonstrated vasopressin activity by bioassay. Vorherr et al.[101] in studying a series of patients with this syndrome, demonstrated that the material extracted from the tumors reacted identically in a radioimmunoassay with arginine vasopressin. Studies on two patients by Hirata et al.[102] using radioimmunoassay, bioassay and gel filtration further confirmed that the extractable material in this syndrome was identical to arginine vasopressin. Finally, George et al.[103] demonstrated synthesis of vasopressin by a human lung carcinoma, by showing incorporation of tritiated amino acids into immunoreactive vasopressin in vitro.

While the most common histologic type of lung cancer associated with vasopressin is, as for ACTH, small cell (oat cell) carcinoma, squamous and anaplastic carcinomas of the lung can also produce this syndrome. Lung cancers in general are the most common neoplasms to be associated with SIADH secretion, but other neoplasms (e.g., prostatic carcinoma, Hodgkins disease, and carcinoma of the adrenal cortex) have also been linked with the syndrome.

The frequency of the syndrome may be estimated from two studies. Gilby et al.[104] reported that 40% of patients with oat cell carcinoma had SIADH secretion. Studies from our laboratory have confirmed at least that a subclinical form of the syndrome may be common[3]. Since proteins produced by normal fetal tissues are often produced by cancers, we selected an antiserum that reacted with the fetal peptide arginine vasotocin (AVT), as well as with arginine vasopressin (AVP). With a radioimmunoassay employing this antiserum, 41% of 41 patients with lung cancer of all histologic types and 37% of 30 patients with colon carcinoma had inappropriately elevated plasma AVT/AVP. These concentrations were higher than the 95% confidence limits for healthy control subjects dehydrated for 18 hours. Many of these patients were not hyponatremic, but presumably would manifest the clinical syndrome if they were water loaded. It is possible in fact that clinical expression of the syndrome in the alert patient requires not only elaboration of a vasopressin-like material by the tumor, but also an abnormal thirst.

Studies have indicated that the highest concentrations of vasopressin in tumors occur in oat cell carcinomas associted with hyponatremia[105,106]. In these studies plasma concentrations of vasopressin have also been significantly elevated in all patients. Plasma vasopressin has also been evaluated as a marker for clinical response and for relapse in small cell carcinoma of the lung. After an objective tumor response, 15 of 19 patients had decreases in plasma vasopressin concentration; the remaining 4 patients had increased levels of vasopressin[81]. Plasma vasopressin levels increased in 11 of 13 patients who exhibited objective evidence of tumor progression.

Vasopressin is normally stored in the posterior pituitary bound to proteins known as neurophysins. A radioimmunoassay study of plasma levels of neurophysins in 26 patients with small cell carcinoma of the lung revealed greatly elevated levels in 11 patients (42%) prior to therapy[107]. Extracts from tumors associated with the hyponatremia syndrome also contained neurophysin by radioimmunoassay.

Growth Hormone (GH) and Growth Hormone Releasing Hormone (GHRH)

Extracts of lung carcinomas[108-112] and gastric carcinomas[111] have been reported to contain immunoreactive GH. Kaganowicz et al.[112] studied a large number of tumors and normal tissues for GH immunoreactivity. None of thirty-three different types of noncancerous tissue (excluding the ovary) were found to contain immunoreactive GH. Of 113 ovaries resected, only one of 76 normal ovaries removed from premenopausal women had GH levels greater than 10 ng/gram tissue, while 7 of 29 ovaries with various types of benign and malignant tumors had GH at levels over 10 ng/gram. Enormous amounts (51,000; 350,000; 5,000 and 4,900 ng/gram) were present in four patients: a breast cancer metastasis in the ovary, skin metastases from breast cancer, an ovary involved by endometriosis, and an ovary containing a serous cystadenoma. Controls were done to show that these tumor or ovarian extracts did not degrade the ^{125}I-labelled GH used in the immunoassay.* From these data, it seems reasonable to conclude that immunoreactive GH may be synthesized by some neoplasms. It is not clear, however, whether this GH is actively secreted and/or whether it is biologically active. None of the patients with elevated tumor GH levels discussed above had clinical evidence of excess GH effect.

In contrast to the lack of clinical findings in these studies, a small number of patients have been reported with bronchial or gastrointestinal carcinoid tumors and acromegaly[113-117]. Although this clinical association might have been fortuitous in some of the patients[104], in at least 5 patients normal GH secretion was restored and/or the clinical syndrome of acromegaly subsided following removal of the bronchial carcinoid[113,115-117]. In most of these cases, no therapy was directed against the hypothalamic-pituitary system; this suggests that the cause of acromegaly was the carcinoid tumor itself. Saeed uz Safer et al.[116] and Leveston et al.[117] demonstrated that extracts of the human carcinoid tumors contained GH releasing factor (GHRF) actuvity using a pituitary cell culture bioassay system. Leveston et al.[117] also demonstrated GHRF in their patient's plasma. Frohman et al.[118] have partially purified and characterized this GHRF from 6 carcinomas (4 lung, and 2 pancreatic). Based on gel filtration it was found to have a molecular weight of 7000-9000 Daltons and was heat stable. Its bioactivity was inhibited by somatostatin, and its releasing activity was destroyed by treatment of the material with trypsin, pronase or chymotrypsin; however, the activity was affected neither by carboxypeptidase A and B, nor by leucine amino-peptidase. Presumably the carcinoids synthesize and ectopically secrete GHRF, a peptide believed to be secreted normally by the hypothalamus as a modulator of pituitary GH secretion. The work of Frohman et al.[118] also offers a possible explanation for the development of GH-secreting pituitary tumors in patients with multiple endocrine neoplasias (MEN type I).

Insulin-like Activity

The histologic types of neoplasms producing hypoglycemia as an ectopic hormonal syndrome are different from those associated with most other ectopic hormonal syndromes. The largest group (64 percent of the cases reported) are soft tissue tumors and include fibrosarcomas, neurofibromas, neurofibrosarcomas, rhabdomyosarcomas, leiomyosarcomas, and mesenchymomas, as well as mesotheliomas. These neoplasms of mesodermal origin are quite large when associated with hypoglycemia, ranging in various reports from 800 to 10,000 grams. About two thirds of these soft tissue tumors develop in the abdomen, both intraperitoneally and retroperitoneally; the remaining one third occur in the thorax[1]. Twenty-one percent of reported patients with the syndrome have hepatic neoplasms (usually hepatoma), and about 6 percent have adrenal cortical carcinomas. The remaining cases have been asociated with a wide variety of carcinomas[1]. The etiology of the hypoglycemia remains incompletely understood. Extracts of 25 neoplasms associated with hypoglycemia have been studied to locate a hypoglycemia-producing factor[1].

---

*It is mandatory in studying tumor content or plasma values of protein hormones, to prove (in samples containing elevated values) that enzymatic degradation of the label does not occur. Such degradation can produce a "high hormone value" as an artifact in the assay.

Using in vitro bioassays (rat diaphragm or epididymal fat pad), insulin-like activity could be demonstrated in 10 of 25 extracts of the neoplasms studied. However, using insulin radioimmunoassays, the extracts from six tumors failed to reveal any detectable insulin. In three instances[1,119], "insulin" activity was present by bioassay but absent by radioimmunoassay in the same extract. These same data suggest that the hypoglycemia-producing material has biological properties similar to insulin but is not identical to insulin structurally. Megyesi et al.[120] studied plasma samples from seven patients who had hypoglycemia associated with extra-pancreatic tumors. Using a radioreceptor assay for soluble nonsuppressible insulin-like activity (NSILA-S), these investigators showed that NSILA-S is a composite of two low molecular weight (5,700 and 5,900) insulin-like growth factors (IGF-1 and IGF-2)[121], which do not react in insulin radioimmunoassays but have biological actions similar or identical to insulin. Two sets of receptors are believed to exist in the liver, one for insulin and one for insulin-like growth factors. All seven patients in this study had blood glucose concentrations below 110 mg/100 ml and very low insulin concentrations by radioimmunoassay. However, five of the seven patients had elevated plasma NSILA-S concentrations; these patients had fibrosarcoma, adrenal cortical carcinoma, hepatoma and malignant pheochromocytoma (two patients). In the remaining two patients (breast carcinoma and reticulum cell sarcoma associated with hypoglycemia) plasma NSILA-S was not elevated. The plasma NSILA-S activity from patients with elevated levels chromatographed on Sephadex G-50 identically with a purified NSILA-S reference preparation. A similar material was extracted from an adrenocortical carcinoma associated with hypoglycemia[122]. The NSILA-S belongs to a family of peptides and proteins (the somatomedins) that possess insulin-like biological properties[123,124]. For example, in contrast to NSILA-S, nonsuppressible insulin-like protein (NSILP) is a glycoprotein, with a molecular weight of 90,000. Several somatomedins that are different from both NSILA-S and NSILP have also been identified[124], and radioimmunoassays have been developed for certain of the somatomedins. Plovink et al.[125] described a woman with a fibrosarcoma and hypoglycemia, whose plasma showed low NSILP has been reported not only in patients who have tumors associated with hypoglycemia, but also in tumor patients without hypoglycemia, and it may prove to be a tumor marker in these patients[126]. The most striking elevations of NSILP have occurred in patients with tumors of mesodermal origin, followed by pulmonary and gastrointestinal neoplasms.

While hypoglycemia associated with extrapancreatic tumors is not always produced by the same substance, it appears likely that these tumors produce one or more of the peptides or proteins from the family of somatomedins. Two examples are NSILP and NSILA-S. The hypoglycemia sometimes associated with hepatoma may not represent a true ectopic hormonal syndrome, but may be a retained activity of the neoplasm which has developed from the tissue (liver) which normally produces somatomedins.

Conclusions

We have discussed a selected group of ectopic hormonal syndromes that are associated with cancers. Many others listed in Table I were not discussed because they are not yet as well characterized. For the hormones ProACTH, lipotropin and hCG, current data suggest that all carcinomas synthesize these proteins. Neoplasms associated with a <u>clinically apparent</u> syndrome have the additional property of metabolizing the protein precursor to a biologically active form. In the case of ProACTH, this consists of enzymatic cleavage to ACTH; in the case of hCG, the precursor is glycosylated. The final metabolic step occurs with histological preference: primarily small cell (oat cell) carcinomas of the lung and carcinomas of the pancreas and thymus for ACTH, and primarily carcinomas of the lung, pancreas and gastrointestinal tract for hCG. We have postulated that all cancers are associated with ectopic protein elaboration, while only those associated with the clinically apparent syndromes produce biologically active substances.

Although the clinical utility of peptide hormones as tumor markers remains investigational, present data suggest that assays specific for the weakly bioactive hormonal precursors secreted by carcinomas have significant clinical potential.

References

1. Odell, WD. Humoral manifestations of non-endocrine neoplasms. In: Williams RD, ed. Textbook of Endocrinology 5th Ed. Philadelphia: Saunders, 1974, 1105-16.

2. Odell WD, Wolfsen AR. Ectopic hormone production by tumors. In: Becker FF, ed. Cancer, A comprehensive treatise. New York: Plenum Publishing Corp. 1975, 3:81-97.

3. Odell WD, Wolfsen AR, Yoshimoto Y, Weitzman R, Fisher DA, Hirose F. Ectopic peptide synthesis: A universal concomitant of neoplasia. Trans Assoc Am Phys 1977; 90:204-27.

4. Bellisario R, Carlson RB, Bahl OP. Human chorionic gonadotropin. Linear amino acid sequence of the   subunit. J Biol Chem 1973; 248:6796-809.

5. Papkoff H, Sairam MR, Farmer SW, Li HL. Studies on the structure and function of interstitial cell-stimulating hormone. Recent Prog Horm Res 1973; 29-563-90.

6. Canfield RE, Morgan FJ, Kammerman S, Bell JJ, Agosto GM. Studies of human chorionic gonadotropin. Recent Prog Horm Res 1971; 27:121-64.

7. Shome B, Parlow AF. Human follicle stimulating hormone (hFSH): First proposal for the amino acid sequence of the α subunit of human luteinizing hormone (hLHα). J Clin Endocrinol Metab 1974; 39:199-202.

8. Odell WD, Hertz R, Lipsett MB, Ross GT, Hammond CB. Endocrine aspects of trophoblastic neoplasms. Clin Obstet Gynecol 1967; 10:290-302.

9. Li MC. Discussion of chemotherapy of choriocarcinoma and related trophoblastic tumors in women. Ann NY Acad Sci 1959; 80-280-4.

10. Fusco FD, Rosen SW. Gonadotropin-producing anaplastic large-cell carcinomas of the lung. N Engl J Med 1966; 275:507-15.

11. Faiman C, Colwell JA, Ryan RJ, Hershman JM, Shields TW. Gonadotropin secretion from a bronchogenic carcinoma. Demonstration by radioimmunoassay. N Engl J Med 1967; 277:1395-79.

12. Rosen SW, Becker CE, Schlaff S, Easton J, Gluck MC. Ectopic gonadotropin production before clinical recognition of bronchogenic carcinoma. N Engl J Med 1968; 297:640-1.

13. Castleman B, Scully RE, McNeely BU. Case Records of Massachusetts General Hospital. Case 13-1972. N Engl J Med 1972; 286:713-9.

14. Matteini M. Su de un caso de gynecomastia associatea a tumore retroperitonele a cellule indifferenziate. Rass Neurol Veget 1952; 9:252-71.

15. McArthur JW.   Para-endocrine phenomena in obstetrics and gynecology. In: Meigs JV, Stugis SH, eds. Progress in gynecology. New York, 1963; 4:146-72.

16. Braunstein GD, Vaitukaitis JL, Carbone PP, Ross GT.   Ectopic production of human chorionic gonadotropin by neoplasms.   Ann Intern Med 1973; 78:39-45.

17. Vaitukaitis JL, Braunstein GD, Ross GT.   A radioimmunoassay which specifically measures human chorionic gonadotropin in the presence of human luteinizing hormone. Am J Obstet Gynecol 1972; 113:751-8.

18. Blackman MR, Weintraub BD, Rosen SW, Kourides IA, Steinwascher K, Gail MH.   Human placental and pituitary glycoprotein hormones and their subunits as tumor markers: A quantitative assessment.   J Natl Cancer Inst 1980; 65:81-93.

19. Yoshimoto Y, Wolfsen AR, Odell WD.   Human chorionic gonadotropin-like substance in nonendocrine tissues of normal subjects.   Science 1977; 197:575-77.

20. Yoshimoto Y, Wolfsen AR, Hirose F, Odell WD.   Human chorionic gonadotropin-like material: Presence in normal human tissues.   Am J Obstet Gynecol 1979; 134:729-33.

21. Yoshimoto Y, Wolfsen AR, Odell WD.   Glycosylation, A variable in the production of hCG by cancers.   Am J Med 1979; 67:414-20.

22. Van Hall EV, Vaitukaitis JL, Ross GT, Hickman JW, Ashwell G. Immunological and biological activity of hCG following progressive desialation.   Endocrinology 1971; 88:456-64.

23. Tsuruhara T, Dufau ML, Hickman J, Catt KJ.   Biological properties of hCG after removal of terminal sialic acid and galactose residues. Endocrinology 1972; 90:296-301.

24. Borkowski A, Maquardt C.   Human chorionic gonadotropin in the plasma of normal, nonpregnant subjects.   N Engl J Med 1979; 301:298.

25. Chen HC, Hodgen GD, Matsuura S, et al.   Evidence for a gonadotropin from nonpregnant subjects that has physical, immunological and biological similarities to human chorionic gonadotropin.   Proc Natl Acad   Sci USA 1976; 73:2885-9.

26. Vaitukaitis JL, Ross GT, Braunstein GD, Rayford PL.   Gonadotropins and their subunits: Basic and clinical studies.   Recent Prog Horm Res 1976; 32:289-321.

27. Bagshawe KD.   Immunological methods in the diagnosis and monitoring of tumors.   In: Bagshawe KD, ed.   Medical Oncology, London, Blackwell Scientific Publications, 1975.

28. Bagshawe KD, Harland S. Immunodiagnosis and monitoring of gonadotropin-producing metastases in the central nervous system. Cancer 1976; 38:112-118.

29. Anderson T, Waldmann TA, Javadpour N, Glatstein E. Testicular germ-cell neoplasms: Recent advances in diagnosis and therapy. Ann Intern Med 1979; 90:373-385.

30. Goldenberg DM, Kim EE, DeLand FH, Van Nagell Jr. JR, Javadpour N, Clinical radioimmunodetection of cancer with radioactive antibodies to human chorionic gonadotropin. Science 1980; 208:1281-1286.

31. Williams RR, McIntire KR, Waldmann TA, Feinleib M, Go VLW, Kannel WB, Dawber TR, Castelli WP, McNamara PM. Tumor associated antigen levels (carcinoembyronic antigen, human chorionic gonadotropin and alpha-fetoprotein) antedating the diagnosis of cancer in the Framingham study. J Natl Cancer Inst 1977; 58:1547-1551.

32. Papapetrou PD, Sakarelou NP, Braouzi H, Fessas PH. Ectopic production of human chorionic gonadotropin (hCG) by neoplasms: The value of measurements of immunoreactive hCG in the urine as a screening procedure. Cancer 1980; 45:2583-2592.

33. Edmonds M, Molitch M, Pierce J, Odell WD. Secretion of alpha and beta subunits of TSH by the anterior pituitary. Clin Endocrinol 1975; 4:525-30.

34. Edmonds M, Molitch M, Pierce J, Odell WD. Secretion of alpha subunits of luteinizing hormoe by the anterior pituitary. J Clin Endocrinol Metab 1975; 41:551-5.

35. Rosen SW and Weintraub ED. Ectopic production of the isolated alpha subunit of the glycoprotein hormones. A quantitative marker in certain cases of cancer. N Engl J Med 1974; 290:1441-7.

36. Kahn CR, Rosen SW, Weingraub BD, Fajans SS, Gorden P. Ectopic production of chorionic gonadotropin and its subunits by islet-cell tumors. A specific marker for malignancy. N Engl J Med 1977; 297:565-9.

37. Stabile BE, Braunstein GD, Hershman JM, Passaro E Jr. Human chorionic gonadotropin alpha subunits as a specific marker for malignancy in the Zollinger-Ellison syndrome. Surg Forum 1978; 24:488-490.

38. Wolfsen AR, Odell WD. Early diagnosis of lung cancer (Ca) using peptide markers. Clin Res 1977; 25:502A.

39. Braunstein GD, Forsythe AB, Rasor JL, Van Scoy-Mosher MB, Thompson RW and Wade ME. Serum glycoprotein hormone alpha subunit levels in patients with cancer. Cancer 1979; 44:1644-1651.

40. MacFarlane LA, Thatcher JN, Seindell R, Beardwell CG, Hayward E, Crowther D. Serum glycoprotein hormone alpha subunit values and survival in metastatic melanoma patients. Eur J Cancer 1979; 15:1497-1501.

41. Wolfsen AR, Odell WD. In: Compendium of assays for immunodiagnosis of human cancer. RB Herberman ed. Developments in Cancer Research Vol. 1, 1979, p. 293-300.

42. Brown VH. A case of plurigelandular syndrome: Diabetes of bearded women. Lancer 1928; 2:1022-3.

43. Liddle GW, Nicholson WE, Island DP. Clinical and laboratory studies of ectopic humoral syndromes. Recent Prog Horm Res 1969; 25:283-314.

44. Kato Y, Ferguson TB, Bennett DE, et al. Oat cell carcinoma of the lung. A review of 138 cases. Cancer 1969; 23:517-24.

45. Ratcliffe JG, Knight RA, Besser GM, et al. Tumor and plasma ACTH concentrations in patients with and without the ectopic ACTH syndrome. Clin Endocrinol 1972; 1:27-44.

46. Bloomfield GA, Holdaway IM, Carrin B, et al. Lung tumours and ACTH production. Clin Endocrinol 1977; 6:95-104.

47. Gewirtz G, Yalow RS. Ectopic ACTH production in carcinoma of the lung. J Clin Invest 1974; 53:1022-32.

48. Wolfsen AR, Odell WD. ProACTH: Use for early detection of lung cancer. Am J Med 1979; 66:765-71.

49. Gasson JC. Steroidogenic activity of high molecular weight forms of corticotropin. Biochemistry 1979; 18:4215-24.

50. Roebuck MM, Jones CT, Holland D, Silman R. In vitro effects of high molecular weight forms of ACTH on the fetal sheep adrenal. Nature 1980; 284:616-8.

51. Eipper BA, Mains RE, Guenzi D. High molecular weight forms of adrenocorticotropin hormone are glycoproteins. J Biol Chem 1976; 251:4121-6.

52. Mains RE, Eipper BA. Biosynthesis of adrenocorticotropic hormone in mouse pituitary tumor cells. J Biol Chem 1976; 251:4115-20.

53. Yalow RS. Ectopic ACTH in carcinoma of the lung. In: Lung Cancer: Progress in Therapeutic Research. F Muggia and M Rozencweig. New York, Raven Press, 1979, p. 209-216.

54. Torstensson S, Thoren M, Hall K. Plasma ACTH in patients with bronchogenic carcinoma. Acta Med Scand 1980; 207:353-357.

55. Gropp C, Havenmann K, Scheuer A. Ectopic hormones in lung cancer patients at diagnosis and during therapy. Cancer 1980; 46:347-354.

56. Hansen M, Hansen HH, Hirsch FR, Arends J, Christensen JD, Christensen JM, Hummer L, Kuhl C. Hormonal polypeptides and amine metabolites in small cell carcinoma of the lung, with special reference to stage and subtypes. Cancer 1980; 45:1432-1437.

57. Hansen M, Hansen HH, Almquist S, Hummer L. Cerebrospinal fluid ACTH and Calcitonin in patients with CNS metastases from small cell bronchogenic carcinoma. Europ J Cancer 1980; 16:855-857.

58. Abe K, Nicholson WE, Liddle GW. Normal and abnormal regulation of beta-MSH in man. J Clin Invest 1969; 48:1580-5.

59. Law DH, Liddle GW, Scott HW Jr., et al. Ectopic production of multiple hormones (ACTH, MSH and gastrin) by a single malignant tumor. N Engl J Med 1965; 273:292-6.

60. Coscia M, Brown HD, Miller M, et al. Ectopic production of anti-diuretic hormone (ADH), adrenocorticotropin (ACTH) and beta-melanocyte stimulating hormone (beta-MSH) by an oat cell carcinoma of the lung. Am J Med 1977; 62:303-7.

61. Bloomfield GA, Scott AP, Lowry PJ, et al. A reappraisal of human beta MSH. Nature 1974; 252:492-3.

62. Bachelot I, Wolfsen AR, Odell WD. Pituitary and plasma lipotropins: Demonstration of artifactual natural of β MSH. J Clin Endocrinol Metab 1977; 44:939-46.

63. Li CH, Barnafi L, Chretien M, Chung D. Isolation and amino-acid sequence of β-LPH from sheep pituitary glands. Nature 1965; 208:1093-4.

64. Ueda M, Takeuchi T, Abe K, Miyakawa S, Ohnami S, Yanaihara N. β-melanocyte-stimulating hormone immunoreactivity in human pituitaries and ectopic adrenocorticotropin-producing tumors. J Clin Endocrinol Metab 1980; 50:550-6.

65. Mains RE, Eipper BA, Ling N. Common precursor to corticotropins and endorphins. Proc Natl Adac Sci USA 1977; 74:3014-8.

66. Odell WD, Wolfsen AR, Bachelot I, Hirose FM. Ectopic production of lipotropin. Am J Med 1979; 66:631-8.

67. Cohen RB, Toll GD, Castleman B. Bronchial adenomas in Cushing's syndrome: Their reltion to thymomas and oat cell carcinomas associated with hyperadrenocorticism. Cancer 1960; 13:812-7.

68. Strott CA, Nugent CA, Tyler FH. Cushing's syndrome caused by bronchial adenomas. Am J Med 1968; 44:97-104.

69. Jones JE, Shane SR, Gilbert E, Flink EB. Cushing's syndrome induced by the ectopic production of ACTH by a bronchial carcinoid. J Clin Endocrinol Metab 1969; 29:1-5.

70. Steel K, Baerg RD, Adams DO. Cushing's syndrome in association with a carcinoid tumor of the lung. J Clin Endocrinol Metab 1967; 27:1285-9.

71. Riggs BL Jr, Sprague RG. Association of Cushing's syndrome and neoplastic disease. Arch Intern Med 1961; 108:841-9.

72. Mason AMS, Ratcliffe JG, Buckle RM, Mason AS. ACTH secretion by bronchial carcinoid tumors. Clin Endocrinol 1972; 1:3-25.

73. Upton GV, Amatruda TT Jr. Evidence for the presence of tumor peptides with corticotropin-releasing-factor-like activity in the ectopic ACTH syndrome. N Engl J Med 1971; 285:419-24.

74. Yamamoto H, Hirata Y, Matsukura S, Imura H, Nakamura M, Tanaka A. Studies on ectopic ACTH-producing tumors. IV CRF-like activity in tumor tissue. Acta Endocrinol (Copenhagen) 1976; 82:183-7.

75. Coombes RC, Hillyard C, Greenberg PB, et al. Plasma-immunoreactive-calcitonin in patients with non-thyroid tumors. Lancet 1974; 1:1080-3.

76. Hillyard CJ, Coombes RC, Greenberg, PB et al. Calcitonin in breast and lung cancer. Clin Endocrinol 1976; 5:1-8.

77. Schwartz KE, Wolfsen AR, Forster B, Odell WD. Calcitonin in non-thyroidal cancer. J Clin Endocrinol Metab 1979; 49:438-44.

78. Silva OL, Becker HL, Primack A, Doppman JL, Snider RH. Hypercalcitonemia in bronchogenic cancer. Evidence for thyroid origin of the hormone. JAMA 1975; 234:183-5.

79. Becker KL, Nash DR, Silva OL, Snider RH, Moore CF. Urine calcitonin levels in patients with bronchogenic carcinoma. JAMA 1980; 243:670-2.

80. Krauss S, Macy S, Ichiki AT. A study of immunoreactive calcitonin and adrenocorticotropic hormone in lung cancer and other malignancies. (Abstract 577) Proceedings of AACR and ASCO, 1980; p. 144.

81. Hansen M, Hammer M, Hummer L. ACTH, ADH and calcitonin concentrations as markers of response and relapse in small-cell carcinoma of the lung. Cancer 1980; 46:2062-7.

82. Albright F. Case Records of Massachusetts General Hospital. Case 27461. N Engl J Med 1941; 225:789-94.

83. Tashjian AH Jr, Levine L, Munson PL. Immunochemical identificatin of parathyroid hormone in non-parathyroid neoplasms associated with hypercalcemia. J Exp Med 1964; 119:467-84.

84. Berson SA, Yalow RS. Parathyroid hormone in plasma in adenomatous hyperparathyroidism, uremia, and bronchogenic carcinoma. Science 1966; 153:907-9.

85. Sherwood LM, O'Riordan JLH, Aurbach GD, Potts JJ. Production of parathyroid hormone by nonparathyroid tumors. J Clin Endocrinol Metab 1967; 27:140-6.

86. Buchle RM, McMillian M, Mallinson C. Ectopic secretion of parathyroid hormone by a renal adenocarcinoma in a patient with hypercalcemia. Br Med J 1970; 4:724-6.

87. Castleman B, McNeely BU. Case Records of the Massachusetts General Hospital. Case 15-1971. N Engl J Med 1971; 284:839-47.

88. Powell D, Singer FR, Murray TM, Menkin C, Potts JT. Nonparathyroid hypercalcemia in patients with neoplastic diseases. N Engl J Med 1974; 289:176-81.

89. Brereton HD, Halushka PV, Alexander RW, Mason DM, Keiser HR, DeVita VT. Indomethacin responsive hypercalcemia in a patient with renal adenocarcinoma. N Engl J Med 1975; 291:83-5.

90. Robertson RP, Baylink DJ, Marini JJ, Adkison HW. Elevated prostaglandins and suppressed parathyroid hormone associated with hypercalcemia and renal cell carcinoma. J Clin Endocrinol Metab 1975; 41:164-7.

91. Ito H, Sanada T, Katayma T, Shimazaki J. Indomethacin responsive hypercalcemia. N Engl J Med 1975; 293:558-9.

92. Seyberth HW, Segre GV, Morgan JL, Sweetman BJ, Potts JT, Oates JA. Prostglandins as mediators of hypercalcemia associated with certain types of cancer. N Engl J Med 1975; 293:1278-83.

93. Tashjian AH Jr. Editorial: H. Prostaglandins, hypercalcemia and cancer. N Engl J Med 1975; 293:1317-8.

94. Benson RC Jr., Riggs BL, Pickard BM, et al. Immunoreactive forms of circulating parathyroid hormone in primary and ectopic hyperparathyroidism. J Clin Invest 1974; 54:175-81.

95. Benson RC Jr., Riggs BL, Pickard BM, Arnaud CD. Radioimmunoassay of parathyroid hormone in hypercalcemic patients with malignant disease. Am J Med 1974; 56:821-6.

96. Drezner MK, Lebovits HE. Primary hyperparathyroidism in paraneoplastic hypercalcemia. Lancet 1978; 1:1004-6.

97. Kukreja SC, Schmeridiak WP, Lad TE, Johnson PA. Elevated nephrogenous cyclic AMP with normal serum parathyroid hormone levels in patients with lung cancer. J Clin Endocrinol Metab 1980; 51:167-9.

98. Schwartz WD, Bennett W, Curlop S, Bartter V. A syndrome of renal sodium loss and hyponatremia probably resulting from inappropriate secretion of antidiuretic hormone. Am J Med 1957; 23:529-42.

99. Amatruda TT, Mulrow PJ, Gallagher JC, Sawyer WH. Carcinoma of the lung with inappropriate antidiuresis. N Engl J Med 1963; 269:544-9.

100. Bower BF, Mason DM. Measurement of antidiuretic activity (ADA) in plasma and tumor in carcinoma of the lung with inappropriate antidiuresis. Clin Res 1964; 12:121 (A).

101. Vorherr RH, Massry SG, Utiger RD, Kleeman CR. Antidiuretic principle in malignant tumor extracts from patients with inappropriate ADH syndrome. J Clin Endocrinol Metab 1968; 28:162-8.

102. Hirata Y, Matsukura, Imura H, Yakura TM, Injima S, Magase C, Itoh H. Two cases of multiple hormone producing small cell carcinoma of the lung. Cancer 1976; 38:2575-82.

103. George JM, Capen CC, Phillips AS. Biosynthesis of vasopressin in vitro and ultrastructure of a bronchogenic carcinoma. Patient with the syndrome of inappropriate secretion of antidiuretic hormone. J Clin Invest 1972; 51:141-8.

104. Gilby ED, Rees LH, Bondy PK. Proceedings of the 6th Internatinoal Symposium on Biology and Characterization of Human Tumours. In: Davis W, Maltoni C, eds. Burch PRJ, linguistic ed. Advances in Tumour Prevention, Detection and Characterization. New York: American Elsevier, 1975; vol. 3, p. 132.

105. Morton JJ, Kelly P, Padfield PL. Antidiuretic hormone in bronchogenic carcinoma. Clin Endocrinol 1978; 9:357-370.

106. Kelly P, Morton JJ. Antidiuretic hormone immunoreactivity in tumour tissue from patients with bronchogenic carcinoma: with and without hyponatremia. Clin Endocrinol 1980; 12:99-101.

107. North WG, LaRochell FT Jr, Melton J, Mills RC, Bolton H, Maure H. Human neurophysins as potential tumor markers for small cell carcinoma. Clin Res 1978; 26:536A.

108. Steiner H, Dahlback O, Waldenstrom J. Ectopic growth-hormone production and osteoarthropathy in carcinoma of the bronchus. Lancet 1968; 1:783-5.

109. Cameron DP, Burger HG, DeKretzer DM, et al. On the presence of immunoreactive growth hormone in a bronchogenic carcinoma. Aust Ann Med 1969; 18:143-6.

110. Sparagana M, Phillips G, Hoffman C, et al. Ectopic growth hormone syndrome associated with lung cancer. Metabolism 1971; 20:730-6.

111. Beck C, Burger HG. Evidence for the presence of immunoreactive growth hormone in cancers of the lung and stomach. Cancer 1972; 30:75-9.

112. Kaganowicz A, Farkouh NH, Frantz AG, Blaustein AH. Ectopic human growth hormone in ovaries and breast cancer. J Clin Endocrinol Metab 1978; 48:5-8.

113. Dabek JT. Bronchial carcinoid tumour with acromegaly in two patients. J Clin Endocrinol Metab 1974; 38:329-33.

114. Weiss L, Ingram M. Ademomatoid bronchial tumors. A consideration of the carcinoid tumors and the salivary tumors of the bronchial tree. Cancer 1961; 14:161-78.

115. Sonksen PH, Ayres AB, Braimbridge M, et al. Acromegaly caused by pulmonary carcinoid tumours. Clin Endocrinol 1976; 5:503-13.

116. Saeed uz Safar M, Mellinger RC, Fine G, Szabo M, Frohman LA. Acromegaly associated with bronchial carcinoid tumor: Evidence for ectopic production of growth hormone releasing activity. J Clin Endocrinol Metab 1979; 48:66-71.

117. Leveston SA, Lee YC, Jaffee BM, Daughaday WH. Massive GH and ACTH hypersecretion associated with metastatic carcinoid tumor. Program of the 60th Annual Endocrine Society Meeting 1978, p. 341 (Abstract).

118. Frohman LA, Szubo M, Berlowitz M. Partial purification and characterization of growth hormone (GH)-releasing factor in extracts of ectopic tumors associated with acromegaly. Program of the VI International Congress of Endocrinology (Abstract #189).

119. Field JB, Keen H, Johnson P, et al. Insulin-like activity of nonpancreatic tumors associated with hypoglycemia. J Clin Endocrinol Metab 1963; 23:1229-36.

120. Megyesi K, Kahn CR, Roth J, Gorden P. Hypoglycemia in association with extrapancreatic tumors: Demonstration of elevated plasma NSILA-S by a new radioreceptor assay. J Clin Endocrinol Metab 1974; 38:931-4.

121. Rinderknecht E, Humbel RE. Polypeptides with nonsuppressible insulin-like and cell-growth promoting activities in human serum: Isolation, chemical characterization and some biological properties of forms I and II. Proc Natl Acad Sci USA 1976; 73:2365-9.

122. Hyodo T, Megyes K, Kehn CR, McLean JP, et al. Adrenocortical carcinoma and hypoglycemia: Evidence for production of nonsuppressible insulin-like activity by the tumor. J Clin Endocrinol Metab 1977; 44:1175-84.

123. Van Wyk JJ, Underwood LE, Hintz RL, et al. The somatomedins: A famiy of insulin-like hormones under growth hormone control. Rec Prog Horm Res 1974; 30:259-318.

124. Poffenbarger PL, Stuart CA, Prince MJ, Medina AT. Chemistry and physiology of a human serum nonsuppressible insulin-like protein (NSILP). In: Giordano G, Van Wyk JJ, Minuto F. eds. Proceedings of the International Symposium on Somatomedins and Growth. New York: Academic Press, 1979.

125. Plovnik H. Non-β-cell tumor hypoglycemia associated with increased nonsuppressible insulin-like protein (NSILP). Am J Med 1979; 66:154-9.

126. Prince MJ, Poffenbarger PL. Elevated serum nonsuppressible insulin-like protein (NSILP) levels in cancer patients. Clin Res 1978; 26:424 A (Abstract).

Chapter 4

Recent Advances in Endoscopy
for Cancer Diagnosis and Staging

George Berci, M.D.

In the last decade endoscopy has contributed significantly to our diagnostic armamentarium in malignant diseases, by providing the ability to obtain tissue samples, stage tumors, and achieve a "second look" at abdominal structures without surgical intervention.

Major considerations in this progress are: a. The physician is able to visualize the organ in question directly, which gives a more accurate display of anatomic detail than any indirect approach (e.g., contrast radiography); and   b. Tissue samples can be obtained under visual control, without surgery.   It is unfortunate that some endoscopic interventional techniques are still being neglected despite convincing evidence of their utility.

Flexible Fiber Endoscopy

The introduction of flexible fiber esophago-gastroscopy has contributed to a higher diagnostic accuracy in the upper gastrointestinal tract.   The value of flexible colonoscopy for the nonoperative removal of polypoid lesions, with particular reference to early-stage carcinomas of the colon, is unquestioned.

The fiberoptic endoscopist is also able to cannulate the pancreatic and common bile ducts (E.R.C.P.), and to display abnormalities affecting the main pancreatic duct and the common bile duct as well as their tributaries (see below, and Chapter 7).

Rigid Endoscopy

Emphasis in succeeding sections will focus upon advances in rigid endoscopy, which are less well appreciated but which parallel the recent progress in flexible endoscopy.   The invention of the Hopkins rod-lens system has opened a new era in endoscopy.   It has resulted in a vastly improved image, and a brighter field of view with smaller instruments.   The miniature electric globes at the distal working end of the telescope have been replaced by fiberglass light-transmitting bundles.   A much stronger light source (with a built-in spare light) can be located externally, and the frustrating problem of internal light source failure during a critical phase of the endoscopic examination has thereby been eliminated.   Standard optic lenses used to be spaced at intervals within the rigid scope this system gave a relatively dim image of poor quality, with a narrow viewing angle.   Hopkins replaced the air interspaces between lenses with glass rods on which small lenses were cemented.   In addition to this, it was possible to miniaturize the entire instrument, which increased safety and convenience.   These improvements have had a major impact in urology, as well as in pediatrics, ENT, neurosurgery, and other areas.[3]

With the Hopkins system, the image is brighter and therefore easier to perceive.   Other parameters like detail resolution, natural color reproduction, viewing angle (size of object perceived) and depth of field are also superior when compared to previous optical systems. As a direct result, examinations can be carried out more easily and expeditiously (Fig. 1). With the traditional lens system, miniaturization was practically impossible, whereas today instruments with an outer diameter of 2.5mm are available. Even these miniaturized endoscopes provide an exquisite image.[4]

Larynx

Mirror examination of the larynx is a century old. In patients in whom there is the slightest suspicion of malignancy, the larynx should be examined by a skilled person with a laryngoscope (telescope) and not solely with the out-dated mirror. The disadvantages of mirror examinations are as follows: Only part of the larynx can be seen, and the mirror has to be moved around to create a "mosaic picture" of the entire larynx. The same object (the mirror) transmits illumination and image simultaneously; therefore slight abnormalities can escape attention because of glare or light reflections. Functional impairment in a moving organ like the larynx can be an important sign of an underlying lesion, and functional abnormalities are often overlooked in mirror examinations because there are only a few seconds available to perceive fast movements. It is also difficult to reconstruct slight impairments in functional appearance, even when accurate descriptions are recorded in the patient's record.

A new telescope has been introduced (Fig. 2) which is smaller than the mirror and is better tolerated by the patient.[5] It allows observation of the entire larynx in a single viewing field without having to move the instrument. The disadvantages of the mirror examination are eliminated. Magnification permits lesions as small as 0.5mm to be appreciated, a fact which assumes great importance when one considers the high curability of early-stage carcinoma of the vocal cords (Figs. 3 and 4). An additional advantage is that one can obtain a permanent record through a cine film strip, videotape, and/or multiple photographs within a few minutes without overtaxing the patient (Fig. 5). A cine recording can be studied at leisure without the patient present, using slow motion analysis with stopframing. The slightest functional impairments can be appeciated in this way, a good example being the often-overlooked entity of a superior laryngeal paralysis.[6] Small lesions hidden in or around inflamed cords are sometimes difficult to see with a mirror even during two or three forced phonations, but a film recording will give the examiner the opportunity to discover a transient abnormality during slow-motion analysis.

Nasopharynx

While lesions in the posterior nasopharynx are relatively rare in this country, this particular area is even more difficult to examine indirectly than the larynx because the mirrors used must be much smaller. On the other hand, the nasopharynx can be visualized extremely well by using the laryngoscope described above and turning it around 180°. It is very important in patients who are being treated by radiotherapy to compare the pre-treatment examination objectively with studies performed during treatment and during the follow-up period, to assess progress or regression of the lesion (Fig. 6).

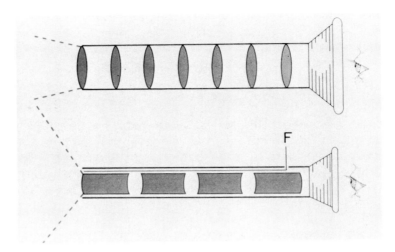

Figure 1. Schematic Diagram of a Conventional Optical System (rigid telescope).

Top: Small lenses are placed at certain intervals, with air separation. This is associated with significant light absorption and a dim image, as well as a narrow viewing angle.

Bottom: · Hopkins rod-lens system. The previous air intervals are replaced by glass rods with tiny lenses attached to each end. Advantages: significantly increased light transmission, a brighter image, easier viewer perception, and a larger viewing angle resulting in better orientation and smaller instruments.

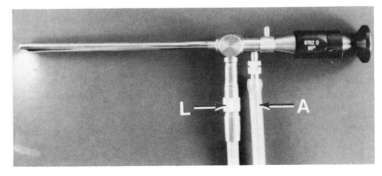

Figure 2. Indirect Laryngoscope, a telescope with 90˙ direction of view and 50˙ viewing angle. External light source provides bright illumination via a fiber optic cable (L). A small amount of air or oxygen is insufflated ahead of the objective (working end) to create positive prssure and avoid fogging (A). Advantages: the entire larynx is een in a single viewing field without moving the telescope. There is a brighter image with enhanced detail.

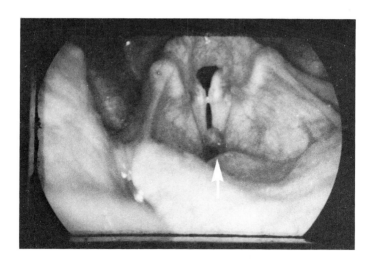

Figure 3. View of the Larynx. A small lesion (arrow) was discovered on the right cord near the anterior commissure. This lesion acted like a "ball valve", being visible transiently during certain phases of forced phonation and disappearing behind the cords. it could easily be overlooked with a mirror.

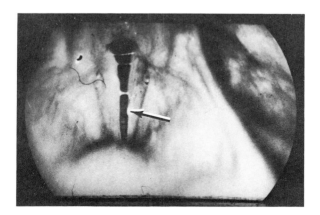

Figure 4. The small lesion on the left cord (arrow) escaped initial detection but was seen on repeated viewing during analysis of a film strip (cine). It proved to be a carcinoma in situ.

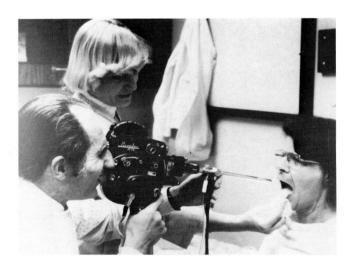

Figure 5. A 16 mm movie camera can be attached and the examination filmed during forced phonation. The entire cycle of movements of the cords is recorded on a film strip which can be analyzed subsequently with slow motion projection. Small lesions or slight functional impairments which would otherwise escape detection are discovered with this technique.

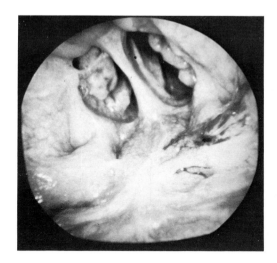

Figure 6. Telescopic view of the posterior nasopharynx and nasal cavity. The entire area can be seen including the posterior nasopharyngeal wall, both choanae, Eustachian tubes, and nasal turbinates. This area is extremely difficult to visualize for the purpose of recognizing small lesions, using a small nasopharyngeal mirror.

Esophagus

While this organ is usually examined with a flexible endoscope, there are still situations in cancer patients where thoracic surgeons prefer the rigid endoscope because of the ability to get a better view of the lesion using a telescope and to obtain a larger specimen using a more substantial biopsy forceps. The rigid scope may be also useful for placing stents within the esophagus in advanced cases, for palliation.

Mediastinum

Mediastinoscopy in skilled hands has become important to assess the operability of certain forms of lung cancer. With a small incision above the sternum, the paratracheal lymph nodes on both sides can be explored and biopsied, and more accurate staging obtained pre-operatively. With paratracheal adenopathy the accuracy of differential diagnosis between carcinoma and granulomatous disease is 100% using mediastinoscopy with appropriate tissue sampling.[7]

Pleural Cavity

Thoracoscopy can be of great assistance in peripheral lung tumors or a pleural efusion of unknown etiology. The thoracoscope (a rigid instrument) is introduced through a small intercostal incision, and the surfaces of the lung and pleura are then inspected and biopsies taken.[8]

Pancreatico-Biliary System

Choledochoscopy at laparotomy with a rigid endoscope has greatly facilitated the process of finding and removing stones from bile ducts. Before the advent of the choledochoscope, much time was spent in irrigating the ducts and performing operating table cholangiograms that were often of poor quality. The originally manufactured choledochoscopes were bulky, whereas the modern right-angle choledochoscope with the Hopkin's rod-lens system is compact and easy to use. The horizontal limb of the choledochoscope is 40 mm in length; a larger version called the nephroscope has a horizontal limb which is 60 mm. It is the horizontal limb which is placed in the bile duct. While the choledochoscope has a limited use in cancer, this is only because neoplasms within the biliary system are rare compared with cholangitis, calculi, and other lesions.

Endoscopic retrograde cannulation of the papilla of Vater via the duodenum (E.R.C.P.) is a noninvasive way of examining the pancreatic and/or the biliary system. This can be most useful in the pre-operative investigation of jaundice. Ductal calculi or narrowing of the bile duct(s) by extrinsic disease (neoplasm; cholangitis; pancreatitis) and pancreatic abnormalities can all be recognized. Cytology can also be obtained, although it is sometimes difficult to interpret. A stone impacted in the ampulla or severe pancreatitis wih edema can make cannulation of the papilla impossible.

Failure of E.R.C.P. to establish the etiology for jaundice, or a strong suspicion of associated peritoneal carcinomatosis or liver involvement, is an indication for laparoscopy. Transhepatic cholecystocholangiography can be added to laparoscopy, with the gallbladder being punctured under direct vision through the laparoscope. Unlike transhepatic percutaneous cholangiography, the success rate with this method does not depend upon dilatation of the ductal system.

Abdominal Cavity

Laparoscopy has been known since the turn of the century, but it has not become popular until recently. The pelvic contents can be examined endoscopically with great precision through a buttonhole incision with much less morbidity than a surgical exploration. This procedure can be an important tool for differential diagnosis of a pelvic mass, for a "second look" in treated ovarian cancer, and in selected patients with pelvic inflammatory disease.[9]

Oncologists and general surgeons have recently become aware of the importance of laparoscopy. This 30-minute procedure performed under local anesthesia can provide important information regarding the actual appearance of an intraperitoneal lesion, and will faciltate directed biopsies with good hemostasis, and without surgical exploration. There is often a significant difference between an aspirated cytology specimen obtained with a percutaneous "skinny needle" approach and an adequate tissue sample obtained during laparoscopy.

Indications for Laparoscopy

Palpable mass: In those cases where the diagnostic workup did not reveal the anatomic site of a mass but merely its secondary effects, such as compression of the rectosigmoid or stomach, laparoscopy can reveal the precise location and extent, as well as facilitate a safe biopsy. In association with large abdominopelvic tumors it is not uncommon to find hugely dilated veins which can be punctured inadvertantly with a percutaneous neelde, resulting in massive bleeding.

Ascites of unknown origin is a good indication for laparoscopy. In patients with ascites it may be difficult to obtain percutaneous liver or other organ biopsies, whereas laparoscopy (after evacuation of some ascitic fluid during the procedure) will provide excellent guidance for a directed biopsy.

In pancreatic carcinoma or other malignant lesions within or adjacent to the abdominal cavity, evidence of peritoneal spread or liver involvement can provide important information which may lead to a change in the treatment plan. In particular, needless surgery may be obviated or a palliative procedure accomplished promptly.

An interesting application for laparoscopy would be a second-look approach to Stage C colon carcinomas, where a large number of patients can be expected to develop liver metastases in a short period of time. Late elevations in serum carcinoembryonic antigen (CEA) in treated colon cancer or the question of continuing or stopping chemotherapy in Stage III ovarian carcinoma could precipitate an exploratory laparotomy; again, this might be made unnecessary by positive findings at laparoscopy (Fig. 7).

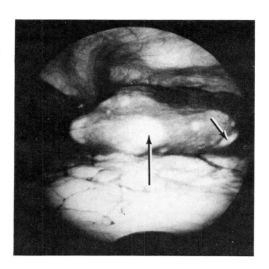

Figure 7. Laparoscopic view of the left lobe of the liver in a patient who had undergone a previous left-sided colectomy for carci noma. Two years postoperatively he was suspected of having dissemination and the left lobe showed several protruding (metastatic) lesions (arrow). A biopsy confirmed the diagnosis.

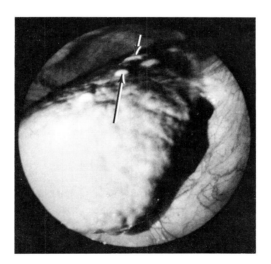

Figure 8. Laparoscopic view of a known cirrhotic patient whose laboratory data did not show significant changes. However, the patient complained of anorexia and weight loss of 3 months' duration. The right lobe exhibited a macronodular appear ance with a few whitish nodules on the anterior surface (arrow); these proved to be hepatocellular carcinoma.

In patients suspected clinically of a hepatic malignancy, with or without a history of cirrhosis or hemachromatosis where laboratory results and imaging studies are borderline or noninformative, laparoscopy can also be used to discover and to verify histologically the presence of carcinoma (Fig. 8).

In summary, laparoscopy can be exceptionally helpful in these as well as in other abdominopelvic disorders. It is therefore unfortunate that this examination has not yet achieved the popularity that it warrants.[10] The accuracy of diagnostic laparoscopy is in the vicinity of 90-92%, as verified by surgery or autopsy.[11] It can be hoped that the technique will occupy in the next few years an ever more important role in the diagnosis and staging of malignancies of the abdominal cavity.

Conclusions

The limited number of endoscopic procedures discussed here are those which have undergone significant improvements in the last decade and for which the results achieved have been extremely promising. Attention is focused on oncologic applications where a simple, fast, inexpensive and safe diagnostic approach is of the highest importance. There are several postgraduate courses currently available where specific endoscopic procedures are taught. Great emphasis is appropriately being given now by various specialty boards to include these important diagnostic tools in teaching programs.

(Editors' Note: Unfortunately, the endoscopic images here are reproduced in black and white rather than in the original color, because of the publication costs attendant upon color reproductions. The author wishes to point out that certain details are better recognized in the original color display.)

References

1.   Wolff, W.I., Shinya, H.:   A new approach to colonic polyps.   Ann. Surg. 178:367, 1973.

2.   Safrany, L.:   Endoscopic retrograde cannulations of the Papilla of Vater.   Chapter 22 in "Endoscopy" edit. by Berci, G., Appleton   Century Crofts, New York, 1976.

3.   Berci, G.:   Rigid endoscopes.   Chapter 5 in "Endoscopy" edit. by Berci, G., Appleton-Century Crofts, New York, 1976.

4.   Hopkins, H.H.:   Optical principles of the endoscopes.   Chapter 1   in "Endoscopy" edit. by Berci, G., Appleton-Century Crofts, New   York, 1976.

5.   Ward, P.H., Berci, G., Calcaterra, T.C.:   Advances in Endoscopic Examination of the Respiratory System.   Ann Oto. Rhino. Laryngol. 83:754, 1974.

6.   Ward, P.H., Berci, G., Calcaterra, T.C.:   Superior Laryngeal Nerve Paralysis: An Often Overlooked Entity. Tr. Am. Acad. Ophth. and   Otol. 84:78, 1977.

7.   Ward, P.H.:   Mediastinoscopy.   Chapter 49 in "Endoscopy" edit. by Berci, G., Appleton-Century Crofts, New York, 1976.

8.   Swierenga, J.:   Thoracoscopy.   Chapter 52 in "Endoscopy" edit. by Berci, G., Appleton-Century Crofts, New York, 1976.

9.   Gomel, V., Corson, S.:   Oncologic (Gyn.) Laparoscopy.   Section 5   in "Laparoscopy", edit. by Phillips, Williams and Wilkins, Baltimore,   1977.

10.   Berci, G.:   Laparoscopy.   Chapter 29 in "Endoscopy" edit. by Berci, G., Appleton-Century Crofts, New York, 1976.

11.   McCallum, R.W., Berci, G.:   Laparoscopy in Hepatic Disease.   Gastroint. Endoscopy. 23:20, 1976.

Chapter 5

Computed Tomography in the Diagnosis and Staging of Thoracic Malignancies

Marshall Bein, M.D.

Computed tomography (CT) has had a significant impact on the diagnosis and staging of neoplasms in many body areas, and the thorax is no exception. This discussion will compare CT with conventional imaging modalities in the following clinical contexts: (1) solitary pulmonary nodule; (2) clinical staging of lung cancer; (3) clinical staging of extrapulmonary neoplasms (e.g., evaluation of pulmonary metastases); and (4) staging of lymphoma.

Solitary Pulmonary Nodule

Chest radiologists and physicians are often confronted with the problem of diagnosing a solitary pulmonary nodule. A reliable criterion of benignancy is the absence of growth for two years or longer[1]. If no previous chest radiographs are available, the presence of calcification on plain radiographs or on conventional tomograms can point toward a benign lesion. Homogeneous, central ("target"), laminated, "popcorn," or punctuate patterns of calcification generally exclude malignancy. Focal calcification located asymmetrically within a nodule does not rule out cancer, since malignancy can originate in an area of previous inflammatory disease[1,2]. There are no other criteria that reliably differentiate benign from malignant nodules. If lack of growth or calcification cannot be established, tissue is usually obtained from a lung nodule for definitive diagnosis using a percutaneous needle approach, fiberoptic bronchoscopy, or thoracotomy.

Siegelman et al have recently described a technique in which CT is performed on noncalcified solitary pulmonary nodules, with the objective of differentiating benign from malignant lesions[3]. Using thin section CT they have shown that CT is more sensitive than standard tomography in assessing the density of pulmonary nodules and that benign and malignant lesions may be distinguished by using the CT (density) numbers. Corroboration of this study is eagerly awaited. In the future it is conceivable that patients might be selected simply for radiographic follow-up to confirm a CT-diagnosed benign nodule, rather than be subjected to a thoracotomy.

Clinical Staging of Lung Cancer

Thoracic imaging modalities can be helpful in defining operability and resectability of lung cancer within the context of the TNM staging system[4-6]. The presence of mediastinal metastases is an important determinant of whether operation is to be performed, since mediastinal nodes alter staging and generally indicate noncurability in lung cancer. However, because nodal enlargement may be malignant or benign (reactive hyperplasia)[7-9], mediastinal exploration is often done for histologic diagnosis. The location of the suspected nodal enlargement determines the surgical approach. Cervical mediastinoscopy can be done to approach paratracheal and, occasionally, large anterior subcarinal nodes, whereas parasternal mediastinotomy is necessary for anterior mediastinal and subaortic (aortic-pulmonic window) nodes[10-12]. A formal thoracotomy is usually necessary to gain access to subcarinal nodes, especially those located posteriorly. In addition to proved mediastinal lymph node involvement by tumor, hematogenous lateral parenchymal metastases also indicate inoperability. However, the latter is less frequently encountered during initial staging of lung cancer[13].

Resectability may be limited by direct extension of the primary tumor into the mediastinum or into other extraparenchymal tissues such as the chest wall or diaphragm. Extranodal extension of neoplasm can also limit resectability in those few patients where a resection of malignant mediastinal nodes is being considered[14-16].

Plain chest radiographs alone are diagnostic in 50-75% of patients with mediastinal lymphadenopathy[9,17,18]. Conventional tomography also will detect nodal enlargement[19,20] and is more sensitive than plain radiography[8,21]. However, it has been reported that tomography will still miss lymphadenopathy in 5-65% of patients when compared with cervical mediastinoscopy and/or thoracotomy[7,9,13,18,22-24].

Radionuclide scanning with 67-gallium may be employed for the detection of mediastinal lymph nodes. Its sensitivity has been reported variously to be between 50 and 100%[13,18,25-28]. False negative results occur with primary lung lesions in paramediastinal locations, where mediastinal lymphadenopathy cannot be separated from the primary tumor itself[27,28].

CT, by virtue of its transaxial anatomic display and the improved contrast resolution it provides between different tissues[29], has several advantages over conventional imaging modalities. It is more sensitive than plain radiography or conventional tomography for the detection of mediastinal lymph node metastases (Figure 1)[13,21,24,30-32]. Nevertheless, false negative results have been reported with CT in 5-20% of patients when compared to mediastinoscopy and/or thoracotomy[13,24,33]. CT can be particularly useful for detecting mediastinal lymphadenopathy when lung cancer occurs in a paramediastinal location and there is no aerated interface to delineate the mediastinal margins[13]. It might also be anticipated that CT could better evaluate the left anterior mediastinum, left paratracheal, and left main stem bronchus regions, which are not well-delineated by conventional imaging modalities because of the lack of immediately contiguous aerated lung. Comparisons between gallium scanning and CT are still inconclusive[13,21], but CT offers the advantage of defining more precisely the anatomic location of lymphadenopathy for possible biopsy.

Direct extraparenchymal extension of the primary tumor cannot be determined reliably by plain radiographs unless rib destruction, an extrathoracic soft tissue mass, an elevated diaphragm from phrenic nerve paralysis[19], or venous distention from superior vena caval obstruction is present. Conventional tomography does not seem to offer any advantages over plain radiography in this respect, and extraparenchymal extension has not yet been evaluated with gallium studies. There is no doubt that extension of lung cancer into the mediastinum or the chest wall can be evaluated better with CT than with conventional modalities (Figure 2)[13,21,24,30-32,34]. Several potential limitations remain, however. CT still cannot differentiate the

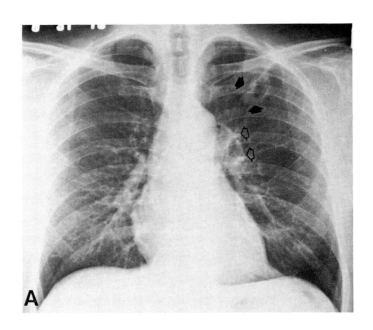

FIGURE 1

Patient with a known cavitating squamous cell carcinoma in the left upper lobe (arrows in (a) and (b)). Both the posteroanterior chest radiograph (open arrows in (a)) and conventional tomography demonstrated left hilar lymphadenopathy, but there were no mediastinal abnormalities. CT (c) demonstrates multiple lymph nodes in the left anterior mediastinum (arrows). A left parasternal mediastinotomy was performed prior to thoracotomy, and biopsy of the nodes demonstrated by CT revealed lymphoid hyperplasia with no evidence of metastases. Thoracotomy was then done and a left upper lobectomy performed. The left hilar nodes were positive for tumor.

Key for Figure C: 1 = right brachiocephalic vein; 2 = left brachiocephalic vein; 3 = innominate artery; 4 = left common carotid artery; 5 = left subclavian artery; T = trachea; E = esophagus.

104

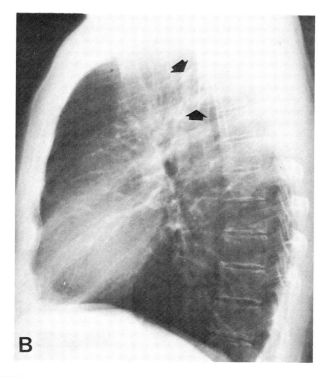

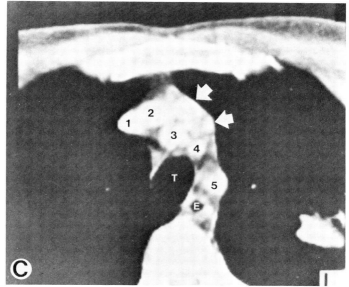

Figure 1, continued.

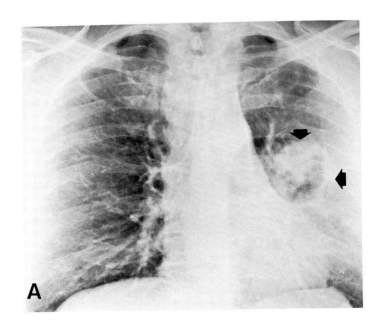

FIGURE 2

A cavitating squamous cell carcinoma (arrows) can be seen in the left upper lobe (a,b). Plain radiography as well as conventional tomography demonstrated that the mass was contiguous with the proximal left pulmonary artery, but it was uncertain whether there was actual vascular or mediastinal invasion. CT (c) demonstrated no cleavage plane between the mass and the proximal left pulmonary artery (arrows). There was also the suggestion of increased density extending along the left pulmonary artery into the region of the aortic-pulmonic window (open arrows). A left parasternal mediastinotomy was performed; tumor was found to have extended along the left pulmonary artery into the aortic-pulmonic window, and there was associated lymphadenopathy which on biopsy proved to be metastatic squamous cell carcinoma. The tumor was unresectable.

Key for Figure C: S = superior vena cava; A = ascending aorta; LPA = left pulmonary artery; DA = descending aorta; C = carina.

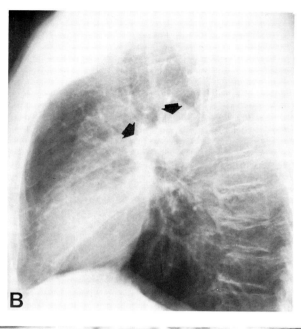

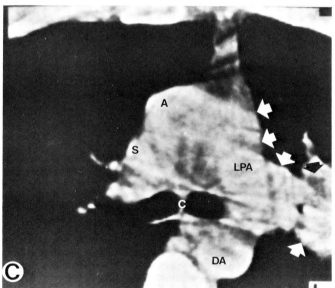

Figure 2, continued.

peripheral margins of a tumor from consolidated or collapsed parenchyma distal to an endobronchial obstruction. Therefore, the absence of aerated lung or a visible tissue plane between a neoplasm and the chest wall, mediastinum or lung hilum does not necessarily indicate unresectability[13,21]. While CT often identifies tumor extension outside of the bony thorax, more experience is needed to determine its efficacy for defining planes of resection between a primary tumor mass and the mediastinum, hilum, pleura, or extrapleural tissues[35]. Motion, volume averaging, or oblique orientations of anatomic parts may often preclude a precise evaluation of resection planes with present CT instruments. Faster scan times and more closely-spaced scanning intervals, with or without multiplanar image reconstruction, could greatly improve the staging accuracy of CT with respect to extraparenchymal extension.

While our experience at UCLA is still limited, we have found that the presence (on CT) of a fat plane between a primary lung tumor and the mediastinum is reliable in predicting resectability. However, failure to demonstrate such a plane suffers from the interpretative limitations that were suggested above. In summary, CT can detect mediastinal lymphadenopathy and extraparenchymal lung extension more effectively than conventional imaging modalities, but there are still substantial limitations. Studies are awaited to determine if increased experience with CT and better pathologic correlation, along with improved instrumentation, can improve results.

Staging of Extrapulmonary Neoplasms - Detection of Pulmonary Metastases

The detection of intrathoracic metastases is important to the staging of many extrathoracic malignancies. Plain chest radiographs are usually performed early. No further evaluation may be needed if metastases are demonstrated and if the patient is not a candidate for a surgical resection. However, selected patients may be amenable to resection of pulmonary metastases[36-38]. In these patients the precise enumeration and localization of metastases may be critical and will dictate the use of more sensitive imaging modalities. In other patients, even if the chest radiograph is normal more sensitive modalities may still be recommended for the exclusion of metastatic disease.

In comparison to standard chest radiography, conventional tomography has been reported to detect additional metastases in 3-60% of patients with a wide spectrum of neoplasms[39-42]. Three-to-five percent are the lower figures usually cited for cancer patients with "normal" chest films in whom metastases are subsequently picked up by tomography[39,42]. Only 1% of breast cancer patients with normal radiographs in one series had lung metastases on tomograms, so the use of tomgraphy is not recommended in breast cancer following a normal chest film[43]. On the other hand, multiple nodules may be found by tomography in 60% of cancer patients who have a solitary pulmonary nodule on routine radiographs[41]. In those cases where additional nodules have been found on tomography following standard radiographs, 55-65% of the newly-found nodules have been metastases[42,44]. Overall, 66% of lung nodules detected by tomography in a group of cancer patients were found to be metastases[44]. The metastatic nodule detection rate or sensitivity for full lung tomography, when compared to thoracotomy and/or to stringent clinical criteria, has been reported to be between 30 and 94%[40-42,44]. The use of a well-penetrated plain film view of the diaphragm along with tomographic cuts of the entire lung at 1 cm intervals, will improve the efficacy of detecting pulmonary nodules[45,46].

Lung nodule detection is even better with CT than with conventional full-lung tomography[24,30,44,47]. Small, subpleural nodules that may go undetected on full-lung tomography are imaged optimally in the transaxial plane by CT. CT has demonstrated a larger number of nodules in up to 50% of cancer patients when compared to conventional tomography[44,47]. However, the clinical utility of this improved sensitivity remains to be proved. In one study, 60% of lung nodules that were detected only by CT were benign[44]. However, in another study, 80% of the additional nodules detected (and resected) were metastases[47]. The majority of patients in whom CT detected a greater number of nodules than full-lung tomography already had one or more nodules present. It will be important to determine how effective CT will be in detecting additional metastatic nodules in a large series of cancer patients who have entirely normal full-lung tomograms.

No definite recommendations can yet be made concerning the indications for CT in detecting parenchymal metastases from extrathoracic malignancies. CT is certainly more sensitive than conventional tomography for detecting nodules, but its specificity needs to be evaluated further. For the moment, chest CT should at least be considered for any patient in whom the more sensitive detection of pulmonary metastases would significantly affect surgical or medical decision-making.

In addition to its role in defining the presence of parenchymal metastases, CT may also be useful to evaluate their resectability. The advantages of transaxial imaging may be used to evaluate the potential resectability of large or critically-situated lesions where less-than-optimal information is obtainable from plain radiography or conventional tomography (Figure 3). CT may also better evaluate the mediastinum for metastases. In highly selected extrapulmonary neoplasms where the resection of mediastinal metastases is being considered, CT might also prove helpful (Figure 4). The use of CT to assess resectability of parenchymal or mediastinal metastases must be individualized for each patient.

Staging of Lymphoma

Hodgkin's disease and non-Hodgkin's lymphoma comprise a broad spectrum of disease entities[48]. Intrathoracic manifestations, most commonly mediastinal lymphadenopathy and/or parenchymal involvement, are frequently found in the lymphomas and often influence the clinical staging and treatment[49]. The exact anatomic extent of mediastinal lymphadenopathy may also be important for localizing lung blocks and radiation treatment ports. Hilar lymphadenopathy contributes to staging, and its presence will determine in some institutions whether the contiguous lung fields receive radiation even in the absence of demonstrable parenchymal disease[50,51]. Parenchymal lymphoma which is separate from the hilum or mediastinum indicates Stage IV disease with consequent therapeutic implications. Extrapulmonary and extranodal thoracic involvement is less commonly found but will also have implications for staging and treatment.

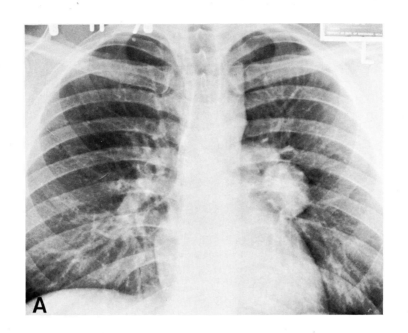

FIGURE 3

This young patient had a previous orchiectomy and retroperitoneal node dissection for embryonal cell carcinoma of the testis. Chest radiographs demonstrated a large solitary nodule (a presumed metastasis) in the left upper lobe contiguous with the left heart border (a) and the left upper lobe bronchus (arrow in (b)). Conventional tomography in multiple projections could not demonstrate a tissue plane between the lung mass and the mediastinum or hilum. There were no other lesions. CT demonstrated a fat plane between the mass and the left upper lobe bronchus (arrow in (c)), and between the mass and main pulmonary artery (arrow in (d)). The metastasis was resected, and no invasion of the hilum or mediastinum was found.

Key for Figures C and D: MPA = main pulmonary artery; RPA = right pulmonary artery; A = aortic arch; DA = descending aorta; LULB = left upper lobe bronchus; LA = left atrium; PV = pulmonary vein; S = superior vena cava.

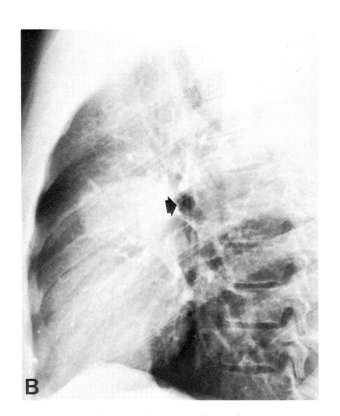

Figure 3, continued.

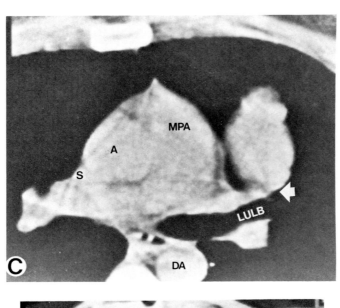

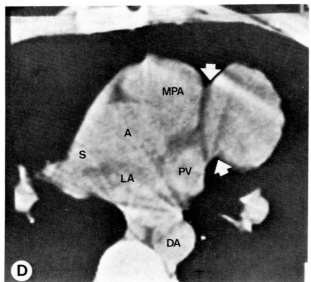

Figure 3, continued.

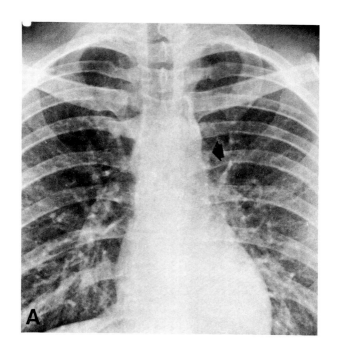

FIGURE 4

Localized left anterior mediastinal lymphadenopathy (arrow in (a)) can be seen in this patient with a past history of orchiectomy and retroperitoneal node dissection for embryonal cell carcinoma. Following chemotherapy, the plain radiograph appeared normal (b) as did conventinal tomography in multiple views. CT demonstrated a single lymph node in the left anterior mediastinum (arrow in (c)) with numerous smaller mediastinal nodes (open arrows). Residual lymphadenopathy was also seen adjacent to the aortic arch (arrow in (d)). The patient was explored, and one of nine mediastinal lymph nodes removed was positive for metastatic neoplasm.

Key for Figures C and D: 1 = right brachiocephalic vein; 2 = left brachiocephalic vein; 3 = innominate artery; 4 = left common carotid artery; 5 = left subclavian artery; S = superior vena cava; A = aortic arch; T = trachea.

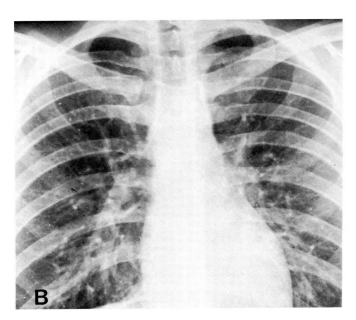

Figure 4, continued.

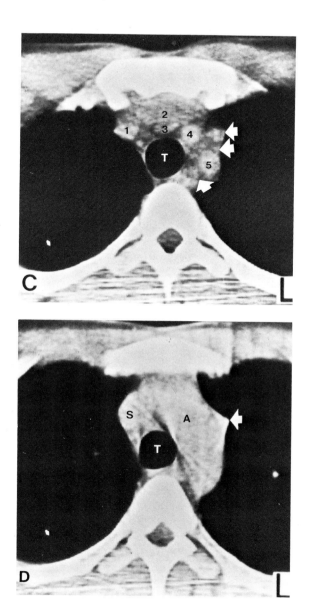

Figure 4, continued.

The standard chest radiograph is of course invaluable for assessing intrathoracic involvement in lymphoma, and the radiographic manifestations in previously untreated patients have been reviewed extensively[52-55]. Initial mediastinal or hilar lymphadenopathy is found more often in Hodgkin's disease than in non-Hodgkin's lymphoma, whereas parenchymal lung involvement is observed somewhat more commonly in non-Hodgkin's lymphoma at first presentation. Pleural effusion is usually secondary to massive central lymphadenopathy, but direct pleural involvement by lymphoma may occur. Thoracic osseous abnormalities are seen infrequently at initial staging. Emphasis has also been placed on the role of periodic routine radiographs for detecting relapse, the sites of which may include the lung parenchyma, mediastinal lymph nodes, pleura and osseous structures[56].

It has been demonstrated that conventional full-lung tomography is more sensitive in demonstrating mediastinal lymph node involvement and parenchymal disease in lymphoma than standard radiographs[57,58]. Although new information was uncovered in approximately 20% of patients, in only 1-3% was the actual disease staging changed and the treatment thereby modified. The use of tomography for demonstrating additional intrathoracic involvement was of greater practical benefit in Hodgkin's disease than in non-Hodgkin's lymphoma.

Imaging with 67-gallium is often employed in patients with lymphoma. The overall sensitivity of gallium for detecting lymphomatous involvement ranges between 35% and 100% and varies with the histologic type of lymphoma and the anatomic location[59-61]. Hodgkin's disease, histiocytic lymphoma, and Burkitt's lymphoma are reported to have the highest detection rates, while mediastinal lymphadenopathy is the location most sensitively detected by this method. It has been suggested that gallium scanning is equal to, complementary to, or better than standard radiography for detecting mediastinal lymphoma[59,60,62]. However, there is a relative paucity of detailed studies to address these comparisons. Gallium scanning may prove to be most useful in evaluating patients for post-treatment recurrences, but it does seem to have an application also during the initial staging process[59].

The use of CT in lymphoma has been studied more extensively for the abdomen than the thorax, but several useful observations have been made[63-66]. CT has been suggested to be sensitive for detecting early or minimal disease in the chest, both nodal and extranodal. It has also been recommended particularly for evaluating recurrent disease. Mediastinal and hilar lymphadenopathy, parenchymal involvement with pulmonary tumor infiltrations or subpleural nodules, effusions or pleural plaques, contiguous extension of mediastinal tumor into the lung parenchyma or the chest wall (Figure 5), and pericardial involvement (Figure 6) have all been demonstrated. While there have been patients with lymphoma in whom CT showed findings that were not appreciated by conventional imaging, there has been no rigorous study comparing CT to conventional examinations, and the role of CT in the thoracic staging of lymphoma still cannot be precise ly defined. CT does appear to have a unique role in delineating mediastinal-hilar involvement for planning radiotherapy portals (Figures 5 and 6)[66]. Particular emphasis has also been given to the contiguous spread of mediastinal lymphoma into the lungs or chest wall and to pericardial involvement; the actual anatomic extent of involvement is better appreciated on CT than on standard radiographs, thereby allowing better treatment localization and dosimetry.

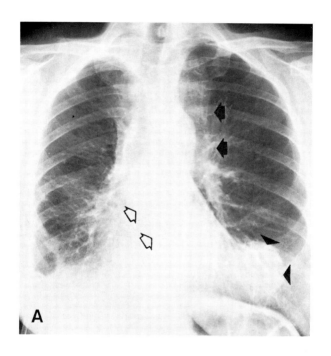

FIGURE 5

This patient with non-Hodgkin's lymphoma has recurrent subcarinal (open arrows in (a)), cardiophrenic angle (arrowheads in (a) and (b)), and internal thoracic (arrows in (a) and (b)) lymphadenopathy. There is also a fibrothorax on the right. The extent of adenopathy is vaguely defined on the posteroanterior chest radiograph. CT demonstrates the precise margins of the thoracic lymphadenopathy (arrows in (c)), with associated extension into the soft tissues anteriorly (open arrow).

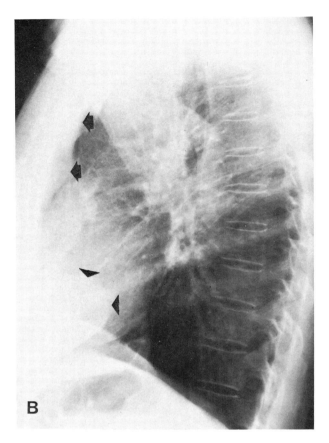

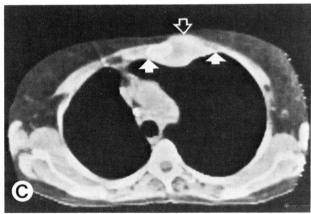

Figure 5, continued.

118

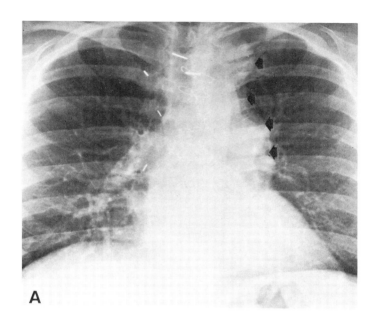

A

FIGURE 6

There is recurrent lymphadenopathy in the left anterior mediastinum (arrows in (a) and (b)) in another patient with non-Hodgkin's lymphoma.   No other lymphadenopathy was evident on plain radiographs.   CT (c) demonstrates cardiophrenic angle (arrows) and chest wall (open arrow) lymphadenopathy.   A gallium scan subsequently was performed and was positive in the same regions, confirming these additional foci of recurrent disease that were important in radiotherapy treatment planning.

Key for Figure C: P = parietal pericardium; I = inferior vena cava; DA = descending aorta.

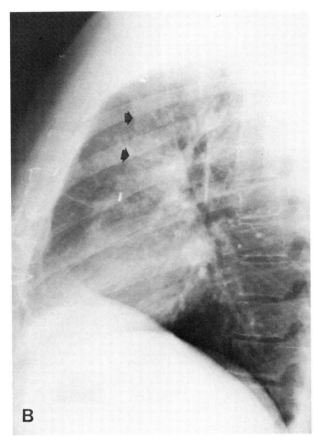

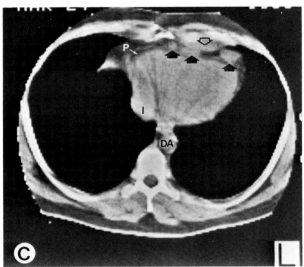

Figure 6, continued.

120

References

1. Siegelman, S.S., Stitik, F.P., Summer, W.R. Management of the patient with a localized pulmonary lesion. In: Pulmonary system: practical approaches to pulmonary diagnosis. Siegelman, S.S., Stitik, F.P., Summer, W.R., eds. New York: Grune and Stratton, 1979: 339-358.

2. O'Keefe, M.E., Good, C.A., McDonald, J.R. Calcification in solitary nodules of the lung. American Journal of Roentgenology 1957; 77:1023-1033.

3. Siegelman, S.S., Zerhouni, E.A., Leo, F.P., Khouri, N.F., Stitik, F.P. CT of the solitary pulmonary nodule. American Journal of Roentgenology 1980; 135:1-13.

4. Clinical staging system for carcinoma of the lung. American Joint Committee for Cancer Staging and End Results Reporting. Chicago, Illinois, 1973.

5. Mountain, C.F., Carr, D.T., Anderson, W.A.D. A system for the clinical staging of lung cancer. American Journal of Roentgenology 1974; 120:130-138.

6. Carr, D.T. The staging of lung cancer. Am Rev Respir Dis 1978; 117:819-823.

7. Peace, P.K., Price, J.L. Preoperative tomographic assessment of the mediastinum in bronchial carcinoma. Thorax 1973; 28:367-370.

8. Greenwell, F.P., Wright, F.W. Rotational tomography. Clin Radiol 1965; 16:377-389.

9. Fishman, N.H., Bronstein, M.H. Is mediastinoscopy necessary in the evaluation of lung cancer. Ann Thorac Surg 1975; 20:678-686.

10. Pearson, F.G. An evaluation of mediastinoscopy in the management of presumably operable bronchial carcinoma. J Thorac Cardiovasc Surg 1968; 55:617-625.

11. Bowen, T.E., Zajtchuk, R., Green, D.C., Brott, W.H. Value of anterior mediastinotomy in bronchogenic carcinoma of the left upper lobe. J Thorac Cardiovasc Surg 1978; 76:269-271.

12. Jolly, P.C., Hill, L.D., Lawless, T.A., West, T.L. Parasternal mediastinotomy and mediastinoscopy. J Thorac Cardiovasc Surg 1973; 66:549-556.

13. Hirleman, M.T., Yiu-Chiu, V.S., Chiu, L.S., Schapiro, R.L. The resectability of primary lung carcinoma: a diagnostic staging review. CT: J Comput Tomog 1980; 4:146-163.

14. Naruke, T., Suemasu, K., Ishikawa, S.   Surgical treatment for lung cancer with metastasis to mediastinal lymph nodes.   J Thorac Cardiovasc Surg 1976; 71:279-285.

15. Naruke, T., Suemasu, K., Ishikawa, S.   Lymph node mapping and curability at various levels of metastasis in resected lung cancer.   J Thorac Cardiovasc Surg 1978; 76:832-839.

16. Rubenstein, I., Baum, G.L., Kalter, Y., Pauzner, Y., Lieberman, Y., Bubis, J.J.   The influence of cell type and lymph node metastases on survival of patients with carcinoma of the lung undergoing thoracotomy. Am Rev Resp Dis 1979; 119:253-262.

17. Whitcomb, M.E., Barham, E., Goldman, A.L., Green, D.C.   Indications for mediastinoscopy in bronchogenic carcinoma.   Am Rev Respir Dis 1976; 113:189-195.

18. Fosburg, R.G., Hopkins, G.B., Kan, M.K.   Evaluation of the mediastinum by gallium-67 scintigraphy in lung cancer.   J Thorac Cardiovasc Surg 1979; 77:76-82.

19. Greene, R.F.   Lungs and mediastinum.   In: Steckel, R.J., Kagan, A.R., eds.   Diagnosis and staging of cancer.   A radiologic approach. Philadelphia: W.B. Saunders, 1976:36-70.

20. Fennessy, J.J.   The radiology of lung cancer.   Med Clin North Am 1975; 59:95-120.

21. Shevland, J.E., Chin, L.C., Schapiro, R.L., Young, J.A., Rossi, N.P.   The role of conventional tomography and computed tomography in assessing the resectability of primary lung cancer: a preliminary report. CT: J Comput Tomogr 1978; 2:1-19.

22. James, E.C., Ellwood, R.A.   Mediastinoscopy and mediastinal roentgenology. Ann Thorac Surg 1974; 18:531-538.

23. Paris, F., Tarazona, V., Blasco, E., Canto, A., Casillas, M., Pastor, J. Mediastinoscopy in the surgical management of lung carcinoma.   Thorax 1975; 30:146-151.

24. Mintzer, R.A., Malave, S.R., Neiman, H.L., Michaelis, L.L., Vanecko, R.M., Sanders, J.H.   Computed versus conventional tomography in evaluation of primary and secondary pulmonary neoplasms.   Radiology 1979; 132:653-659.

25. De Meester, T.R., Bekerman, C., Joseph, J.G., et al.   Gallium-67 scanning for carcinoma of the lung.   J Thorac Cardiovasc Surg 1976; 72:699-708.

26. Alazraki, N.P., Ramsdell, J.W., Taylor, A., Friedman, P.J., Peters, R.M., Tisi, G.M.   Reliability of gallium scan chest radiography compared to mediastinoscopy for evaluating mediastinal spread in lung cancer. Am Rev Respir Dis 1978; 117:415-420.

27. De Meester, T.R., Golomb, H.M., Kirchner, P., et al. The role of gallium-67 scanning in the clinical staging and preoperative evaluation of patients with carcinoma of the lung. Ann Thorac Surg 1979; 28:451-464.

28. Lesk, D.M., Wood, T.E., Carroll, S.E., Reese, L. The applicability of 67-gallium scanning in determining the operability of bronchogenic carcinoma. Radiology 1978; 128:707-709.

29. Ter-Pogossian, M.M. Some physical aspects of computed tomography. Syllabus on Computed Tomography 1979. Oak Brook: The Radiological Society of North America, 1979:109A1-11

30. McLoud, T.C., Wittenberg, J., Ferrucci, J.T. Jr. Computed tomography of the thorax and standard radiographic evaluation of the chest: a comparative study. J Comput Assist Tomogr 1979; 3:170-180.

31. Emami, B., Melo, A., Carter, B.L., Munzenrider, J.E., Piro, A.J. Value of computed tomography in radiotherapy of lung cancer. American Journal of Roentgenology 1978; 131:63-67.

32. Crowe, J.K., Brown, L.R., Muhm, J.R. Computed tomography of the mediastinum. Radiology 1978; 128:75-87.

33. Underwood, G.H. Jr., Hooper, R.G., Axelbaum, S.P., Goodwin, D.W. Computed tomographic scanning of the thorax in the staging of bronchogenic carcinoma. N Engl J Med 1979; 300:777-778.

34. Heitzman, E.R., Goldwin, R.L., Proto, A.V. Radiologic analysis of the mediastinum utilizing computed tomography. Radiol Clin North Am 1977; 15:309-329.

35. Bein, M.E., Holmes, E.C. Pulmonary mass in a smoker (preoperative imaging studies in the intrathoracic staging of lung cancer). Diagnostic Oncology Case Studies. Kagan, A.R., Steckel, R.J., eds. American Journal of Roentgenology (In press).

36. Holmes, E.C., Ramming, K.P., Eilber, F.R., Morton, D.L. The surgical management of pulmonary metastases. Semin Oncol 1977; 4:65-69.

37. Takita, H., Merrin, C., Didolkar, M.S., Douglass, H.O., Edgerton, F. The surgical management of multiple lung metastases. Ann Thorac Surg 1977; 24:359-363.

38. Morrow, C.E., Vassilopoulos, P.P., Grage, T.B. Surgical resection for metastatic neoplasms of the lung: experience at the University of Minnesota Hospitals. Cancer 1980; 45:2981-2985.

39. Polga, J.P., Watnick, M. Whole lung tomography in metastatic disease. Clin Rad 1976; 27:53-56.

40. Neifeld, J.P., Michaelis, L.L., Doppman, J.L. Suspected pulmonary metastases. Correlation of chest x-ray, whole lung tomograms, and operative findings. Cancer 1977; 39:383-387.

41. Didolkar, M.S., Cedermark, B.J., Goel, I.P., Takita, H., Moore, R.H. Accuracy of roentgenograms of the chest in metastases to the lungs. Surg Gynec and Obst 1977; 144:903-905.

42. Sindelar, W.F., Bagley, D.H., Felix, E.L., Doppman, J.L., Ketcham, A.S. Lung tomography in cancer patients. Full-lung tomograms in screening for pulmonary metastases. JAMA 1978; 240:2060-2063.

43. Curtis, A.M., Ravin, C.E., Collier, P.E., Putman, C.E., McLoud, T., Greenspan, R.H. Detection of metastatic disease from carcinoma of the breast: limited value of full lung tomography. Am J Roentgenology 1980; 134:253-255.

44. Schaner, E.G., Chang, A.E., Coppman, J.L., Conkle, D.M., Flye, M.W., Rosenberg, S.A. Comparison of computed and conventional whole lung tomography in detecting pulmonary nodules: a prospective radiologic-pathologic study. Am J Roentgenology 1978; 131:51-54.

45. Bein, M.E. Plain film diaphragm view as adjunct to full lung tomography. Am J Roentgenology 1979; 133:217-220.

46. Bein, M.E., Greenberg, M., Liu, P-Y., Ohara, J., Bassett, L.W., Schaefer, C.J., Steckel, R.J. Pulmonary nodules: detection in 1 and 2 cm full lung linear tomography. Am J Roentgenol 1980; 135:513-520.

47. Muhm, J.R., Brown, L.R., Crowe, J.K., Sheedy, P.F., Hattery, R.R., Stephens, D.H. Comparison of whole lung tomography and computed tomography for detecting pulmonary nodules. Am J Roentgenology 1978; 131:981-984.

48. Callihan, T.R., Berard, C.W. The classification and pathology of the lymphomas and leukemias. Semin Roentgenol 1980; 15:219-226.

49. Kaplan, H.S. Essentials of staging and management of the malignant lymphomas. Semin Roentgenol 1980; 15:219-226.

50. Hoppe, R.T., Rosenberg, S.A., Kaplan, H.S., Cox, R.S. Prognostic factors in pathological stage IIIA Hodgkin's disease. Cancer 1980; 46:1240-1246.

51. Palos, B., Kaplan, H.S., Kargmark, C.J. The use of thin lung shields to deliver limited whole-lung irradiation during mantle-field treatment of Hodgkin's disease. Radiology 1971; 101:441-442.

52. Blank, N., Castellino, R.A. The intrathoracic manifestations of the malignant lymphomas and the leukemias. Semin Roentgenol 1980; 15:227-245.

53. Filly, R., Blank, N., Castellino, R.A. Radiographic distribution of intrathoracic disease in previously untreated patients with Hodgkin's disease and non-Hodgkin's lymphoma. Radiology 1976; 120:277-281.

54. Steckel, R.J., Kagan, A.R. Hodgkin's disease. In: Steckel, R.J., Kagan, A.R., eds. Diagnosis and Staging of Cancer. A radiologic approach. Philadelphia: W.B. Saunders, 1976:1-18.

55. Kagan, A.R., Steckel, R.J.   Non-Hodgkin's lymphoma.   In: Steckel, R.J., Kagan, A.R., eds.   Diagnosis and staging of cancer.   A radiologic approach. Philadelphia: W.B. Saunders, 1976:1-18.

56. Castellino, R.A., Blank, N., Cassady, J.R., Kaplan, H.S.   Roentgenologic aspects of Hodgkin's disease.   II.   Role of routine radiographs in detecting initial relapse.   Cancer 1973; 31:316-323.

57. Castellino, R.A., Filly, R., Blank, N.   Routine full lung tomography in the initial staging and treatment planning of patients with Hodgkin's disease and non-Hodgkin's lymphoma.   Cancer 1976; 38:1130-1136.

58. Davidson, J.W., Clarke, E.A.   Influence of modern radiological techniques on clinical staging of malignant lymphomas.   Canad Med Assoc J 1968; 99:1196-1204.

59. Turner, D.A., Fordham, E.W., Ali, A., Slayton, R.E.   Gallium-67 imaging in the management of Hodgkin's disease and other malignant lymphomas. Semin Nucl Med 1978; 8:205-218.

60. Hoffer, P.   Status of gallium-67 in tumor detection.   J Nucl Med 1980; 21:394-398.

61. Silberstein, E.B.   Cancer diagnosis.   The role of tumor-imaging radiopharmaceuticals.   Am J Med 1976; 60:226-237.

62. Kay, D.N., McCready, V.R.   Clinical isotope scanning using ^{67}Ga citrate in the management of Hodgkin's disease.   Br J Radiol 1972; 45:437-443.

63. Ellert, J., Kreel, L.   The role of computed tomography in the initial staging and subsequent management of the lymphomas.   J Comput Assist Tomogr 1980; 4:368-391.

64. Jones, S.E., Tobias, D.A., Waldman, R.S.   Computed tomographic scanning in patients with lymphoma.   Cancer 1978; 41:480-486.

65. Kreel, L.   Computed tomography of the lung and pleura.   Semin Roentgenol 1978; 13:213-225.

66. Pilepick, M.V., Rene, J.B., Munzenrider, J.E., Carter, B.L.   Contribution of computed tomography to the treatment of lymphomas.   Am J Roentgenol 1978; 131:69-73.

Chapter 6

Computed Tomography in the Diagnosis and Evaluation
of Primary Head and Neck Cancer

Anthony A. Mancuso, M.D.

INTRODUCTION - CT vs. CONVENTIONAL RADIOGRAPHIC STUDIES

Computed tomography (CT) has already revolutionized neuroradiology. Its effect on the diagnostic evaluation of patients with diseases elsewhere in the body (e.g., abdomen, chest, spine) has been slower to evolve, and its early impact in the evaluation of patients with cancer of the paranasal sinuses, nasopharynx, oropharynx, parotid gland, larynx and neck lies somewhere in between. With head and neck cancer, the categorical problem for the clinician is straightforward: those planning therapy need to know the full extent of the primary lesion and its regional spread. It has become clear that CT, while it cannot diagnose cancer, does show the local extent of the lesion better than any other imaging study applied to these anatomic areas.

CT's superior contrast resolution provides details about the soft tissues surrounding the upper aerodigestive tract that were heretofore impossible to obtain by any means, including direct inspection at surgery.[1-5] It also happens that in most circumstances the axial imaging plane is ideal for evaluating the extracranial head and neck structures. Combining the usual axial views with direct coronal scans or multiplanar reconstructed images may provide confirmatory data in some instances, as with orbital and sellar lesions. The bone detail on second through fourth generation CT scanners is more than adequate for diagnosis, and recourse to conventional pluridirectional tomograms for "a better look at the bone" is simply not necessary.[2] CT has, in fact, completely replaced pluridirectional tomography in the laryngopharynx[8-11], and CT-assisted sialography has replaced the conventional contrast sialogram for mass lesions of the parotid[3,12] and submandibular glands. It eliminates the need for angiography in detecting intracranial extension of extracranial malignancies, and sometimes for the diagnosis of benign lesions (e.g., juvenile angiofibromas, neuromas, and paragangliomas). In summary, CT has revolutionized the radiologic approach to extracranial head and neck cancer in the same way as it has revolutionized neuroradiology, by reducing the quantity of less informative conventional studies and, in particular, invasive special procedures.

LARYNGEAL CANCER

Mucosal detail in the larynx may be studied by direct laryngoscopy, with appropriate biopsies confirming the nature of pathologic changes. CT directly complements the clinical examination, because it shows all of the deep tissue planes of the larynx (paralaryngeal space) and the cartilages, none of which can be adequately assessed clinically or by other radiologic studies. While observed fixation of a vocal cord and/or the visible extent of the primary

128

tumor do provide some evidence of deep extension, CT alone demonstrates invasion of soft tissue planes unequivocally, and the potential tumor-free margins.[13,14]

In the infraglottic region, CT shows the relationship of tumor to the cricoid cartilage which may be all-important in planning partial laryngectomy.[11,13] At the glottic level, CT shows the local extent of lesions relative to the anterior commissure, to both true cords and to the cricoarytenoid joint (Figure 1). Dynamic scans made during phonation can be used to document function.[8]

Supraglottically, extensions of tumor within the paralaryngeal and pre-epiglottic spaces can now be seen in detail because these spaces are normally of fibrofatty density and infiltrating lesions are of higher density (Figure 2). Early tumor extension can be appreciated in these areas. However, one must always remember that CT does not confirm histology and that infiltration may be due to tumor, infection, reactive edema or bleeding (Figure 3).[11]

Pyriform sinus malignancies have a high incidence of exolaryngeal extension through the cricothyroid and thyrohyoid membranes. CT easily shows these extensions, which even when they are massive are difficult to detect clinically (Figure 4).[11] A bulky primary tumor which is confined to the pyriform sinus can simulate exolaryngeal extension or regional lymph node disease clinically, but CT can help to make the distinction, which is a critical one. CT is also more sensitive than other radiologic studies in showing cartilage invasion by tumor.[11] Subtle invasion may sometimes be more difficult to detect because of inhomogeneities in thyroid cartilage mineralization.

OTHER NECK TUMORS (OUTSIDE THE LARYNGOPHARYNX)

CT can be very useful in selected patients with other primary tumors involving the neck.[15] These are usually carcinomas of the thyroid or the cervical esophagus, or soft tissue sarcomas. With one study, CT will show the relationship of a tumor to all of the important structures of the neck, including: carotid sheath, thyroid gland, esophagus, larynx, trachea, scalene muscles, brachial plexus, and the spinal column and cord (Figure 6). This single study, if done first, will often obviate the need for several other, perhaps more invasive examinations.

The role of CT in the evaluation of cervical lymph node metastases will be discussed in the next chapter.

MALIGNANCIES OF THE PARANASAL SINUSES

There are four critical routes of spread for primary paranasal sinus tumors: orbital, intracranial, nasopharyngeal, and infratemporal fossa. Spread into any of these areas, except the orbit, will preclude a surgical cure.

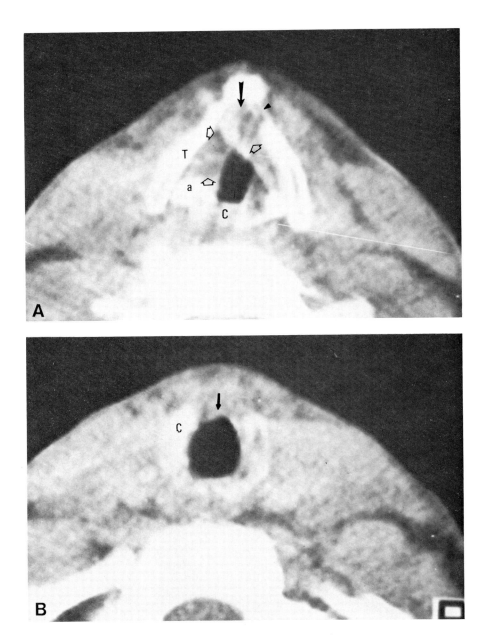

Figure 1. (A) Glottic level. Tumor (open arrows) involves cord and spreads contralaterally across anterior commissure (arrow). Lack of motion artifact on left indicates fixation of arytenoid (a). Thyroid cartilage is calcified (T). Small defect (arrowhead) in thyroid cartilage was caused by tumor invasion, but it may also have been a normal variant (see text). (B) Anterior subglottic extension (arrow) to the cricoid ring (c) level.

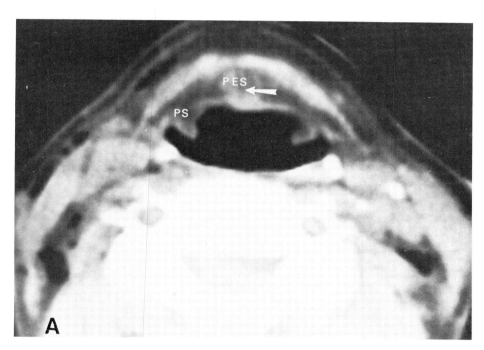

Figure 2. (A) Normal supraglottic larynx. PES-preepiglottic space; PS-paralaryngeal space; hypoepiglottic ligament (arrow). (B) in another patient, anterior epiglottic lesion invades preepiglottic and paralaryngeal spaces (arrowheads) and narrows airway (   ). H = hyoid. (C) Marginal supraglottic lesion invades right aryepiglottic fold (black arrow), and metastatic nodes obliterate planes around carotid sheath (arrowheads). C = carotid; J = jugular; white arrow denotes normal aryepiglottic fold.

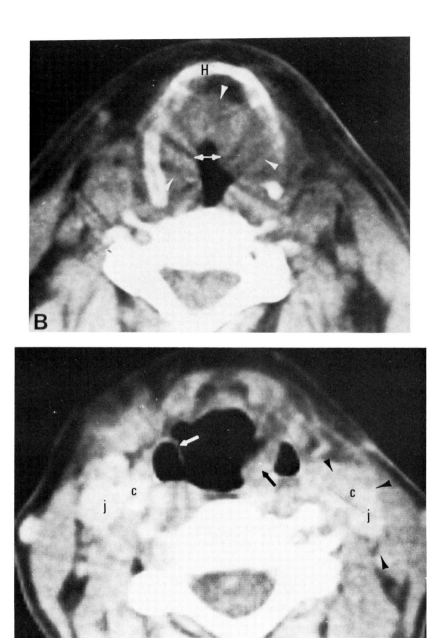

Figure 2, continued.

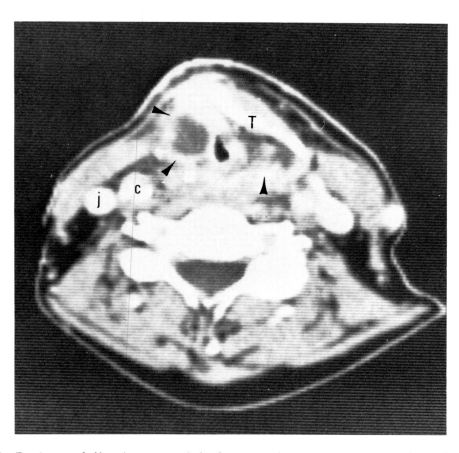

Figure 3. Patient following partial laryngopharyngectomy and radiation for pyriform sinus cancer. On I.V. contrast scan staining mass with low density center fills the remaining larynx (arrowheads). It was an abscess but could just as well have been recurrent tumor. T = thyroid cartilage; C = carotid; J = jugular.

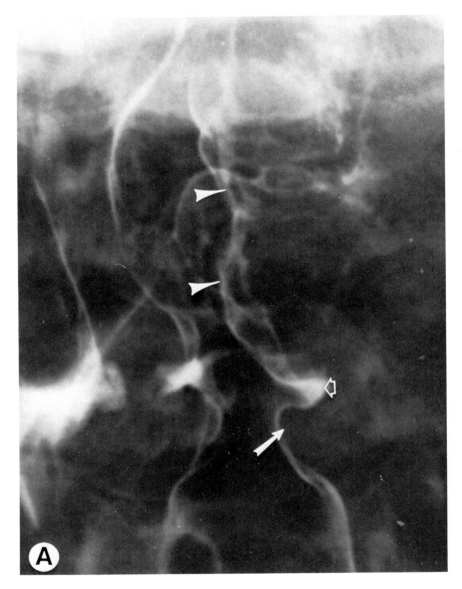

Figure 4. (A) Laryngogram from patient with pyriform sinus cancer shows no filling of left pyriform sinus and displacement of ipsilateral aryepiglottic fold (arrowheads). Left true cord (arrow) and laryngeal ventricle (open arrow) appear normal, although CT showed pathologically confirmed paralaryngeal extension to the true cord level. (B) CT of same patient shows exolaryngeal extension (arrowheads) and spread into preepiglottic space (arrow).

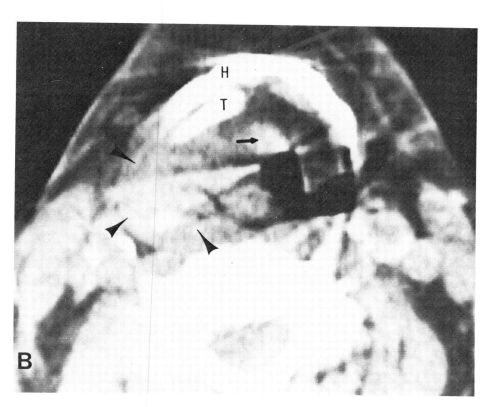

Figure 4, continued.

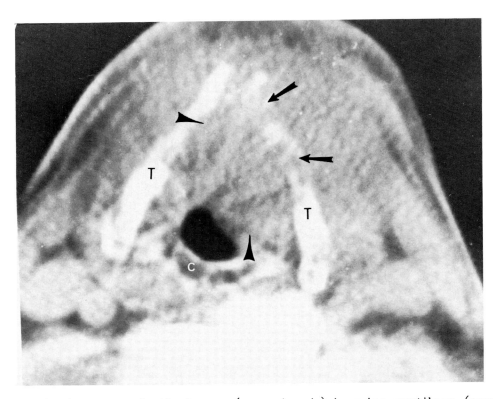

Figure 5. Massive transglottic tumor (arrowheads) invades cartilage (arrow). T = thyroid cartilage; C = cricoid cartilage.

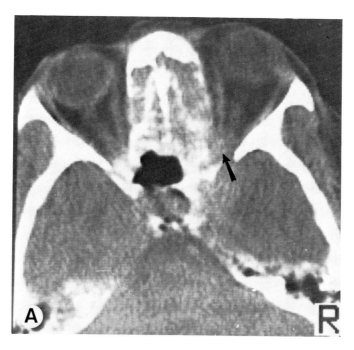

Figure 7. Orbital extensions of paranasal sinus tumors. A and B are of the same patient. (A) Axial section at cribiform plate. Tissue density fills superior ethmoids, destroys medial wall of orbit (arrowhead), displaces medial rectus muscle and infiltrates orbital apex (arrow). (B) Section through inferior orbital tissue shows orbital apex extension (arrow) and proptosis. (C) A different patient with an antral carcinoma and subtle involvement of the orbital floor (arrow) which could only be shown definitively on coronal sections.

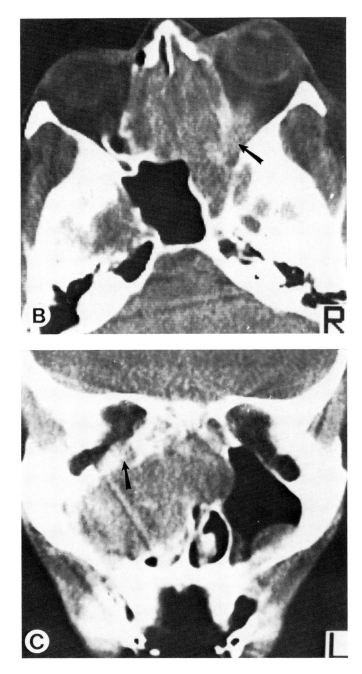

Figure 7, continued.

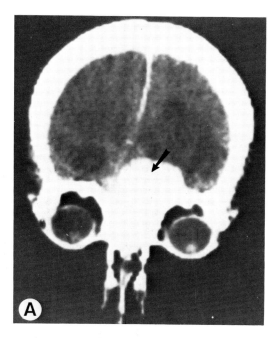

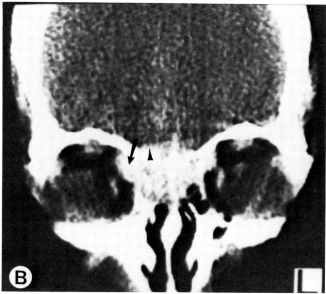

Figure 8. Intracranial extensions of paranasal sinus malignancies. (A) Massive extension through the cribiform plate (arrow), enhances with contrast infusion. (B) Minimal extension into the olfactory bulb and subfrontal regions (arrowhead) and orbit (arrow).

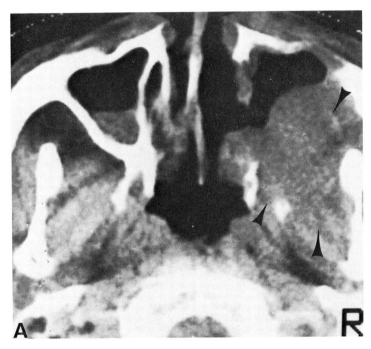

Figure 9. Posterior extensions of paranasal sinus malignancies. (A) Antral tumor with massive infratemporal fossa spread (arrowhead). (B) Coronal section showing nasopharyngeal involvement in a different patient. The mass (arrowheads) obliterates the eustachian tube orifice when compared with the normal side (arrow). (C) Same patient as in B. Tumor destroys the anteromedial wall of the antrum (arrow) and extends into the soft tissues of the face.

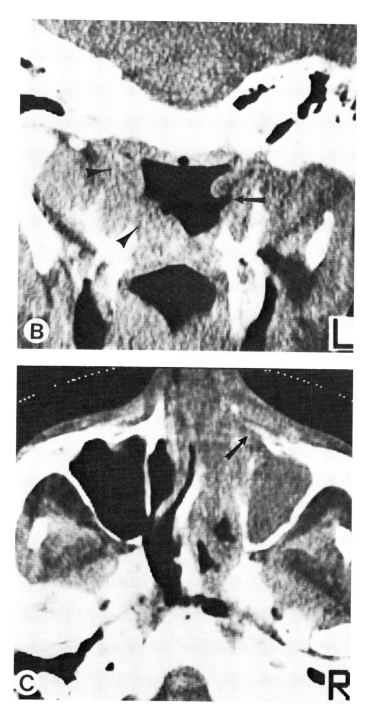

Figure 9, continued.

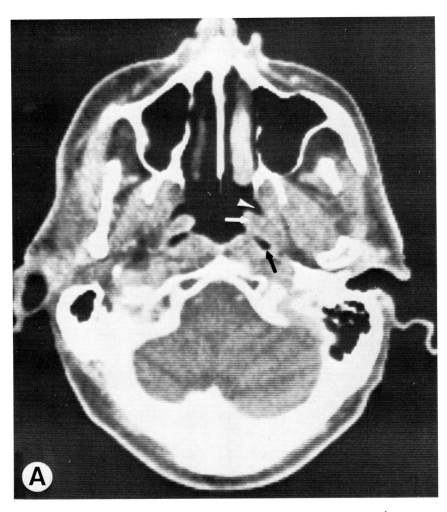

Figure 10A. Normal nasopharynx. Eustachian tube orifice (white arrowhead); Torus tubarius (white arrow); lateral pharyngeal recess (black arrow). Deep tissue planes are normal and symmetric.

144

distention of the fossae of Rosenmueller or slight differences in the size of the eustachian tube orifices if the deep tissue planes are normal. If the deep tissue planes are normal on CT and the mucosal surfaces appear normal on direct examination, then the nasopharynx is normal. All superficial noninfiltrating masses in the nasopharynx we have studied have turned out to be normal lymphoid tissue; this is usually confirmed on physical examination, but sometimes biopsy is required because of an atypical appearance or clinical presentation.[6,7,16]

CT is also the preferred imaging examination for following progress during and after therapy, in lesions of the oropharynx and nasopharynx (Figures 10B-C). Progression or response of the primary tumor and its nodal metastases may be documented accurately. Subsequent intracranial, orbital and paranasal sinus spread are precisely delineated by CT (Figure 11).

Some tumors grow entirely submucosally within the nasopharynx, giving no mucosal evidence of their presence. Even repeated biopsies may miss the lesion. On several occasions, CT has revealed submucosal masses (adenocystic primaries, solitary myelomas, chordomas) under such circumstances, and a deeper, CT-directed biopsy has revealed the tumor (Figure 12). For this reason, we always recommend CT as an adjunct to endoscopy and biopsy for the evaluation of the "unknown head and neck primary" (see Chapter 14: ed.).

SALIVARY GLANDS

CT-assisted sialography is now the imaging examination of choice for evaluating parotid[3,12] and submandibular gland lesions. In the parotid, CT can determine: a) whether a mass is intrinsic or extrinsic to the gland; b) the relationship of the mass to the plane of the facial nerve; c) other clues which help predict the likelihood of malignancy (Figure 13).[3,12] In the submandibular gland, it determines principally whether the mass is intrinsic or extrinsic to the gland.

CONCLUSION

CT has replaced or strongly complements the older contrasted tomographic studies for evaluating primary tumors in the larynx, sinuses, and salivary glands. It can also show tumor extension to the skull base and brain as well as cervical adenopathy.

COMPUTED TOMOGRAPHY IN THE EVALUATION OF CERVICAL LYMPH NODE METASTASES

CT is now a prime imaging examination for evaluating intra-abdominal, retroperitoneal, pelvic and mediastinal lymph nodes in cancer. Although CT

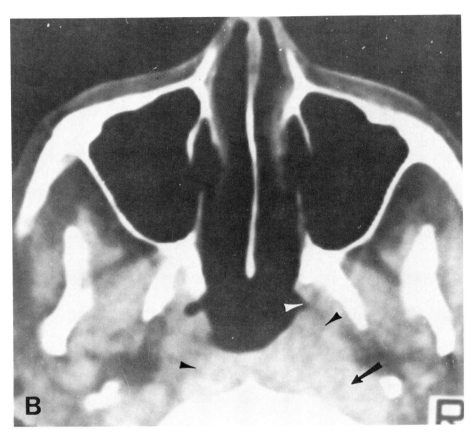

Figure 10B. Nasopharyngeal cancer undergoing radiation therapy. Mass infiltrates deep tissue planes and extends slightly across midline (black arrowheads). Right eustachian tube orifice is partially occluded (white arrowhead) and nodes or primary tumor surround right carotid sheath (arrow).

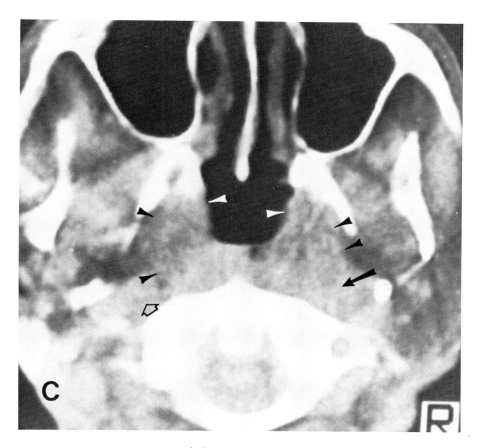

Figure 10C. Same patient as in (B). Six months after completion of therapy, tumor (black arrowheads) surrounds the nasopharyngeal airway bilaterally. There was no visible (mucosal) evidence of recurrence. Both eustachian tube orifices are now obliterated (white arrowheads). Cervical node involvement may also be bilateral (arrow, and open arrow).

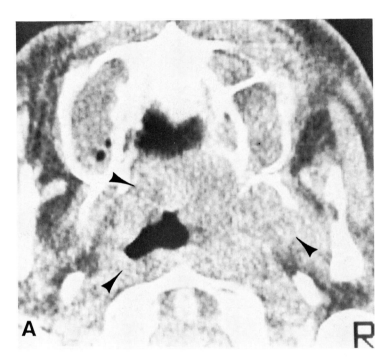

Figure 11. (A) Massive circumferential growth of a nasopharyngeal cancer (arrowheads). (B) The clivus (arrow), skull base about the foramen lacerum (arrowheads) and right pterygoid processes (open arrow) are destroyed. (C) Massive intracranial extension and secondary edema (arrowheads) in a non-contrast study.

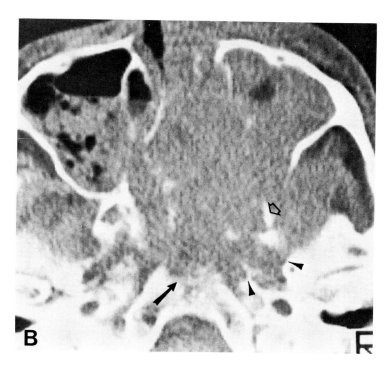

Figure 11, continued.

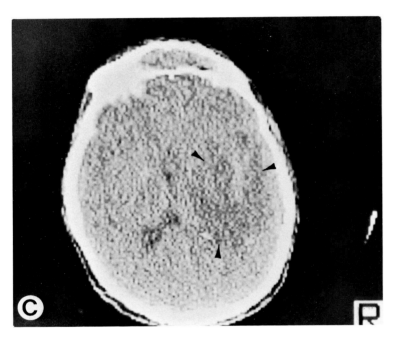

Figure 11, continued.

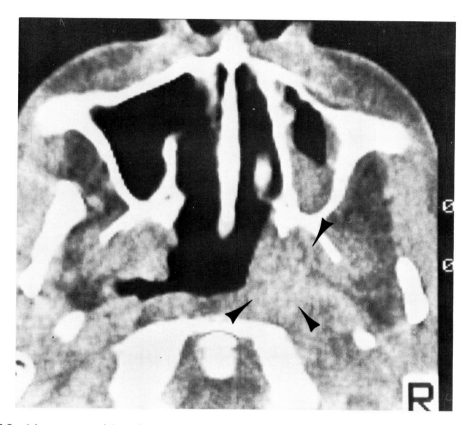

Figure 12. Numerous biopsies in this patient failed to show evidence of tumor. On direct examination the mucosa appeared normal. Deep biopsy finally confirmed the submucosal mass (arrowheads) was nasopharyngeal carcinoma.

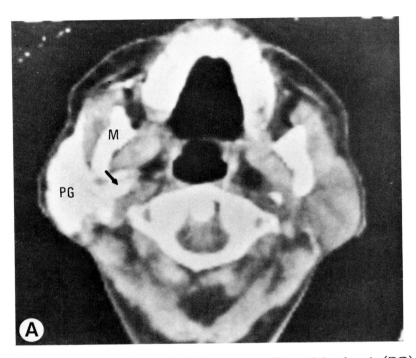

Figure 13. (A) Normal CT-assisted sialogram. Parotid gland (PG) stains with contrast; its deep lobe (arrow) wraps around the mandible (M). (B) Same patient as in (A). Clinical examination now revealed a "parotid mass". CT shows parapharyngeal mass (arrows) displacing the parotid which was intrinsically normal. Mass was later proved to be an oropharyngeal carcinoma with nodal metastases. (C) A different patient with an intrinsic, irregular parotid lesion (arrowheads), together with enlarged nodes suggesting malignancy. Mucoepidermoid carcinoma with enlarged "reactive" nodes were found at surgery.

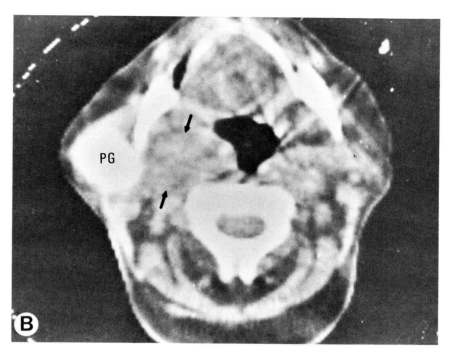

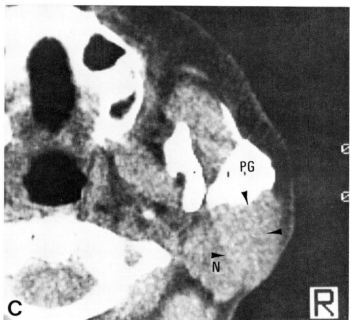

Figure 13, continued.

diagnosis of lymph node metastases in each of these regions has pitfalls, it still provides useful data that can prove pivotal in patient management. The need for lymphoangiography may be correspondingly reduced.

Before CT, physical examination was the only widely applied diagnostic method for evaluating cervical nodes. McGavran et al[17] reported that 11 of 68 patients (16%) with carcinoma of the larynx undergoing elective radical neck dissection had <u>clinically inapparent</u> nodal metastases, and that patients with supraglottic and transglottic tumors were at high risk for clinically "occult" contralateral metastases. Nasopharyngeal primaries metastasize first to high posterior cervical nodes, which are difficult to palpate when small. We reported in 1978 that CT was capable of detecting clinically inapparent nodal metastases.[18] Miller and Norman also reported a case of cervical metastatic disease from a pharyngeal primary in an article describing the general value of CT in detecting neck lesions.[19] We subsequently reported a prospective (10 cases) and retrospective (52 cases) study which showed that CT is helpful in assessing a variety of clinically significant factors which relate to the question of cervical metastases[20], including:

1) CT's ability to detect nodal metastases that are between 2.0 and 2.5 cm and are still clinically inapparent because they lie deep to the sternocleidomastoid muscle and are not palpable, particularly in stocky individuals.

2) CT findings usually correlate well with the clinical impression of normal-sized nodes when they are palpable clinically, although microscopic tumor may still be present in such nodes.

3) CT may give an indication of extranodal (extracapsular) extension of tumor and carotid fixation.

4) In midline primaries in the head and neck (soft palate, posterior tongue, nasopharynx), CT can predict bilateral nodal disease with the same accuracy as unilateral metastases.

CT has the same limitations in diagnosing cervical lymph node cancer as it has in other regions of the body: the study is anatomic, not histologic. Conceivably, nuclear magnetic resonance imaging may have more to offer eventually in terms of tissue specificity. At present, we use the following CT criteria for predicting the likelihood of lymph node metastases in the neck:

1) A solitary nonenhancing or rim-enhancing mass greater than 1.5 cm in diameter in the nodebearing regions (Figure 1).

2) More than three nodes 6-15 mm in size which cannot be separated from one another, which appear as a lobulated mass or have indistinct margins.

3) Obliteration of the normal fat-fascial planes around the carotid sheath in a non-operated, nonradiated neck (or one in which a change can be seen following a normal "baseline" post-therapy scan) (Figure 14).

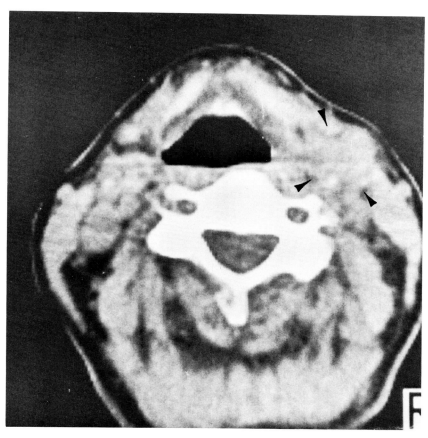

Figure 14.   Middle-aged female with a primary supraglottic lesion. Palpable nodal mass obliterates planes around carotid sheath on one side (arrowheads); palpable contralateral metastases are also visualized.

4) A nodal mass of any size with a low-density center.

Signs of extranodal tumor extension and/or carotid fixation (Figure 15) are:

1) Indistinct margins of a nodal mass (an equivocal sign by itself).

2) Obliteration of normal tissue planes, with diffuse or rim enhancement (best sign).

3) Absence of clear tissue planes between an otherwise discreet, well circumscribed nodal mass and the carotid artery (not too reliable).

As more soft tissue studies of the neck are done, these CT criteria will undoubtedly be revised. For now, they should serve as guidelines for evaluating node metastases. Finally, it is important to be aware of differences in the biologic behavior of head and neck tumors at different primary sites, in order to be certain that appropriate levels in the neck have been covered by scans in searching for regional node metastases: for instance, primaries in the nasopharynx metastasize early to posterior cervical nodes near the foramen magnum, whereas primaries within the oral cavity metastasize to submaxillary and jugulodigastric nodes, and oropharynx/hypopharynx and laryngeal primaries metastasize to mid-jugular as well as to jugulodigastric nodes.

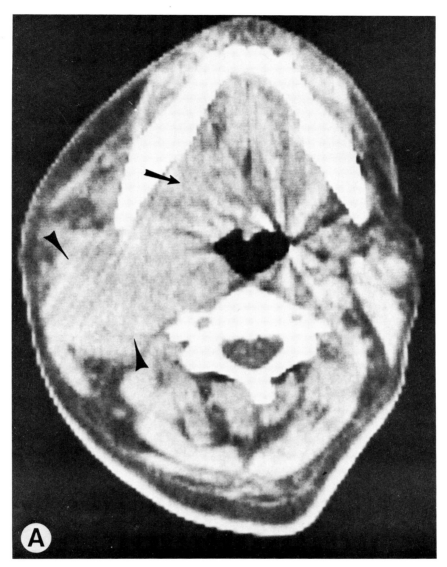

Figure 15. (A) Large nodal mass (arrowheads) surrounds carotid sheath, encroaches on the soft tissues of the floor of the mouth and tongue base (arrow), and obliterates the planes between the mas and the deep and superficial neck musculature. (B) A slightly lower section shows a central low density area (arrow) in the matted notal mass (arrowheads). Surgery confirmed a necrotic nodal mass with extranodal extension and carotid and brachial plexus fixation.

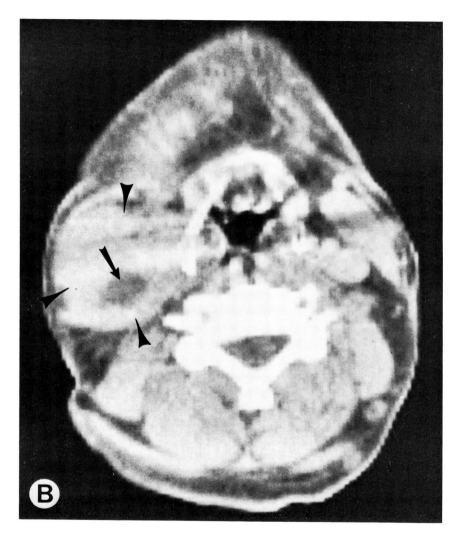

Figure 15, continued.

158

References

1. Carter, B.L., Karmody, C.S.: Computerized tomography of the face and neck. Semin Roentgenol 13:257-266, July, 1978.

2. Mancuso, A.A., Hanafee, W.N., Winter, J., et al: Extensions of paranasal sinus tumors and inflammatory disease as evaluated by CT and pleuridirectional tomography. Neuroradiology 16:449-453, 1978.

3. Som, P.M., Biller, H.G.: The combined CT-sialogram. Radiology 135:387-390, May, 1980.

4. Mancuso, A.A., Calcaterra, T.C., Hanafee, W.N.: Computed tomography of the larynx. Rad CINA 16:195-208, August, 1978.

5. Nicholson, R.L., Kreel, L.: CT anatomy of the nasopharynx, nasal cavity, paranasal sinuses and infratemporal fossa. CT 3:13-23, March, 1979.

6. Mancuso, A.A., Bohman, L.G., Hanafee, W.N., Maxwell, D.: Computed tomography of the nasopharynx-Normal and variants of normal. Radiology 137:113-121, October, 1980.

7. Bohman, L.G., Mancuso, A.A., Thompson, J., Hanafee, W.N.: CT approach to benign nasopharyngeal masses. AJR 136(1):173-180, January, 1981.

8. Gamsu, G., Webb, W.R., Shallit, J.B., Moss, A.A.: Computed tomo graphy in carcinoma of the larynx and pyriform sinus: The value of phonation CT. In press AJR, to appear March, 1981.

9. Mancuso, A.A., Tamakawa, Y., Hanafee, W.N.: CT of the fixed vocal cord. AJR 135:429-434, September, 1980.

10. Archer, C.R., Yearger, V.L., Friedman, W.H., et al: Computed tomography of the larynx. J CAT 2:404-411, September, 1978.

11. Mancuso, A.A., Hanafee, W.N.: A comparative evaluation of computed tomography and laryngography. Radiology 133:131-138, October, 1979.

12. Stone, D.N., Mancuso, A.A., Rice, D., Hanafee, W.N.: CT parotid sialography. In press (Radiology)

13. Ogura, J.H., Heeneman, H.: Conservation surgery of the larynx and hypopharynx: Selection of patients and results. Can J Otolaryngol 2:11-16, 1973.

14. McGavran, M.H., Bauer, W.C., Ogura, J.H.: The incidence of cervical lymph node metastases from epidermoid carcinoma of the larynx and their relationship to certain characteristics of the primary tumor. Cancer 14:55-56, January/February, 1961.

15. Miller, E.M., Norman, D.: The role of computed tomography in the evaluation of neck masses. Radiology 133:145-149, 1979.

16. Hanafee, W.N., Mancuso, A.A., Jenkins, H.A., Winter, J.:   Computer
    ized tomographic scanning of the temporal bone.   Annals of Otorino
    laryngology 88(5):721-727, September/October, 1979.

17. McGavran, M.H., Bauer, W.C., Ogura, J.H.:   The incidence of cervical
    lymph node metastases from epidermoid carcinoma of the larynx and
    their relationship to certain characteristics of the primary tumor.
    Cancer 14:55-56, January/February, 1961.

18. Mancuso, A.A., Hanafee, W.N., Ward, P.:   Correlated CT Anatomy and
    Pathology of the Larynx: Scientific Exhibit.   RSNA, Chicago, 1978.

19. Miller, E.M., Norman, D.:   The role of computed tomography in the
    evaluation of neck masses.   Radiology 133:145-149, October, 1979.

20. Mancuso, A.A., Maceri, D., Rice, D., Hanafee, W.N.:   CT of cervi   cal
    lymph node cancer.   In press AJR, to appear February, 1981.

Chapter 7

Early Diagnosis and Accurate Staging
of Abdominal Cancers

Frederick S. Keller, M.D.
Josef Rösch, M.D.

Early diagnosis and accurate staging of abdominal cancers is essential for optimal management. In the past several years substantial progress has been made in the radiological diagnosis of abdominal malignancies. The intorduction and technical improvement of newer imaging modalities such as ultrasound and computerized axial tomography (CT) has had a significant impact on the radiological work-up of patients with suspected malignant disease. Technical innovations and refinements in pre-existing radiologic modalities have also improved diagnostic accuracy. The introduction of the Chiba or "skinny needle" has made percutaneous transhepatic cholangiography a safer and more efficient procedure. Furthermore, percutaneous skinny needle aspiration of cytological material from suspicious mass lesions or lymph nodes has recently become a well accepted procedure (a description of percutaneous abdomino-pelvic biopsy techniques is presented in Chapter 10.) The introduction of iminodiacetic acid (IDA) derivatives promises to give radio-nuclide imaging a more important role in the diagnosis of biliary disease, since these compounds can be labelled with Tc^{99} and can provide crucial information regarding the patency of the biliary system (see Chapter 7). The use of superselective catheterization of vessels supplying a tumor during visceral angiography combined with direct magnification, and pharmacological studies with the injection of vasoactive drugs have also contributed to increased diagnostic accuracy.

Armed with all of these techniques, the radiologist in the 1980's is in a strong position to render early and accurate diagnoses in most patients with suspected malignant disease in the abdomen. When abdominal cancer is found, the radiologist should determine its size and extent. Radiologic evaluation should be performed expeditiously with the least number of tests, minimum expense, and without reduplication of already obtained information.

Hepatic Malignancies

The radiologic evaluation of hepatic tumors has been substantially improved in recent years. With the selection of appropriate radiologic modalities and careful evaluation of the findings it is possible to detect most hepatic masses, even in their early stages, and frequently to determine their nature. There is, of course, a significant difference between the detection of a liver mass and the diagnosis of that mass. Benign and often innocuous hepatic tumors may be detected by multiple radiologic modalities but unless they can be accurately diagnosed pre-operatively, patients may undergo a surgical procedure accompanied by substantial morbidity or even mortality. A suggest diagnostic algorithm for liver masses is given in Figure 1.

The non-invasive imaging modalities, including nuclear medicine, ultrasound, and occasionally CT scanning, are used mainly as screening procedures. While they are sensitive and can detect hepatic lesions, they

162

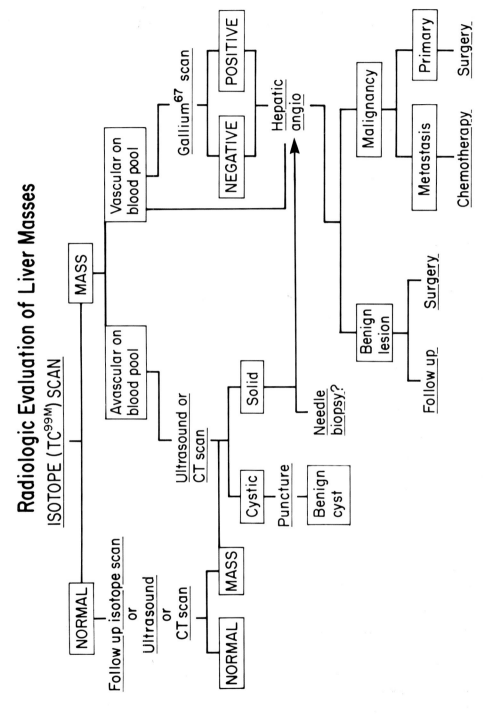

Fig. 1 Flow chart for radiologic work-up of hepatic masses.

163

often do not give detailed information about the nature of the lesions. Radionuclide scans give a good view of the entire liver, are inexpensive, are sensitive for lesions larger than two or three centimeters, and are easily reproducible. In our opinion, they are the preferred screening method and are also excellent for following patients with known metastatic disease (Chapter 8).

Ultrasound and CT scanning as screening methods, in addition to imaging the liver, may offer excellent information about adjacent organs and structures. The wide availability, low expense, and lack of ionizing radiation favor the initial use of ultrasound over CT. Both of these modalities may give information about the nature of a liver mass, particularly whether it is cystic (ultrasound) and whether it contains significant amounts of fat (CT).

Definitive diagnosis of liver masses, however, is usually achieved with angiography. Selective hepatic angiography in the form of a conventional bolus injection or - when necessary - an infusion study, can detect most vascular lesions, even small ones a centimeter or less in diameter. For avascular masses angiography is slightly less sensitive and is limited to somewhat larger lesions (2 cm or more in diameter). The pattern of vascular changes in the intrahepatic arteries and neovascularity within a lesion may occasionally enable the radiologist to make a specific tissue diagnosis. Furthermore, angiography is critical to assess the operability of liver tumors and to demonstrate the vascular anatomy when a hepatic resection is considered. In the latter instances, angiography is often complemented by portography, usually indirect (arterial pharmacoportography) but occasionally direct (transhepatic portography), as well as venographic studies of the inferior vena cava and hepatic veins.

Hepatocellular Carcinoma

Hepatocellular carcinoma is the most common primary liver tumor and its association with the more common forms of cirrhosis is well known.[1-3] Hemachromatosis and Clonorchis Sinensis (liver fluke) infestation are also associated with an increased incidence of hepatocellular carcinoma. Orientals have a predilection for hepatomas and acquire them at a relatively young age.[3]

The primary objectives of the diagnostic radiologist in hepatoma are its discovery, differentiation from other benign or malignant masses, and determination of resectability.

Radionuclide scanning with ^{99}Tc sulfur colloid is usually recommended as the initial step in patients suspected of having a hepatocellular carcinoma. An area of decreased radionuclide uptake invariably is present in a region containing gross tumor, while the surrounding liver is normal (Figure 2). If underlying cirrhosis is present (approximately 67% of all cases of hepatocellular carcinoma in the United States), however, a patchy or diffusely mottled uptake of isotope occurs throughout the liver, making it difficult and sometimes impossible to reach an accurate diagnosis.[1] [67]Gallium citrate may be helpful in these patients in arriving at a diagnosis of hepatoma, since approximately 80-90% of primary liver tumors have a marked affinity for

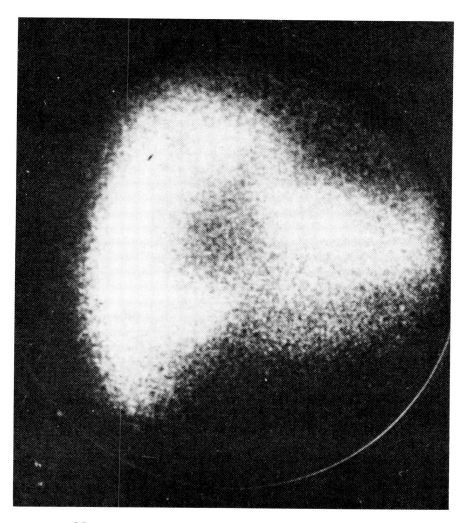

Fig. 2 Technetium^{99} sulfur colloid scan in a patient with hepatocellular carcinoma: A large focal area of decreased isotope uptake is noted in the center of the right liver lobe. A ^{67}gallium scan demonstrated increased radionuclide uptake in the same area.

gallium and a focal "hot" area is present on the gallium scans in the exact location of a "cold" area on the sulfur colloid scans. However, it must be remembered that although a positive [67]gallium scan is suggestive of hepatocellular carcinoma, other hepatic lesions such as abscesses, sarcoid granulomata, metastases, and lymphomas may also concentrate gallium and cause a false positive diagnosis of hepatoma.[1]

The appearance of hepatocellular carcinoma on ultrasound is quite variable and includes sonodense as well as sonolucent masses, diffusely abnormal parenchymal patterns, and even normal-appearing liver.[4] These sonographic patterns may also be seen in a variety of other hepatic lesions, both benign and malignant.

The CT scan pattern of hepatocellular carcinoma is usually a low density area within the liver. CT scanning has been proven to be quite sensitive in detecting hepatoma, and in one study of 47 patients with known hepatomas the CT scans were abnormal in 78%; the scans were equivocal in 11% and negative in the remaining 11%.[5] However, the changes detected by CT are also not specific for hepatoma and can be seen in benign tumors and in other primary and secondary liver malignancies.[5]

Angiography has been generally accepted as the most sensitive modality for the diagnosis of hepatocellular carcinoma.[3,5] Depending upon presentation either as a focal, multifocal, or diffuse tumor, the angiographic findings in hepatoma may vary. However, in all these types of hepatoma bizarre tumor neovascularity, consisting of irregular vascular networks and lakes, is present. The major vessels feeding the tumor often are enlarged, and there frequently is diversion of blood flow into tumor and away from areas of normal liver parenchyma. Shunting of hepatic arterial blood directly into the portal venous system is also seen frequently in association with hepatocellular carcinoma (Figure 4). Sheafs of arterial tumor vessels within the lumens of hepatic veins and sometimes extending into the inferior vena cava (the "thread and streak sign") are highly specific for hepatoma and delineate intravascular extensions.[3] Angiography can also determine with high accuracy the peripheral extent of the tumor and its resectability.[3]

Rarely, hepatocellular carcinoma invades the major bile ducts causing obstructive jaundice.[6] In these instances direct cholangiography will demonstrate a smooth or lobulated filling defect within the bile duct(s) and help to exclude other causes of obstructive jaundice which are occasionally associated with hepatomas such as metastatic nodes in the porta hepatis or blood clots from tumor-induced hemobilia.

Angiosarcoma is a rare tumor, accounting for less than 2% of primary liver malignancies.[7,8] Although its cause remains obscure, increased frequency of this tumor has been noted in association with exposure to thorium dioxide, vinyl chloride, and arsenic.[7,8] While typical sonographic or CT appearances have not yet been described, angiographically amputation and encasement of large hepatic arterial branches is present. The parenchymal phase of the arteriogram often demonstrates extensive avascular regions (necrotic areas?) interspersed with hypervascular regions consisting of irregular vascular lakes.[7]

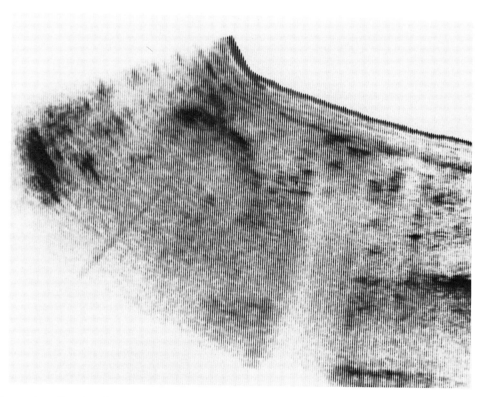

Fig. 3 Longitudinal abdominal ultrasound scan in a patient with hepatocellular carcinoma: An echodense mass (mark) is present in the right liver lobe. This sonographic appearance indicates a solid mass but is not specific for any particular type of lesion. (Sonogram courtesy of S.C. Henderson, M.D.)

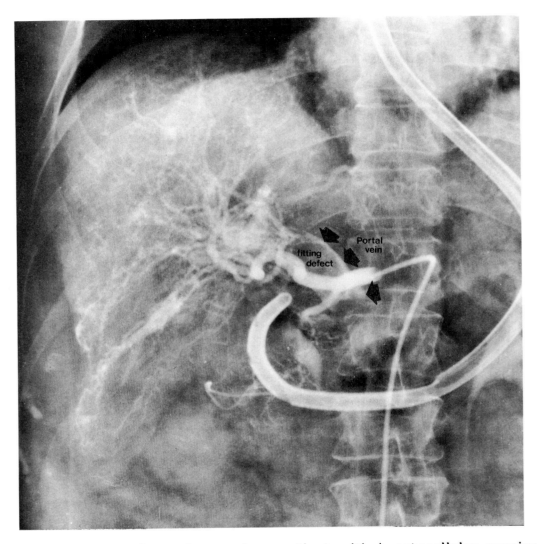

Fig. 4 Selective hepatic angiogram in a patient with hepatocellular carcinoma:
There is marked hypervascularity with disorganized vessels in the liver
hilus. Arterial-portal shunting is present with early abnormal filling of
the portal vein (mark). A lucent filling defect is present in the portal
vein.

Hepatic Metastases

Detection of hepatic metastases may be of utmost importance in the management of patients with known abdominal malignancies. As with primary tumors, hepatic radionuclide scintigraphy is the preferred screening method and is also excellent for following patients with known metastatic disease. If a discrepancy exists between the clinical findings and the ^{99}Tc sulfur colloid scan, further evaluation with either hepatic sonography or CT scanning is indicated (Figure 5).[9-13]

With the advent of accurate non-invasive imaging modalities, the screening role of angiography has diminished substantially. However, angiography is still indicated if the results of the noninvasive tests are conflicting (Figure 6), and angiography is critical if a partial hepatic resection is contemplated.[14] In a series from one large cancer institute, numerous patients considered for hepatic resection of a presumed solitary liver metastasis (as judged by a combination of ultrasound, nuclear medicine, and CT scans) were found by angiography to have, in addition to the known metastatic lesion, several smaller metastases elsewhere in the liver.[14] Angiography with subsequent selective hepatic artery infusion of chemotherapeutic agents and/or tumor embolization may also play an important role in the therapy of metastatic disease (see Chapter 14).

PANCREATIC, BILIARY, AND AMPULLARY CANCER

Obstructive jaundice is usually the major presenting sign in patients with biliary and ampullary tumors, and also with cancer of the head of the pancreas. Numerous radiologic modalities, invasive as well as noninvasive, are currently available for imaging the biliary system and the pancreas in these situations. Radiologic differentiation of obstructive from non-obstructive jaundice is usually not required because an experienced clinician can make the distinction approximately 85% of the time on the basis of a careful history, physical examination, and an analysis of the laboratory data. However, when the radiologist is consulted to differentiate obstructive from non-obstructive jaundice adequate tools are now available to confirm the diagnosis.

Radioisotope scanning with ^{99}Tc-IDA (iminodiacetic acid) compounds often will diagnose obstructive jaundice; however, because of poor excretion of the compound, the number of non-diagnostic examinations is high when serum bilirubin levels are above 7-8 mg/100 ml[15-17] (see also, Chapter 7.) Sonographic as well as CT evaluation of the biliary tree rely primarily on the recognition of ductal dilatation. Both modalities are quite sensitive in detecting dilated intrahepatic and extrahepatic ducts, and often the level of the obstruction can be determined.[18-26]

Usually, however, for complete and detailed evaluation of the biliary system prior to surgical therapy some form of direct cholangiography such as endoscopic retrograde cholangiopancreatography (ERCP), percutaneous transhepatic cholangiography (PTC) with the "skinny needle", or occasionally transjugular cholangiography is required.

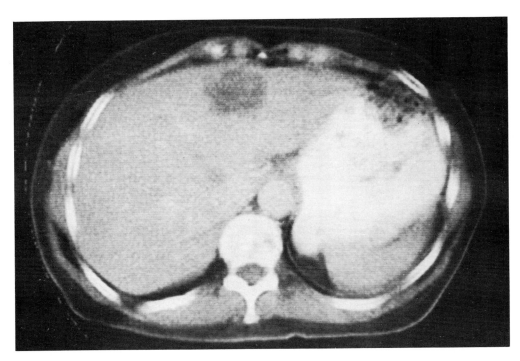

Fig. 5 CT scan of the liver in a patient with previous colon resection for adenocarcinoma: An area of decreased tissue attenuation (mark) in the anterior part of the medial segment of the left liver lobe represents a metastasis. Two smaller metastases are also visible in this section. (CT scan courtesy of R. VanKolken, M.D.)

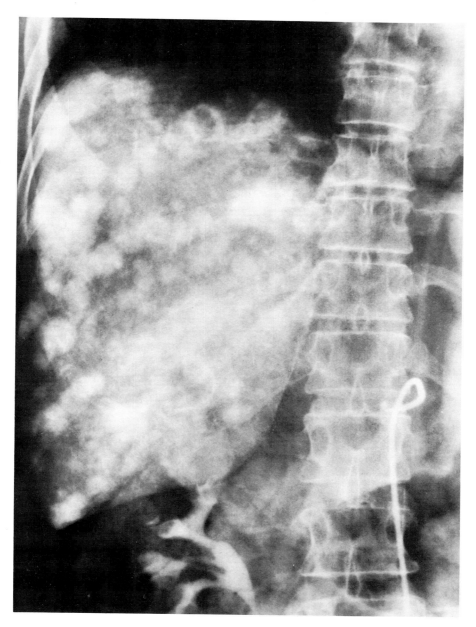

Fig. 6 Selective hepatic angiogram (parenchymal phase) in a 63 year old woman following right mastectomy for adenocarcinoma: Multiple hypervascular metastases are noted. A radionuclide scan had revealed diffuse mottling and was not diagnostic of metastases.

Endoscopic retrograde cholangiopancreatography (ERCP) was first performed in Japan in the late 1960's.[27]   The technique was introduced into the
United States several years later, and soon achieved fairly wide acceptance.
In this examination the gastroenterologist and radiologist combine their efforts
to visualize the biliary and pancreatic ducts.   A special side-viewing endoscope
is used to cannulate the papilla of Vater.   Ideally, both the common bile duct
and the pancreatic duct are injected with contrast material and when they are
opacified, radiographs are obtained.   ERCP is quite accurate in diagnosing
cancers of the biliary system and pancreas (see below); however, its successful
performance requires an experienced and highly-skilled endoscopist.

The Chiba or "skinny needle" was introduced by Okuda in 1974 and has
revolutionized percutaneous transhepatic cholangiography (PTC), making it a
simpler, more efficient, and safer procedure.[28]   Conventional cholangiography
prior to the introduction of the Chiba needle was performed with a large
gauge stylet covered by an outer teflon sheath.   The examination had to be
done immediately before surgery because a high incidence of bile leak or
hemoperitoneum occurred as a result of the procedure.   Skinny needle PTC is
done with a 22 or 23 gauge flexible stainless steel needle, does not require
immediate surgical intervention, and has many fewer complications.
Furthermore, success in demonstrating an obstructed biliary system ranges from
92-100%, even in relatively inexperienced hands.[29,30]

Since the introduction of the Chiba needle, transvenous (transjugular)
cholangiography has been used infrequently.   In this examination an
angiographic catheter is introduced percutaneously into the internal jugular
vein and is advanced through the right atrium retrogradely into a hepatic
vein.   A special needle is then introduced through the catheter, and entrance
into the biliary system is accomplished by puncture of the liver parenchyma
between the catheterized hepatic vein and a dilated intrahepatic bile duct.[31]
Since transcutaneous puncture of the peritoneum and liver capsule are avoided
with this "internal" biliary opacification technique, it is potentially useful for
those patients with a coagulopathy or ascites in whom PTC is contraindicated
and ERCP has been unsuccessful.   The disadvantages of this technique include
its relative complexity, and the necessity for considerable angiographic
experience to perform it successfully and without complication.

Which of the above imaging methods should be used first in suspected
obstructive jaundice?   In our opinion, the method of choice in individual
institutions depends upon which modalities are performed with expertise and
what specific information is required pre-operatively by the surgeon.   Few
surgeons feel comfortable operating with only a diagnosis of "obstructive
jaundice," and the majority now demand to know the exact level of obstruction
and the condition of the biliary system proximal to it in order to plan an
effective strategy for surgical decompression.   Often ERCP and PTC are used
in the same patient as complementary examinations: ERCP will demonstrate
the biliary system distal to a complete obstruction, and PTC will show the
proximal biliary tree.   Furthermore, if one method is unsuccessful the other
frequently can still be employed to obtain essential information about the
biliary system pre-operatively.

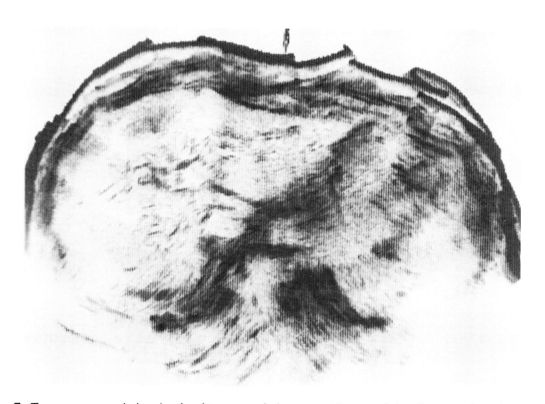

Fig. 7 Transverse abdominal ultrasound in a patient with obstructive jaundice: Dilated intrahepatic bile ducts are present and appear as multiple sonolucenices bordered by parallel strips of dense echos. The dilated ducts are arranged in a stellate distribution (sonogram courtesy of S.C. Henderson, M.D.).

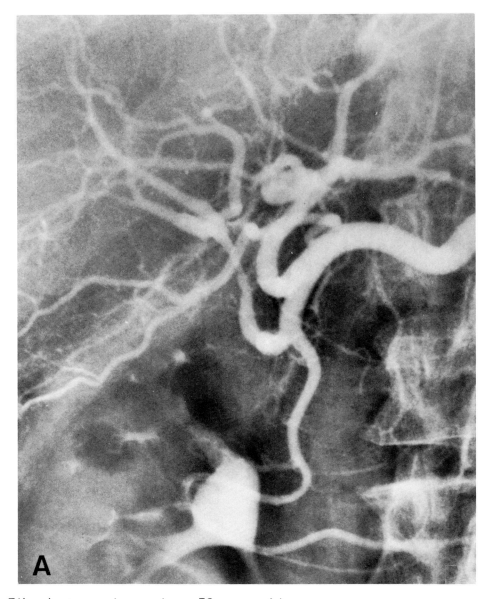

Fig. 8 Bile duct carcinoma in a 38 year old woman:

A.   Selective hepatic angiogram reveals tumor encasement of the proximal right hepatic artery.   The portal vein (seen on the venous phase of a superior mesenteric angiogram) was also encased, indicating nonresectability.

B.   Transhepatic cholangiogram demonstrates irregular narrowing of the common hepatic duct extending from the confluence of the left and right hepatic ducts down to the common bile duct.   The pancreatic duct is filled minimally.

174

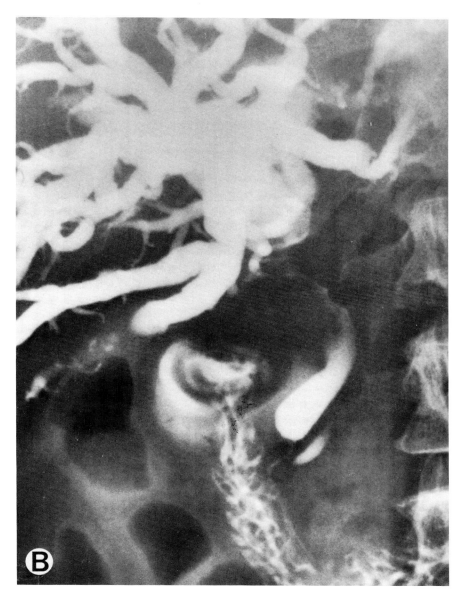

Figure 8, continued

Primary bile duct carcinoma is not uncommon, and anatomically it usually presents as a small, localized nodular or annular tumor. Occasionally, however, these neoplasms may occur as lumenal, polypoid or papillary masses.[32] The anatomic locale most frequently involved is the common hepatic duct including the confluence of the left and right hepatic ducts (Figure 8). The second most frequent site of involvement is the common bile duct.[32] Since these carcinomas may be located high in the porta hepatis, exploratory laparotomy for obstructive jaundice without an adequate pre-operative cholangiogram may easily result in the tumor being missed at surgery. The cholangiographic findings are often fairly specific for biliary carcinoma; however, some pitfalls do exist. Infiltrating-type mural tumors which spread along the bile ducts may have an appearance form of bile duct carcinoma is not frequent. Similarly, a polypoid intraluminal tumor may rarely be mistaken for an obstructing gallstone. An algorithm for the diagnosis of biliary malignancies is given in Figure 9.

The radiologic diagnosis of carcinoma of the pancreas has improved substantially in recent years. Until the late 1960's the conventional upper GI series was the basic screening procedure.[33] Its accuracy was low, and since the criterion for a positive study was displacement of the gastric antrum or the duodenum by a mass, usually only far-advanced and unresectable cancers could be detected. In the mid-1960's hypotonic duodenography was introduced.[34] This study is performed after pharmacologic relaxation of the duodenum with either glucagon or an anticholinergic drug. The duodenum is then outlined with barium and air, and its medial wall is carefully examined for nodular irregularity or a double contour often seen with pancreatic carcinoma (Figure 10). Sometimes the medial wall of the duodenum is fixed and retracted because of the scirrhous character of a pancreatic carcinoma, causing irregular spiculation.

With the introduction of ultrasound and CT scanning, the upper GI series and hypotonic duodenography are rarely used now as screening tests for pancreatic malignancy. The latter studies can sometimes be helpful, nevertheless, for assisting in differential diagnosis and for assessing gastric and duodenal lesions. Both ultrasound and CT scanning are capable of producing good anatomic images of the pancreas (Figure 11). Since they are noninvasive, are not stressful for the patient, and can usually visualize the pancreas accurately, they have now become the primary screening procedures for detection of pancreatic carcinoma. However, for an intrapancreatic mass to be detected by these modalities it must be large enough (3-4 cm in diameter) to deform the contour of the pancreas (Figure 13). The specificity of these two modalities is also low, and it is frequently impossible to distinguish between inflammatory and neoplastic pancreatic masses by ultrasound or CT scanning. Some secondary signs such as pseudocyst formation or pancreatic calcifications in inflammatory disease, or the presence of liver metastases in patients with pancreatic carcinoma, may help to make this crucial differentiation. Recently, guided fine needle biopsies of suspicious pancreatic masses which have been discovered and localized by ultrasound and/or CT, have been extremely valuable in determining their nature. It must be remembered, however, that a negative percutaneous biopsy cannot exclude the presence of pancreatic carcinoma.

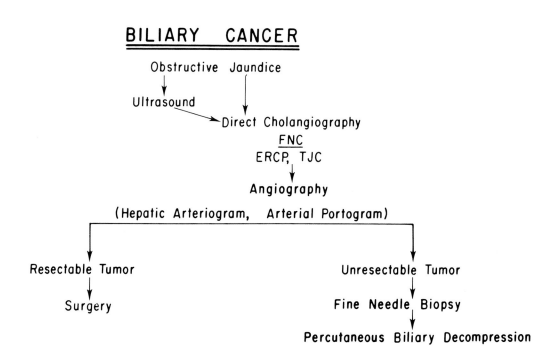

Fig. 9 Flow chart for the radiologic work-up of biliary cancer.

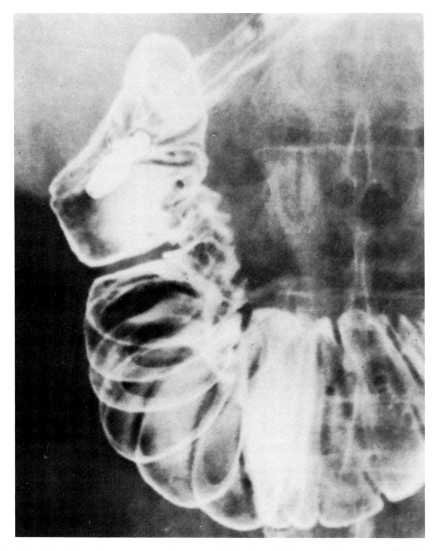

Fig. 10 Hypotonic duodenogram in a patient with carcinoma of the pancreatic
head: There is a double contour spiculation and nodular irregularity
along the medial aspect of the descending portion of the duodenum
caused by neoplastic compression and invasion.

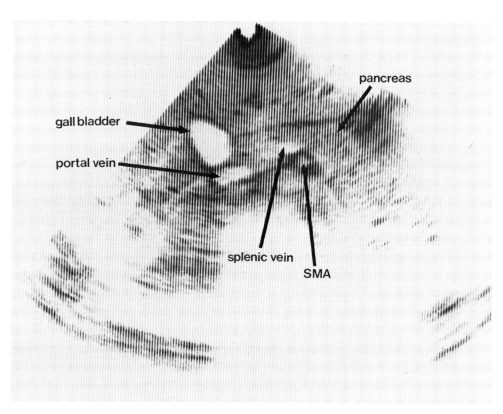

Fig. 11 Transverse abdominal sonogram demonstrating a normal appearing
       pancreas: The normal-sized pancreas is anterior to the splenic vein
       and superior mesenteric artery. The gall bladder also has a normal
       appearance (sonogram courtesy of S.C. Henderson, M.D.).

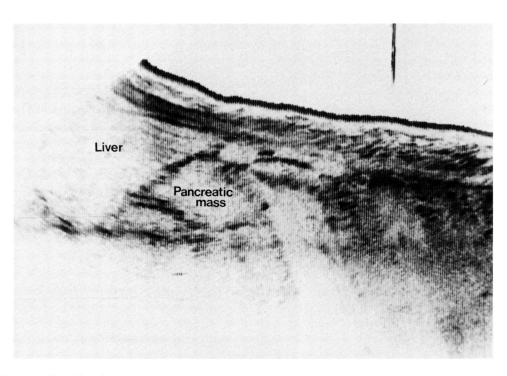

Fig. 12 Longitudinal ultrasound scan in a patient with jaundice: A prominent mass (mark) is seen in the pancreatic head (sonogram courtesy of S.C. Henderson, M.D.).

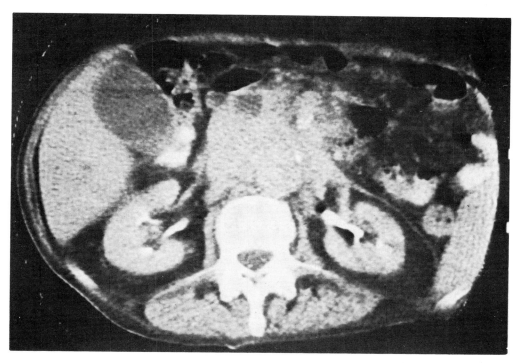

Fig. 13 CT scan of a patient with painless jaundice and a prominent epi-
gastric mass: A large mass (mark) is present involving the pancreatic
head and body. The dilated common bile duct within the pancreas
and the gallbladder are seen as low density areas. (CT scan courtesy
of R. VanKolken, M.D.)

Carcinoma of the head of the pancreas typically encases the intra-pancreatic portion of the common bile duct, resulting in irregular narrowing or complete obstruction which can readily be demonstrated by some form of direct cholangiography. Pancreatic cancers which are located close to the common bile duct, and ampullary carcinomas causing biliary obstruction (with resultant jaundice) early in their course, can sometimes be detected while still small and potentially resectable. Usually, dilated biliary ducts can be demonstrated by ultrasound or CT scans, even if the obstructing tumor is too small to be visualized. In these instances, some form of direct cholangiography (PTC or ERCP), with or without angiography, can accurately localize the site of obstruction and can frequently determine its nature (Figure 14). For lesions of the ampulla and pancreatic head, ERCP has the added advantages of direct endoscopic visualization of the papilla and the opportunity to evaluate an opacified pancreatic duct.

The ERCP findings of pancreatic carcinoma are quite specific; furthermore, it is usually possible to distinguish between pancreatic, inflammatory, and neoplastic disease using this modality.[35-39] Since almost all pancreatic cancers originate frm the pancreatic ducts, ERCP has the potential to detect tumors when they are still small and possibly resectable. Irregular obstruction of the pancreatic duct is the most common finding when ERCP is performed in patients with pancreatic carcinoma (Figure 15). If the tumor is located in the pancreatic head, the common bile duct is usually involved also, with either encasement or occlusion, giving the "double-duct sign."[38]

In addition to ERCP, properly performed superselective pancreatic cholangiography is capable of detecting small and potentially resectable pancreatric cancers with a high degree of accuracy. Nevertheless, review of the current literature on angiography in the diagnosis of pancreatic malignancies reveals considerable controversy, with reported diagnostic accuracies in the range of 40% to 95%.[40-47] These conflicting reports have resulted from the different angiographic techniques used in these studies and, in particular, from the different degrees of success in visualizing the intrapancreatic arteries -- the prime requisite for an accurate diagnosis of pancreatic lesions. Put in another way, the degree of visualization of small intrapancreatic arteries is an indication of the adequacy of the angiogram and will correlate highly with its accuracy in diagnosing pancreatic cancer and other diseases of the pancreas.

Catheterizations of the celiac and superior mesenteric arteries are the basic techniques underlying the performance of pancreatic angiograms. Injections into these two arteries will opacify the larger arterial branches surrounding the pancreas and will permit diagnosis of large (advanced) lesions that have extended to the borders of, or outside the pancreas (Figure 16). Rarely, selective angiograms of the celiac and superior mesenteric arteries will also fill the small intrapancreatic branches and make possible the diagnosis of smaller cancers. When celiac and superior mesenteric arteriograms are the only studies performed, overall diagnostic accuracy is in the range of 60%. However, the use of superselective catheterization with injection into second and third order branches such as the hepatic, splenic, gastroduodenal, dorsal pancreatic, and pancreaticoduodenal arteries increases the diagnostic accuracy

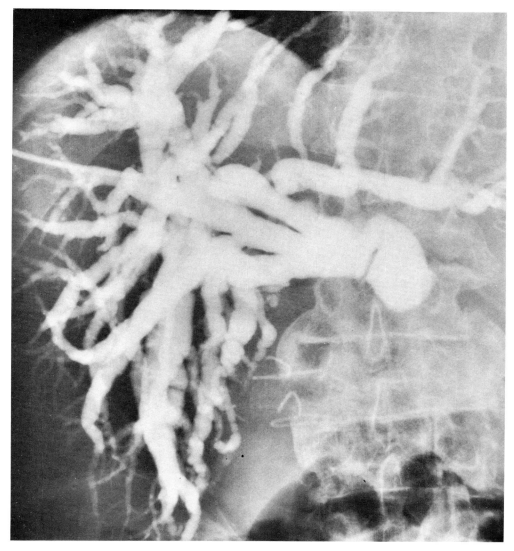

Fig. 14 Percutaneous transhepatic cholangiogram in a patient with pancreatic carcinoma: The intrahepatic ducts are markedly dilated. There is abrupt occlusion of the dilated common bile duct where it enters the pancreas.

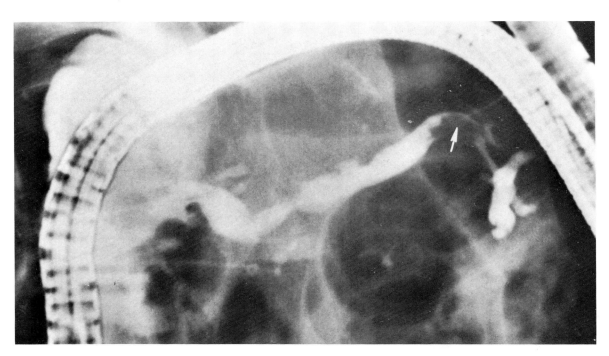

Fig. 15 ERCP in a patient with carcinoma of the pancreas: An irregularly
        narrowed segment (arrow) is seen in the pancreatic duct near the
        junction of the body and tail of the pancreas.   This finding is highly
        specific for pancreatic carcinoma.

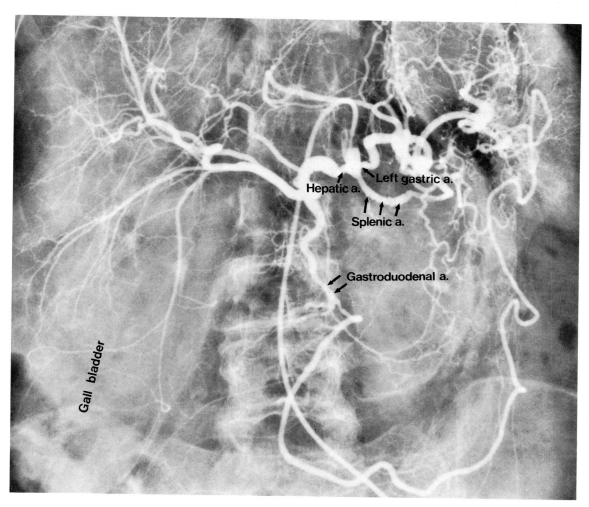

Fig. 16 Celiac angiogram in a patient with a large, unresectable pancreatic cancer: There is tumor encasement of the splenic, left gastic, hepatic and gastroduodenal arteries (arrows). The gallbladder is greatly distended as the result of occlusion of the common bile duct by tumor.

of pancreatic angiography to more than 90%, leading to the detection of small (1-2 cm) pancreatic carcinomas when they are still localized within the pancreas and potentially resectable (Figure 17A, B).[48-50]

In patients with pancreatic carcinoma, angiography is also extremely useful in determining the local extent of tumor, the involvement of adjacent organs, the presence or absence of liver metastases, and resectability. Patients with involvement confined to the intrapancreatic arteries usually have resectable tumors. When major peripancreatic arteries such as the splenic, hepatic or gastroduodenal, or the superior mesenteric, splenic, or portal veins are involved the tumor is unresectable.

For those patients with a resectable tumor, pancreatic angiography can demonstrate vascular anomalies in the upper abdomen which may complicate surgical removal, thus giving the surgeon additional knowledge on which to base his operative approach. Angiography is also useful and accurate for differentiating pancreatic carcinoma from other (non-neoplastic) pancreatic lesions, particularly chronic pancreatitis.

Typically scirrhous in nature, pancreatic carcinoma incites considerable desmoplastic reaction which accounts for the characteristic angiographic findings of arterial and venous encasement or occlusion. The encased arteries often have a serpiginous or serrated ("saw-tooth") appearance. In the late phases of the angiogram, venous occlusion is frequently evidenced by opacification of prominent collateral veins.[48,50] A diagnostic decision tree for the radiological work-up of a patient with suspected pancreatic carcinoma is given in Figure 18.

In addition to pancreatic adenocarcinomas, islet cell carcinomas and cystadenocarcinomas are other forms of pancreatic malignancy. However, they are rare and each has a fairly distinctive angiographic appearance. Islet cell carcinomas exhibit abundant tumor vessels and are hypervascular with a circumscribed tumor blush. Cystadenocarcinomas are also hypervascular, but exhibit multiple lucent areas on the parenchymal phase of the angiogram which represent the cystic components of these tumors.

Renal Carcinoma

The radiologic diagnosis of renal masses has also undergone considerable change in the past decade. In the 1950's and 1960's, renal masses were often surgically explored to determine whether they were cysts or tumors. Since a large number of elderly patients have asymptomatic, simple renal cysts that are serendipitously discovered on excretory urography for other conditions, many otherwise unneeded operations were being performed on elderly, high-risk patients.

Using the radiologic modalities now available, including percutaneous cyst puncture, the crucial distinction between a renal cyst and renal cancer can be made in approximately 92% of patients.[51] Eight percent of patients with a renal space-occupying lesion still require an operation because of indeterminate results from their radiologic evaluation.[51]

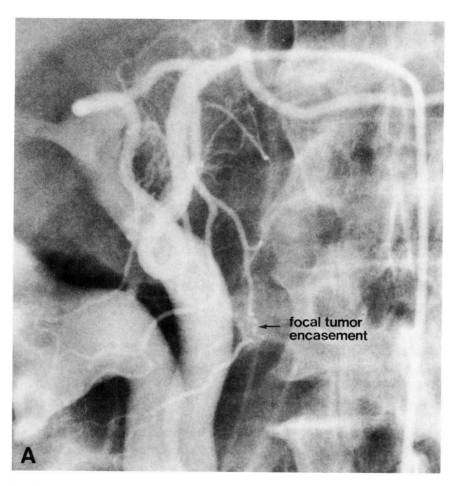

focal tumor
encasement

A

Fig. 17 A & B

Selective gastroduodenal (A) and inferior pancreaticoduodenal (B) angiograms in a patient with a small (1.0 cm x 1.5 cm) cancer in the pancreatic head. The patient presented with obstructive jaundice, and ultrasound and CT scans demonstrated dilated bile ducts but no obstructing lesion. The lesion was successfully resected. The angiograms revealed highly localized tumor encasement (arrows in the pancreatic head. The normal pancreatic body is well outlined on the inferior pancreaticoduodenal angiogram.

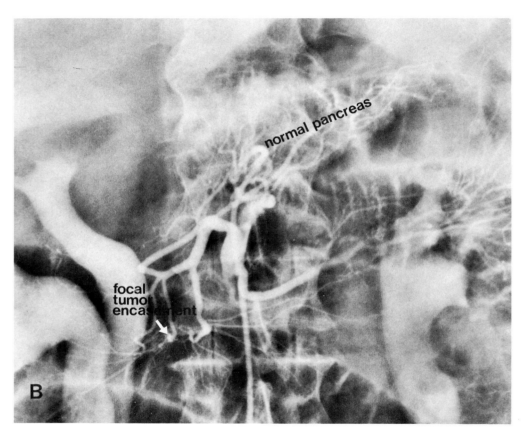

Figure 17, continued

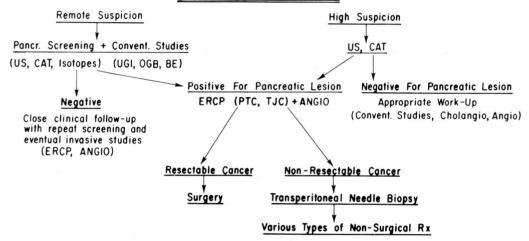

Fig.18 Flow sheet for the radiologic work-up of pancreatic carcinoma.

A suggested approach to the patient with a renal mass is illustrated in Figure 19. Excretory urography with nephrotomography is the primary screening method for evaluation of the urinary tract. In pregnant patients or in those with renal failure or an earlier documented allergic reaction to contrast material, renal ultrasonography will provide a good morphologic impression of the kidneys. If a space-occupying lesion is discovered (during an excretory urogram) which is lucent during the nephrogram phase compared to the remainder of the kidney, has thin walls, and is sharply defined from the remainder of the renal parenchyma, it is most likely a cyst. The patient will then ordinarily undergo ultrasonography, and if the lesion fulfills all the criteria for a simple cyst, cyst puncture with aspiration and analysis of the fluid for malignant cells is performed (Figure 20). If the aspirated fluid is clear and without malignant cells, the work-up is terminated. Recently, some radiologists have advocated replacing cyst puncture with a CT scan.[52] In their opinion, if the renal mass has all the CT characteristics of a simple cyst, no more diagnostic procedures need be done.

On the other hand any mass that "blushes" during the nephrotogram is likely to be solid, and the patient should therefore undergo renal angiography for further study (Figure 21). In addition, masses that appear to be cystic on the nephrotomograms but do not fulfill the criteria of a simple cyst by ultrasound or CT scanning should also be evaluated with angiography (Figure 22). Selective renal angiography with the addition of magnification and pharmacologic techniques is highly accurate in diagnosing renal masses, even very small intrarenal tumors. Furthermore, with this modality it is frequently possible to differentiate benign kidney tumors such as oncocytomas, adenomas, and angiomyolipomas from malignant lesions (angiomyolipomas containing foci of fat can be diagnosed definitively by CT scanning because of the low attenuation which is typical of fat tissue). When the angiographic findings indicate the possibility of a benign tumor, the surgeon can plan on a possible heminephrectomy or wedge resection, depending upon the results of a frozen section biopsy (Figure 23). Conversely, if the angiographic findings are those of a renal cell carcinoma (Figure 24), a radical nephrectomy can be planned. In large, inoperable renal carcinomas, therapeutic embolization of the primary tumor has sometimes been useful for palliation and has been reported to promote regression of pulmonary metastases[53] (see also, Chapter 14).

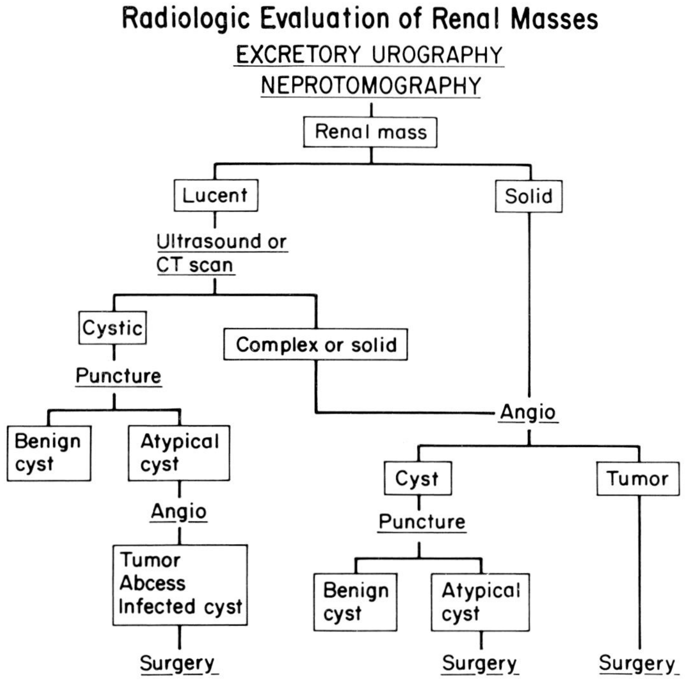

Radiologic Evaluation of Renal Masses

EXCRETORY UROGRAPHY
NEPROTOMOGRAPHY

Fig. 19 Flow sheet for radiologic work-up of renal masses.

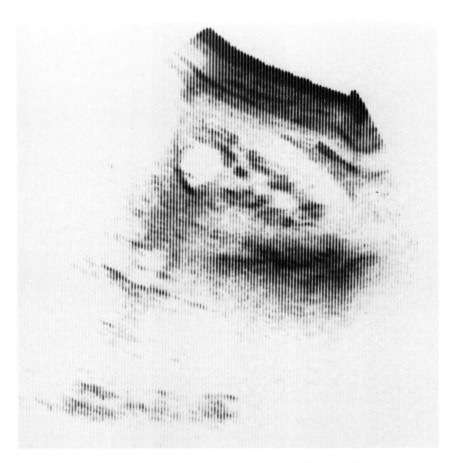

Fig. 20 Ultrasound scan of a simple renal cyst: A sonolucent space-occupying lesion with dense echoes ("through transmission") along its posterior border is noted in the superior portion of the left kidney. This is the charateristic ultrasonic appearance of a simple renal cyst (sonogram courtesy of S.C. Henderson, M.D.).

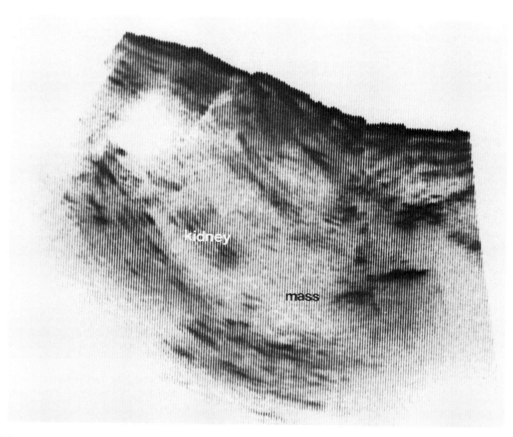

Fig. 21 Sagittal ultrasound scan in a patient with renal carcinoma: A
        prominent solid mass extends from the inferior aspect of the left
        kidney (sonogram courtesy of S.C. Henderson, M.D.)

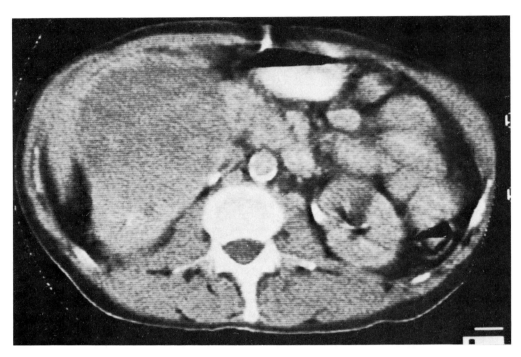

Fig. 22 CT scan of a complicated renal cyst: A large thick-walled mass arises from the anterior portion of the right kidney. Inside the mass are areas that have enhanced after administration of intravenous contrast material. A hemorrhagic cyst was found at surgery. The CT appearance of this complicated cyst is the same as that seen in many renal carcinomas (CT scan courtesy of R. VanKolken, M.D.).

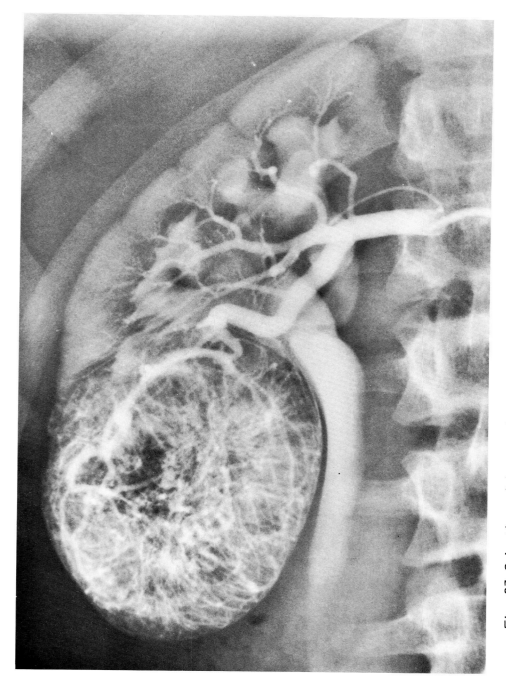

Fig. 23 Selective right renal angiogram in a 35 year old male with a renal mass: A vascular mass is seen in the lower pole of the right kidney. Typical tumor vessels or encasement are not present, but the vessels are arranged in an orderly, spoke-wheel fashion. The angiographic diagnosis was "possible oncocytoma," and a hemi-nephrectomy was done after frozen sections at surgery confirmed this diagnosis.

195

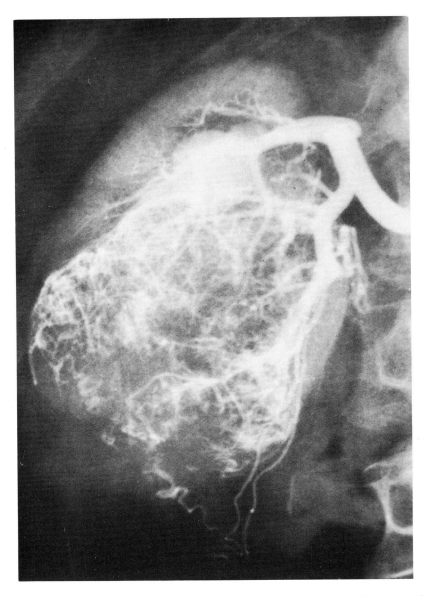

Fig. 24 Selective right renal angiogram in a patient with renal carcinoma:
Bizarre irregular vessels with puddling of contrast material and
displacement of major arterial branches are present throughout most of
the kidney. A thin rim of normal parenchyma is noted on the superior
lateral aspect. Contrast with Figure 23.

REFERENCES

1. Alpert, E., Ferrucci, C., Athanasoulis, R., et al.: Primary hepatic tumor. Gastroenterology 74:759-769, 1978.

2. Scully, R.E., Galdabini, J.J., McNeely, B.U.: Case records of the Massachusetts General Hospital. New Engl J Med 300:484-489, 1979.

3. Marks, W.M., Jacobs, R.P., Goodman, P.C., et al.: Hepatocellular carcinoma: Clinical and angiographic findings and predictability for surgical resection. AJR 132:7-11, 1979.

4. Kamin, P.D., Bernardino, M.E., Breen, B.: Ultrasound manifestations of hepatocellular carcinoma. Radiology 131:459-461, 1979.

5. Itai, Y., Nishikawa, J., Tasaka, A.: Computed tomography in the evaluation of hepatocellular carcinoma. Radiology 131:165-170, 1979.

6. Van Sonnenberg, E., Ferrucci, J.T.: Bile duct obstruction in hepatocellular carcinoma (hepatoma) - clinical and cholangiographic characteristics. Radiology 130:7-13, 1979.

7. Velaquez, G., Katkov, H., Formanek, A.: Primary liver tumors in the pediatric age group; an angiographic challenge. RoFo 130:408-417, 1979.

8. Scully, R.E., Galdabini, J.J., McNeely, B.U.: Case records of the Massachusetts General Hospital. New Engl J Med 300:1148-1154, 1979.

9. Petasnick, J.P., Ram, P., Turner, D.A., et al.: The relationship of computed tomography, gray-scale ultrasonography and radionuclide imaging in the evaluation of the hepatic masses. Semin Nucl Med 9:8-21, 1979.

10. Wooten, W.B., Green, B., Goldstein, H.M.: Ultrasonography of necrotic hepatic metastases. Semin Nucl Med 128:447-450, 1978.

11. Moss, A.A., Schrumpf, J., Schneyder, P., et al.: Computed tomography of focal hepatic lesions: A blind clinical evaluation of the effect of contrast enhancement. Radiology 131:427-430, 1979.

12. Vicary, F.R., Shirley, I.: Ultrasound and hepatic metastases. Br J Radiol 51:596-598, 1978.

13. Snow, J.H., Goldstein, H.M., Wallace, S.: Comparison of scintigraphy, sonography, and computed tomography in the evaluation of hepatic neoplasms. AJR 132:915-918, 1979.

14. Berk, R.N.: Progress in clinical radiology: Diagnostic imaging of the liver and bile ducts. Invest Radiol 13:265-278, 1978.

15. Weissman, H.S., Frank, M., Rosenblatt, R., et al.: Cholescintigraphy, ultrasonography and computerized tomography in the evaluation of biliary tract disorders. Semin Nucl Med 9:22-35, 1979.

16. Wistow, B.W., Subramanian, G., Gagne, G.M., et al.: Experimental and clinical trials of new ^{99m}Tc-labeled hepatobiliary agents. Radiology 128:793-794, 1978.

17. Rosenthall, L.: Clinical experience with the newer hepatobiliary radiopharmaceutics. Can J Surg 21:297-300, 1978.

18. Wheeler, P.G., Theodossi, A., Pickford, R., et al.: Non-invasive techniques in the diagnosis of jaundice - ultrasound and computer. Gut 20:196-199, 1979.

19. Vallon, A.G., Lees, W.R., Cotton, P.B.: Grey scale ultrasonography in cholestatic jaundice. Gut 20:51-54, 1979.

20. Weill, F., Marmier, A., Paronneau, P., et al.: Ultrasonography in jaundice: Signs and results in 199 cases (author's transl). J Radiol Electrol Med Nucl 59:659-668, 1978.

21. Taylor, K.J., Rosenfield, A.T., Spiro, H.M.: Diagnostic accuracy of gray scale ultrasonography for the jaundiced patient. A report of 275 cases. Arch Intern Med 139:60-63, 1979.

22. Cooperberg, P.L.: High-resolution real-time ultrasound in the evaluation of the normal and obstructed biliary tract. Radiology 129:477-480, 1978.

23. Morris, A., Fawcitt, R.A., Wood, R., et al.: Computed tomography, ultrasound, and cholestatic jaundice. Gut 19:685-688, 1978.

24. Goldberg, H.I., Filly, R.A., Korobkin, M., et al.: Capability of CT body scanning and ultrasonography to demonstrate the status of the biliary ductal system in patients with jaundice. Radiology 129:731-737, 1978.

25. Raskin, M.M.: Hepatobiliary disease: A comparative evaluation by ultrasound and computed tomography. Gastrointest Radiol 3:267-271, 1978.

26. Shanser, J.D., Korobkin, M., Goldberg, et al.: Computed tomographic diagnosis of obstructive jaundice in the absence of intrahepatic ductal dilatation. AJR 131:389-392, 1978.

27. Salmon, P.R.: Re-evaluation of endoscopic retrograde cholangiopancreatography as a diagnostic method. Clin Gastrointerol 7:651-666, 1978.

28. Okuda, K., Tanikawa, K., Emura, T., Juratomi, S., Jinnouchi, S., Urabe, K., Sumikoshi, T., Danda, Y., Fukuyama, Y., Musha, H., Mori, H., Shimokawa, Y., Yakushiji, F., and Matsuura, Y.: Nonsurgical percutaneous transhepatic cholangiography: Diagnostic significance in medical problems of the liver. Dig Dis 19:21-36, 1974.

29. Redeker, A., Karvountzis, G., Richman, R., and Horisawa, M.: Percutaneous transhepatic cholangiography. An improved technique. JAMA 231:386-387, 1975.

30. Ferrucci, J., Wittenberg, J., Sarno, R., and Dreyfuss, J.: Fine needle transhepatic cholangiography: A new approach to obstructive jaundice. AJR 127:403-407, 1976.

31. Rosch, J., Lakin, P.C., Antonovic, R., et al.: Transjugular approach to liver biopsy and transhepatic cholangiography. New Engl J Med 289:227-231, 1973.

32. Berk, R.N., Clemett, A.R.: Radiology of the Gallbladder and Bile Ducts. W.B. Saunders Co., Philadelphia, PA, 1977, pp. 316-318.

33. Swart, B.: Value and limitation of examination of the gastrointestinal tract in pancreatic disease, in Anacker, H. (ed.): Efficiency and Limits of Radiologic Examination of the Pancreas. Stuttgart, G. Thieme, 1975, pp. 42-53.

34. Bilbao, M,K., Rosch, J., Frische, L.H., et al.: Hypotonic duodenography in the diagnosis of pancreatic disease. Semin Roentgenol 3:280-287, 1968.

35. Goldberg, H.I., Bilbao, M.K., Stewart, E.R., et al.: Endoscopic retrograde cholangiopancreatography. Am J Dig Dis 21:270-278, 1976.

36. Anacker, H., Weiss, H.D., Kramann, B.: Das Pankreaskarzinom im endoskopischen retrograden Pankreaticocholangiogramm. RoFo 122:238-242, 1975.

37. Anacker, H., Weiss, H.D., Kramann, B.: Endoscopic Retrograde Pancreaticocholangiography (ERCP). Berlin, Springer-Verlag, 1977.

38. Freeny, P.C., Bilbao, M.K., Katon, R.M.: "Blind" evaluation of endoscopic retrograde cholangiopancreatography in the diagnosis of pancreatic carcinoma. Radiology 110:271-274, 1976.

39. White, T.T., Silverstein, F.E.: Operative and endoscopic pancreatography in the diagnosis of pancreatic cancer. Cancer 37:449-461, 1976.

40. Lunderquist, A.: Angiography in carcinoma of the pancreas. Acta Radiologica Suppl 235, Stockholm, 1965.

41. Boijsen, E.: Selective pancreatic angiography. Br J Radiol 39:481-487, 1966.

42. Nebesar, R.A., Pollard, J.L.: A critical evaluation of selective celiac and superior mesenteric angiography in the diagnosis of pancreatic diseases, particularly malignant tumor: Facts and "Artefacts." Radiology 1017-1027, 1967.

43. Bookstein, J.J., Reuter, S.R., Martel, W.: Angiographic evalution of pancreatic carcinoma. Radiology 90:757-764, 1969.

44. Baum, L., Athanasoulis, C.A.: Angiography, in Eaton, S.B., Ferrucci, J.T.: Radiology of the Pancreas and Duodenum. Philadelphia, Saunders, 1973, pp. 227-260.

45. Reuter, S.R., Redman, H.C., Bookstein, J.J.: Differential problems in the angiographic diagnosis of carcinoma of the pancreas. Radiology 96:93-99, 1970.

46. Tylen, U.: Accuracy of angiography in the diagnosis of carcinoma of the pancreas. Acta Radiol Diag 14:449-466, 1973.

47. Kaude, J.W., Wirtanen, G.W.: Celiac epinephrine enhanced angiography. AJR 110:818-826, 1970.

48. Rosch, J., Holman, D.C.: Superselective arteriography of the pancreas, in Anacker, H. (ed.) Efficiency and Limits of Radiologic Examination of the Pancreas. Stuttgart, G. Thieme, 1975, pp. 159-168.

49. Herlinger, H., Finlay, D.B.L.: Evaluation and follow-up of pancreatic arteriograms. A new role for angiography in the diagnosis of carcinoma of the pancreas. Clin Radiol 29:277-284, 1978.

50. Reuter, S.R.: Superselective pancreatic angiography, in Anacker, H. (ed.) Examination of the Pancreas. Stuttgart, G. Thieme, 1975, pp. 149-158.

51. Abrams, H.L.: Renal mass lesions: A diagnostic approach to tumors and cysts. JCE Radiol 1:11-51, 1979.

52. McClennan, B.L., Stanley, R.J., Melson, G.L., Leavitt, R.G., Sagel, S.S.: CT of the renal cyst: Is cyst aspiration necessary? AJR 133:671, 1979.

53. Swanson, D.A., Wallace, S., Johnson, D.E.: The role of embolization and nephrectomy in the treatment of metastatic renal carcinoma. Urol Clin North Am 7:719-730, 1980.

Chapter 8

Recent Advances in
Nuclear Medicine Scanning Techniques
(with Particular Attention to the Diagnosis and Staging
of Abdominal Malignancies)

Thomas P. Haynie, M.D.*

INTRODUCTION

Nuclear scanning is widely used in cancer diagnosis, staging and follow-up. Nuclear medicine procedures can substitute for less advantageous procedures, or they can serve as adjuncts to newly introduced techniques. Our nuclear medicine clinic at the University of Texas M.D. Anderson Hospital (UTMDAH) injects over 1 curie of activity during the average working day. In the United States, some 7 million nuclear medicine procedures are performed each year, and there are instrumentation sales of $80 million per year and radiopharmaceutical sales of $50 million per year.[1]

The power of nuclear medicine to reveal disease is accomplished through the high degree of contrast achieved with minute amounts of radiopharmaceuticals. This high contrast is the result of the differential concentration of administered radionuclide in diseased versus non-diseased tissues. Through the use of a variety of radiopharmaceuticals, different variables in the same organ or structure can be measured.

Although the availability of ultrasound and computed tomography has reduced emphasis on some aspects of radioisotope imaging, particularly brain and pancreas studies, other areas exist where radionuclide imaging remains active such as in the liver and lung, or is even increasing as in the heart and bone.[2]

ADVANCES IN NUCLEAR INSTRUMENTATION AND RADIOPHARMACEUTICALS

Some short-term directions are evident in nuclear medicine at the moment. (1) Technetium-99m has retained its pre-eminence as a radiopharmaceutical because of convenience, low cost and good physical and chemical properties; (2) Iodine-123, while not yet economic, is producing a mini-revival of interest in iodine; (3) Rubidium-81/krypton-81 and germanium-68/gallium-68 generators are being used, but costs and distribution logistics are still a problem; (4) Cyclotron-produced radionuclides are providing labels for tumor-localizing compounds; and (5) sodium iodide thalium-activated crystals are being challenged in specialized applications by gas-filled, cesium iodide, or bismuth germanium detectors, particularly in the construction of positron emission tomographic devices.

Nuclear medicine image quality is determined by (1) contrast resolution (lesion-to-background counts), and (2) spatial resolution and sensitivity of the instrumentation. While high count test phantom images may give 3 to 4 mm spatial resolution, in actual practice full-width half maximum is on the order

*The author acknowledges with gratitude the helpful criticism of Howard J. Glenn, Ph.D., Monroe F. Jahn, Ph.D., and Edmund E. Kim, M.D.

of 8 to 12 mm. Since energy resolution is of the order of 15 to 20% at 140 kev, this forces the acceptance of scattered photons which further decrease spatial resolution. If nuclear images are to be improved, spatial resolution will have to be optimized, and some tomographic imaging techniques must come into general use to mitigate overlap.[3] Also with tomographic imaging a lower target to non-target ratio can be detected ($\sim$2:1) as compared to planar imaging ($\sim$8:1).

Tomography in nuclear medicine is presently in its infancy. One method of performing nuclear tomography is longitudinal tomography, where a plane of interest is maintained in focus while overlying and underlying activity is blurred, contributing to an increased background level. Another method is transverse emission computed tomography which collects data from a plane of interest, and activity away from this plane does not degrade image contrast.[4] Two obstacles to the application of computed tomography techniques to gamma ray emitters are (1) the field of view of the collimator varies with depth; and (2) reconstruction requires sampling from different angles, while variations in anatomy influence image fidelity. For this reason, positron emitters are well suited for tomographic imaging.[5]

There are now four main approaches to positron camera construction: (1) planar arrays of sodium iodide thalium activated crystals; (2) rotating dual opposed scintillation cameras operating in coincidence mode; (3) a ring of sodium iodide thalium activated crystals, and (4) a multiwire proportional chamber positron camera.[3] Although there are still formidable cost and logistical problems to be overcome, the future can be contemplated with some optimism.

The requirements for spatial resolution (small statistical error) are not as severe when the difference between radionuclide concentration between lesion and background are large (e.g., several hundred percent). The relatively large contrast differences seen in some radiopharmaceutical studies as compared to tissue absorption differences, may point to a potential advantage for emission computed tomography over x-ray computed tomography.[4] However, approaches to enhance contrast are available for transmission modalities also.

ADVANCES IN DETERMINING THE USEFULNESS OF DIAGNOSTIC TESTS

Nuclear medicine was originally used to image structures invisible with conventional x-rays; however, ultrasound and computed tomography presently provide alternative imaging procedures for the same tissues as does nuclear medicine, and conflicting results can be anticipated.[6] Who is to resolve such dilemmas, and how this is to be done without introducing bias into the interpretation are current problems of considerable interest.

Increased application of sophisticated (and expensive) imaging systems has moved the specialty of nuclear medicine in a short time into an age of enhanced accountability. Emphasis on cost containment is stimulating us to determine the least amount of diagnostic imaging that is clinically applicable and necessary.[7] A large number of factors must be given consideration, such as <u>technical output,</u> meaning reproducibility, reliability, <u>information content</u> including sensitivity, and specificity, likelihood ratio, receiver operating characteristics and <u>prior probability determination.</u> Also to be considered is whether treatment is dependent on confirmation or exclusion of disease, the definition of disease extent, and/or absolute confidence in the diagnostic results, and what health outcomes are anticipated (including mortality and morbidity, and the quality of life).[8] The clinician must determine the ultimate efficacy of a diagnostic test but decisions are also influenced by the perceptions of patients, causing a dilemma for cost containment.[9]

Healthy and diseased patient populations overlap to some extent, whereas accuracy determinations for diagnostic tests often imply only one true-negative and one true-positive fraction. The sensitivity and specificity of a diagnostic test will of course change if the diagnostic criteria are changed. The criteria may be easily controlled when tests have numeric results, but may be difficult to control with subjectively interpreted tests.[10] Observers alter their criterion levels to suit clinical settings, and sensitivity and specificity fluctuate in clinical practice; a receiver-operating-characteristic (ROC) curve is the result. Therefore, in comparing two or more tests, we should compare observer performances in terms of ROC curves and consider the influence of prior probability of disease on overall accuracy.[11]

ROC curves can be generated in several ways, but the most common way is the rating method, whereby an observer indicates a level of confidence on a multi-category scale that abnormality is present.[10] It should be noted that no entirely satisfactory statistical method has been described for determining the significance of ROC curve separation. At the present time, experimentally determined points are fitted with error bars representing the square root of the binominal variance. No statement can be made about relative detectability of disease with two diagnostic tests if one appears more sensitive but less specific than the other. It is even difficult to judge how much better a more sensitive and specific test may be, since a change in criterion may cause a large change in sensitivity while causing a small change in specificity. Overall percentage accuracy (OPA) is also faulty in comparing diagnostic tests, since this parameter is sensitive to disease prevalence and may be insensitive to changes in lesion detectability when disease prevalence is very high or very low.

Situations in which conflicting reports are generated about separate imaging techniques may benefit from direct comparison of the techniques with the following questions: (1) was each study technically satisfactory?; (2) was the anatomic region in question adequately visualized?; (3) is an abnormality by one technique confirmed by another?; and (4) are two abnormal studies visualizing the same object?[6]

A statement of the problem in using staging procedures in the pre-operative search for occult metastatic disease is as follows: given the known sensitivity and specificity of pre-operative staging examinations, and given survival data suggesting that surgery is the therapy of choice in patients without metastatic disease, should pre-operative examinations be performed on patients with presumably operable carcinoma? To answer that question properly it helps to diagram the steps in decision analysis, and thereby to establish a quantitative method for making diagnostic and therapeutic judgements incorporating both probabilistic data and value judgements.[12] First, we structure the decision-making process using a "decision tree"; decision nodes are dispatched as squares, chance nodes as circles. Chance occurrences are each assessed for their probability and the utility of each potential outcome is considered. A value assessment is reached by considering factors pertinent to the patient, the physician, as well as to society, and we must finally combine the probability of each outcome with its utility.[13]

In order to use the values derived from decision analysis, we can introduce threshold concepts which suggest three types of solutions to clinical problems: (1) to withhold treatment without testing; (2) to go ahead and treat without diagnostic testing; or (3) to perform a diagnostic test that may determine the subsequent treatment approach.[14] The diagnostic testing threshold is the probability of disease at which there is no difference between the value of withholding treatment and performing the test. The test-treatment threshold is the point at which no difference exists between the value of performing the test and of administering the treatment. In certain circumstances, a test may provide information that is essential for directing therapy. In these circumstances, a test treatment threshold does not exist because therapy cannot be administered without the diagnostic test. The concept of a testing threshold, however, remains valid. The impact of the accuracy of a test on the threshold is to broaden its range of use as diagnostic accuracy increases, and to narrow its range of usefulness as the risk increases. It is apparent that the risk of the test must also be weighed against the risk of exposing patients without disease to the risks of unnecessary treatment or of withholding treatment. Thus the risk and reliability of a diagnostic test are counterbalancing forces. For a patient suspected of a disease, the best choice is to withhold therapy if the probability of disease is less than the testing threshold, to administer therapy if the disease probability is greater than the test treatment threshold, and to perform the test if the probability lies between the two thresholds.

Defining the clinical role of a new nuclear medicine technique or radiopharmaceutical is not an activity in which nuclear medicine has traditionally excelled. The short history of the specialty includes examples of exaggerated and innappropriate claims which had to be modified or withdrawn later. The clinical role of any diagnostic test must be defined in relation to other relevant procedures already in existence. Useful new procedures will provide unique information or the same information more safely, reliably, or economically.[15] With this background let us look at some specific diagnostic uses of nuclear medicine in abdominal malignancies.

RECENT ADVANCES IN LIVER SCANNING

Although continuing technological changes make consensus difficult to establish on the choice of an imaging procedure for the liver, the following strengths and weaknesses can be identified for radionuclide imaging. The strengths are that it is simple to perform, all patients are examinable, there are no "blind" spots, the cost is moderate, there is minimal waiting for the result, the procedure is reasonably sensitive, and it can provide information about reticuloendothelial function. The weaknesses of radionuclide imaging of the liver are that it is only a dual organ exam (liver-spleen), there is poor delineation of lesions adjacent to the liver, spatial resolution is only adequate (especially for deep lesions) and it is usually ineffective for characterizing lesions as to their etiology.[2]

Radionuclide liver imaging with technetium-99-m sulfur colloid specifically is useful as a screening procedure. It can be performed on virtually any patient without preparation and with a low radiation burden, is technologically easy to reproduce, and gives both structural and functional information about the entire organ. It can also increase the utility and accuracy of a subsequent computed tomography or ultrasound examination.[16] At present, scintigraphy remains the primary initial imaging procedure for hepatic parenchymal disease, and for screening for metastatic malignancy. Ultrasonography should be the initial diagnostic procedure for suspected biliary tract disease and perihepatic abscesses. Computed tomography is especially valuable in distinguishing extrinsic from intrinsic hepatic lesions when ultrasound results are equivocal, and for examining patients who for various reasons cannot be studied adequately with ultrasound.[17]

In recent years, we have seen a number of approaches to improving the results from radionuclide imaging of the liver which include: (1) minimizing motion artifacts by breath holding, using the upright position, analog circuitry, respiratory gating, and computer techniques; (2) using emission multiplane tomography; (3) emphasizing correlations of different scintigraphic patterns with different disease states; (4) combining liver scanning with ultrasound and/or CT imaging; and (5) combining results of liver scanning with serologic studies such as CEA, alkaline phosphatase, and SGOT.[18] The reported true-positive rates for liver scanning in disease vary because of differing percentages of patients with early versus late disease, the use of instruments with different scanning resolutions, and differences in observer performance.

The sensitivities for the three major imaging procedures employed at UTMDAH in 94 cases with metastatic disease to the liver were computed tomography 96%, scintigraphy 94%, and ultrasound 77%. Specificities of these procedures were computed tomography 86%, scintigraphy 67% and ultrasound 50%.[19] It would appear that the most accurate combination of screening tests in this study was computed tomography and scintigraphy. Specificity was defined as the differentiation of malignancy from benign disease. Cases of focal nodular hyperplasia, cavernous hemangioma, and amebic abscess could not be differentiated by these three procedures. The large volume of cases, as well as cost considerations dictate the following sequence of procedures at our institution. Liver scintigraphy is performed as the initial examination and is often used to follow the course of disease since it is very sensitive, it is the least expensive procedure, and it can be performed on a large number of patients (Figure 1). Sonography is used to confirm nuclear medicine findings and to resolve problems. Computed tomography is reserved for those cases where there is a conflict between scintigraphy and ultrasound.

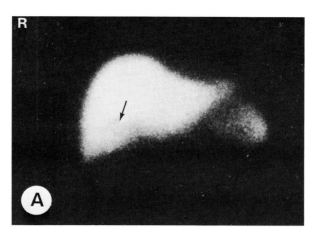

Figure 1A. True negative liver scan (anterior view); 55-year-old woman with bronchogenic carcinoma. Defect in lower right lobe (arrow) is in gallbladder region and was judged a normal variant. CT scan revealed gallstones, but the liver was within normal limits.

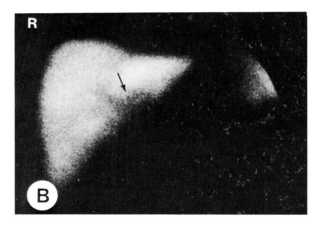

Figure 1B. False negative liver scan (anterior view); 45-year-old man presented with pulmonary nodules and mass in left kidney. Defect in lower left lobe (arrow) is in region of porta hepatis and was judged a normal variant. Arteriogram revealed a hypernephroma of the left kidney and diffuse, small metastatic nodules in the liver.

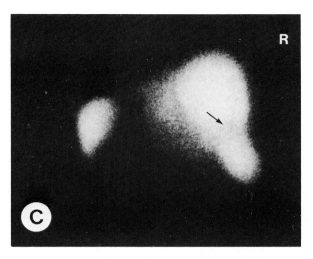

Figure 1C. False positive liver scan (posterior view); 63-year-old woman with breast cancer, post-mastectomy and radiotherapy, presented with malignant pleural effusion and bone metastases. Defect in lower right lobe was interpreted to be suggestive of metastases; however, liver sonogram was within normal limits and follow-up liver scans showed no change in appearance.

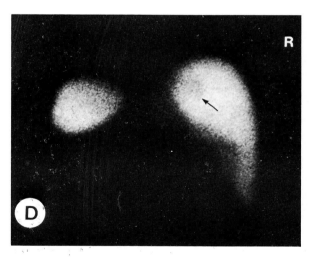

Figure 1D. True positive liver scan for "benign" lesion (posterior view); 62-year-old woman with malignant melanoma removed from toe with subsequent metastases to right groin nodes and left eye. Defect in upper right lobe (arrow) was interpreted as possibly metastatic, and ultrasound and CT scan confirmed a solid lesion. However, serial studies over the next 4 years showed no change and the patient is currently off therapy for 2 years with no evidence of disease. Clinical impression is hamartoma.

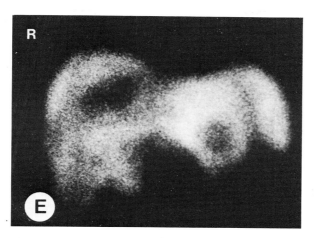

Figure 1E. True positive liver scan for metastatic lesions (anterior view); 65-year-old man with colon carcinoma resected 3 years previously, presenting with pulmonary nodules. Liver function tets were markedly abnormal and liver scan shows widespread involvement. Patient expired 3 months later of liver failure.

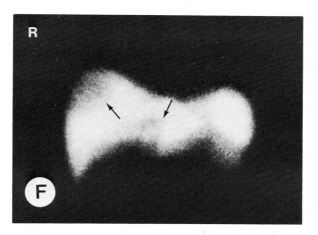

Figure 1F. True positive liver scan for biliary obstruction caused by metastatic lesions (anterior view). 47-year-old man with jaundice and pruritis, and a mass in right upper lung. Liver scan demonstrates defects in porta hepatis and right upper lobe (arrows). Ultrasound demonstrated biliary obstruction and metastatic nodules. Bronchoscopy diagnosed a small cell undifferentiated primary tumor in the lung. Transhepatic biliary drainage, chemotherapy and radiotherapy relieved the obstructive jaundice, but the patient expired 8 months later of brain metastases.

Recently in an article from the University of Texas M.D. Anderson Hospital concerned with non-invasive imaging modalities in malignant melanoma, the use of radionuclide liver scanning as the basic screening test in the evaluation of metastatic melanoma has been questioned.[19B] This study revealed a higher false-positive rate for radionuclide scans than for ultrasound or computed tomography. Patient selection may have played a part in this, since most equivocal radionuclide liver scans are submitted for ultrasound and/or CT examinations, while obviously normal or abnormal studies are not so frequently referred. The recommendation in the latter paper is that sonography of the liver, abdomen, and pelvis be the primary screening procedure based on cost and availability of equipment and the ability to reveal lesions not only in the liver but elsewhere in the abdomen and pelvis. CT scanning was recommended if the sonogram is technically inadequate, although computed tomography was considered much more reliable than either radionuclide liver scanning or ultrasonography and may largely replace both of these studies in the future.

Aburano et al have combined the results of liver scanning and carcinoembryonic antigen (CEA) determinations in 327 patients with a variety of gastrointestinal cancers.[20] Only discrete focal defects were called abnormal on liver scanning, and 70% of 113 patients with hepatic metastasis were detected by liver scanning. Only 1% false-positives were called in 214 normal livers. CEA levels above 5 ng% were found in 72% of metastatic disease patients and in 16% of normal patients. The predictive value of focal defects on liver scans for metastatic cancer in this series was 97%. A composite of high CEA with high serum alkaline phosphatase or hepatomegaly had a predictive value of 92%. As a single test, the liver scan was superior to the CEA assay; however, CEA may be useful as an adjunct to the liver scan in the evaluation of patients. CEA may also detect recurrences in locations other than the liver.

Scintiangiography is often added to the standard liver scanning procedure, but its usefulness in differentiating benign from malignant disease is limited.[21] In 554 patients in which scintiangiography was abnormal in 104, 47 had chronic liver disease, 29 neoplastic liver disease, 15 aortic aneurysms, 8 extrahepatic masses, 3 increased collateral circulation, and 2 congestive heart failure. Diffuse early liver perfusion in the arterial phase has proved reliable as a sign of chronic hepatic disease, although interpretation may be difficult.

Focal areas of increased uptake of radiocolloid on the liver scan have been reported in superior vena caval obstruction, hepatic venocclusive disease, hamartoma, hemangioma, abscess and on an iatrogenic basis.[22] The mechanism proposed is a focal increase in blood flow which presents the reticuloendothelial cells locally with a greater dose of colloid, producing a hot spot. A "warm" spot may be related to venous collaterals near adenomata and areas of interstitial fibrosis.

In patients with hepatoma, three gross pathologic patterns have been identified: (1) well encapsulated tumors; (2) poorly-encapsulated but solitary tumors; and (3) diffuse parenchymal involvement.[23] This leads to variable patterns on liver scanning, and the isodense appearance of some tumors may result in a false negative either with ultrasound (28%) or with computed tomography (21%). In patients with a predisposition to hepatoma, including those with postnecrotic cirrhosis, previous thoratrast administration, or alcoholic liver disease, and those with persistently elevated alphafetoprotein levels, technetium sulfur colloid scanning has been found to be highly sensitive but not specific for hepatoma. The combination of liver defects on sulfur colloid scanning with increased gallium uptake suggests hepatoma, abscess, or rarely metastatic disease, and some investigators recommend that patients suspected of hepatocellular carcinoma undergo both studies for initial evaluation.

Liver cell adenoma and focal nodular hyperplasia are distinct pathologic entities; one of the chief differences is the presence of bile ducts and Kupffer cells in focal nodular hyperplasia, whereas both are absent in liver cell adenomata. For this reason, a mass showing uptake of technetium sulfur colloid is more likely to be focal nodular hyperplasia.[24]

The effect of chemotherapy on the liver scan has been investigated in 15 patients undergoing therapy with a variety of agents.[25] Eight showed changes in radiocolloid distribution in the liver, including uneven uptake in 3, hepatomegaly in 2, and shift of radiocolloid to the spleen and/or bone marrow in 6. Four of these 8 patients also showed moderate elevations in their serum enzymes. Changes occurred as early as the third day. Two of the 8 returned to a normal pattern despite continued chemotherapy. Four of the patients were on a regimen which included a nitrosourea. The conclusion is that scan alterations induced by chemotherapy are minor and transient. No examples of focal hepatic defects were seen.

RECENT ADVANCES IN SPLEEN SCANNING

Radionuclide imaging is probably the best modality for spleen imaging, but diffuse infiltrative disease is poorly detected and discrete metastases are uncommon in this organ.[2] The normal-sized spleen is poorly imaged with ultrasound because of overlying ribs, and insufficient data are available to compare radionuclide scanning and computed tomography for tumor imaging in the spleen. The technetium sulfur colloid scan is an effective method initially to evaluate spleen size, position, and focal or diffuse alterations (Figure 2). Sonography can be a useful next step to determine if focal defects are solid or cystic and to show the relationship of the spleen to adjacent organs. Computed tomography may be reserved for instances in which diagnostic questions still remain. Angiography is used mainly for evaluating splenic trauma.[26]

Of 900 patients evaluated with radionuclide imaging for liver/spleen abnormalities, 835 had normal-sized spleens without defects.[26] In the remaining 65 (7%) the spleen was AB normal, 41 with splenomegaly and 24 with focal defects. Splenomegaly was secondary to liver disease in 39 patients and to leukemia in 2 patients. The 24 patients with focal defects were evaluated further with ultrasound. Five studies proved inadequate because of rib or lung artifact. In the remaining patients focal defects ultimately were shown to be caused by multiple myeloma, lymphangiomatosis, metastatic carcinoma with hemorrhage, abscess and lymphoma.

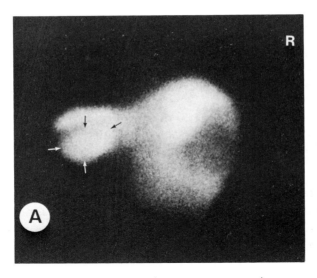

Figure 2A. True negative spleen scan (posterior view); 29-year-old woman with "splenomegaly" and swelling of left neck. Liver-spleen scan reveals normal-sized spleen (arrows), but there is a large defect in right lobe of liver suggestive of metastatic disease. Laparatomy revealed a large Wilms' Tumor of the left kidney and metastatic liver disease.

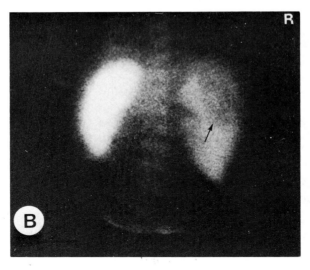

Figure 2B. True positive spleen scan secondary to liver disease (posterior view). 72-year-old man with transitional cell carcinoma of the bladder, post-cystectomy and radiotherapy, presented with abnormal liver function tests and pulmonary nodules. Liver-spleen scan reveals a defect in right lobe of liver (arrow), and splenic enlargement with increased uptake in spleen and bone marrow. Ultrasound confirmed metastasis in right lobe.

212

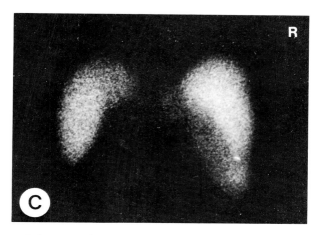

Figure 2C. True positive spleen scan, for enlargement (posterior view); 62-year-old woman with chronic lymphatic leukemia, progressive in spite of chemotherapy. Spleen not palpable clinically, but spleen scan and ultrasound showed enlargement that was progressive.

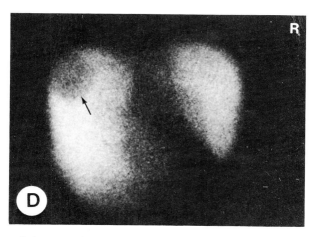

Figure 2D. True positive spleen scan, for enlargement and a mass lesion (posterior view); 74-year-old man with massive splenomegaly secondary to myelofibrosis and myeloid metaplasia. Spleen scan showed marked enlargement and a defect in the upper pole (arrow). Sonogram confirmed a solid mass, and splenectomy was performed demonstrating extramedullary hematopoiesis and a splenic hamartoma.

Accessory spleens may appear on computed tomography as left upper quadrant masses and may be difficult to differentiate from tumors.[27] In six patients whose spleen had been removed 4 to 33 years earlier, the identity of the accessory spleen was confirmed by technetium sulfur colloid scanning in 4 cases, and by angiography in two. Their diameters ranged from 3.5 to 5.0 cm. The clinical significance of the accessory spleens in these patients was the possibility that they might be mistaken for more significant masses arising from adjacent organs such as the kidney, adrenal gland, and pancreas. Heat-damaged Tc-99m red blood cells may also be used to visualize the spleen without interference from the liver, in selected cases.

Disorders which may cause a reversal of the liver:spleen uptake ratio on sulfur colloid scans include parenchymal liver disease, diabetes, congestive heart failure, anemia, sepsis, and (as previously noted) chemotherapy. Increased macrophage activity and/or increased splenic blood flow may be responsible, but the exact pathophysiology is not known. Forty-seven of 147 malignant melanoma patients (32%) were reported to have increased splenic update.[28] Patients with lymph node metastases and nodular melanoma had an increased frequency of enhanced uptake, and the group with increased splenic uptake had earlier and more frequent tumor recurrences.

RECENT ADVANCES IN GALLIUM SCANNING FOR TUMORS

Caution must be exercised in applying earlier sensitivity and specificity studies for gallium scanning to current clinical techniques. Gallium scans produced in early studies were limited by low count densities. Multiple pulse analyzers, large field-of-view cameras and tomographic scanners, and higher doses of radioactivity have significantly improved the image quality of gallium scans[29] (Figure 3). Ordinarily, in scanning for tumors 5-10 mCi of gallium-67 is administered and scanning is carried out 48 and/or 72 hours after injection, using a scanning camera or planar tomographic scanner on the 93, 184, and 296 kev photopeaks.

Gallium scanning as a staging modality is highly sensitive for the detection of mediastinal involvement in Hodgkin's disease, where its sensitivity is over 95%. However, it is only moderately sensitive (approximately 80% true positive) for cervical and other superficial nodes, and much less sensitive in the para-aortic and iliac regions (about 50%).[29] For the detection of para-aortic adenopathy, gallium imaging as reported by the older methods is less sensitive than lymphography, computed tomography, and perhaps also ultrasound.

Direct comparison of the accuracy of gallium scanning and lymphangiography for detecting para-aortic nodes in non-Hodgkin's lymphoma was reported in 45 patients.[31] In 17 of these patients, biopsy-proved disease was detected by lymphangiography but was missed by gallium scan. In no patient did the gallium scan correctly predict tumor involvement of para-aortic nodes that was missed by lymphangiography, and in three patients the gallium scan was falsely positive.

Tumors of the gastrointestinal tract and related organs, except for the liver, are detected with a low sensitivity by gallium-67, averaging less than

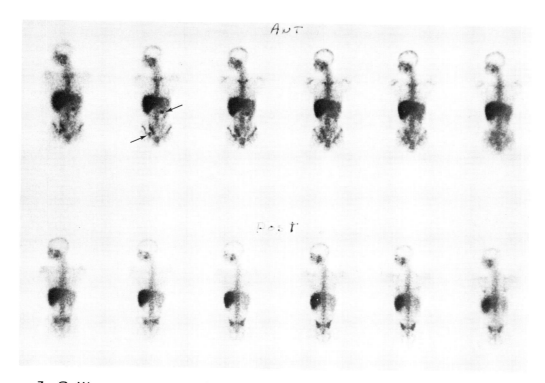

Figure 3. Gallium tomoscans for testicular malignancy; 20-year-old man post-right orchidectomy for endodermal sinus tumor with mass in left abdomen. Gallium scan reveals abnormal focus of uptake in left abdomen, with adjacent area of reduced activity and another area of increased uptake in right inguinal region (arrows). Abdominal CT scan revealed a 6 cm mass in left paraaortic region and iliac node enlargement. Lymphangiogram and arteriogram confirmed these findings. Patient treated with chemotherapy.

Courtesy of Medical Communication, the University of Texas at Houston, M.D. Anderson Hospital and Tumor Institute.

50%.[29]   The sensitivity for pancreatic lesions is only about 15%, and for colon primaries 20 to 40%.   In the genitourinary tract, with the possible exception of testicular tumors, sensitivity is in the range of 50% or less, and hence the use of gallium is not considered justifiable.

RECENT ADVANCES IN OTHER TUMOR SCANNING AGENTS

Cobalt-57 bleomycin has been used to image patients for abdominal and pelvic tumor deposits.   The most encouraging results were seen in lung cancer, where liver and adrenal metastases were detected on scans and all known sites were demonstrated in 15 of 17 patients.[35]   Next were gastrointestinal tract tumors, where primary and metastatic liver lesions were seen and local recurrences identified in the pelvis in 12 of 17 patients.   Unfortunately, commercial availability of this preparation is probably not going to materialize because of difficulties associated with the long physical half-life of cobalt-57.

Indium-111 has been used in place of cobalt-57 for labeling bleomycin, and in a study of 14 lymphoma patients with 25 histologically positive sites using indium-bleomycin followed by gallium citrate, indium-bleomycin detected 56% and gallium 84%.[36]   When both scans were compared in each patient, gallium was clearly superior in 12 out of 14, and the other two showed equal detectability.   It was concluded that indium-111 bleomycin is not useful either as a substitute for or as a complement to gallium-67 citrate in evaluating patients with lymphoma.

Recently thallium-201 has been studied in cancer patients from six institutions in Japan.[37]   Imaging was performed with either rectilinear scanners or gamma cameras following the administration of 0.7 to 2 mCi of thallium chloride, 5 to 10 minutes after injection.   Sensitivity was good in primary liver cancer (70%), but zero for liver metastases.   In lymphomas as in liver cancer, sensitivity was lower than for gallium (54%).

Radioiodinated anti-carcinoembryonic antigen immunoglobulin G has been injected and background subtracted with technetium-99m pertechnetate labeled albumin, using a large field-of-view camera and imaging at 4, 8, 24, and 48 hours.   In one series of 18 patients in which a variety of primaries was studied, radioantibody imaging detected 10 of 11 primary tumors (91%), and 15 of 18 metastatic lesions (83% sensitivity).[38]   In one colon tumor, the radioactivity ratio in the tumor relative to adjacent normal colon was 2.5.   In a more recent series of 24 tumor patients injected with purified goat anti-CEA antibody, photoscanning was definitely abnormal in 11 patients, equivocal in 8, and normal in 8.[39]   The smaller percentage of positive cases in the second group might be the result of differences in photoscanning techniques or the interpretation of results, but it seems unlikely to be attributable to differences in the properties of the antibody.   Presently, this method of "tumor immuno-detection" is not available for routine clinical use.   The use of monoclonal antibodies or of antibody fragments against CEA may render the method more sensitive and more reliable in the future.

Carbon-11 amino acids have been investigated as tumor localizing agents, particularly aminocyclopentanecarboxylic acid (ACPC), a derivative of cycloleucine which was studied as a cancer chemotherapy agent years ago.[40] Although carbon-11 ACPC detected 30 lesions in 38 patients with a variety of active malignancies, simultaneously performed gallium-67 scans detected 50 lesions in these patients. One case of cancer in the abdomen was well seen with C-11 ACPC, but was uncertain with gallium-67 because of interference from bowel contents.

RECENT ADVANCES IN SCANNING FOR INFLAMMATORY DISEASE

Since inflammatory lesions are often differential possibilities in the diagnosis and staging of malignancies, a brief summary of recent progress in their detection by nuclear medicine techniques is presented here.

Abscess localization, when localizing signs are present, is generally best accomplished with ultrasound or computed tomography. However, when localizing signs are not present radioisotope studies can be helpful[2] (Figure 4). A 4-to-6 hour gallium scan may be performed with follow-up at 24, 48, 72 hours and beyond if necessary.[30] Although gallium-67 is now the established agent for routine use, recent investigation with indium-111 white blood cells has given encouraging results, and if technical problems of production and stability can be solved, this radiopharmaceutical could be used routinely in the future. Frequently, gallium scans reveal the kidney to be the true site of infection in a suspected abdominal or retroperitoneal abscess.

Activity in the lumen of the colon is one of the principal problems in the evaluation of abdominal abscess using gallium. In 132 patients examined, 63 had colon activity.[32] In 36 of these 63, the activity was observed to change in location and intensity and the scan was therefore thought to be normal. In 25 of the remaining 27 patients, the charts were reviewed and 13 were shown to have no evidence of colonic diseae, whereas 3 had undergone abdominal surgery and could not be prepared adequately with colon cleansing. The remaining 9 all had colonic inflammatory disease. Colonic gallium activity which persists over 48 hours without change in location or appearance may indicate colonic disease, provided thorough bowel preparation has been carried out.

Combining data from several series, the sensitivity of gallium-67 for the detection of abscess was 91% with a specificity of 93%.[33] Although gallium-67 cannot differentiate fluctuant abscesses from inflammatory masses (as is often possible with ultrasound or CT), gallium does have one striking advantage and that is its capability of evaluating the entire body to identify a cause for cryptogenic fever and sepsis. After localizing a lesion with gallium-67, ultrasound or CT can be employed for further characterization of the process.

Indium-111 oxine, used in the preparation of labeled white blood cells, is not available for routine use. The technique involves separation of the white blood cells, labeling with indium-111, and re-injection of 1 mCi of the labeled cells. Indium-111 labeled white cells seem to have a high degree of specificity for abscesses, and the absence of elevated uptake of indium-111 white cells makes a neoplasm much more likely, especially when a technetium sulfur colloid scan (liver) demonstrates a photopenic lesion.[34]

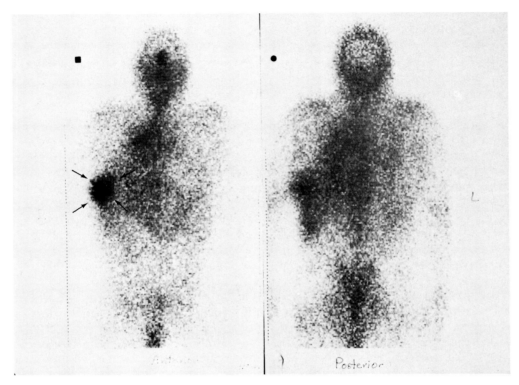

Figure 4. Gallium scan in liver abscess; 64-year-old man with disseminated oat cell carcinoma of the lung and obstructive jaundice. Liver scan and sonogram revealed liver metastases, with biliary tract obstruction at the level of the distal common bile duct. Percutaneous transhepatic bile drainage was initiated and chemotherapy begun. He experienced severe neutropenia with fever, and several gram negative organisms were cultured from the bile. Gallium scan revealed localized area of increased uptake (arrows) suggestive of an abscess, confirmed with CT scan. Patient was treated with antibiotics.

Courtesy of Medical Communication, the University of Texas at Houston, M.D. Anderson Hospital and Tumor Institute.

RECENT ADVANCES IN PANCREATIC SCANNING

Despite fifteen years of use, the pancreas scan with selenomethionine is still not generally accepted an an efficacious procedure.[41] When used, it is usually reserved for patients in whom no abnormality has been seen on ultrasound or CT and the suspicion of pancreatic disease remains high. A normal pancreas scan rules out pancreatic disease with 90 to 95% certainty, but an "abnormal" study has less certain significance.

Radionuclide pancreatic studies are frequently of poor diagnostic quality because of factors such as the overlying liver and varying degrees of selenium-75 concentration in the pancreas and surrounding viscera. Multiplane tomographic scanning offers improved spatial resolution in this organ at different depths.[42] A 250 uCi dose of selenium-75 selenomethionine is injected and tomographic scanning carried out 30 minutes later. Tomographic scans have been judged superior to camera images in 10 of 20 cases, and inferior in 3.

The substitution of carbon-11 for carbon-12 in amino acids inspires hope for improved pancreatic imaging, and studies have demonstated pancreatic concentration of carbon-11 valine, carbon-11 tryptophan, and carbon-11 aminocyclobutane carboxylic acid (ACBC). A positron emission tomographic device was used and scans were started 5 minutes after the injection of 6 to 45 mCi. Twenty-four patients were examined and 10 were normal.[43] Of the fourteen abnormal patients on scans, 8 had carcinoma of the pancreas, 3 abdominal lymphoma, and 3 pancreatitis. Unexpectedly, 4 cancers of the pancreas specifically showed increased isotope concentration. In addition, one lymphoma showed increased uptake of ACBC. Resolution and contrast of emission computed tomography (ECT) were superior to conventional scans, but inferior to ultrasound and CT.

RECENT ADVANCES IN ADRENAL IMAGING

Adrenal scintigraphy has a unique role in adrenal diagnosis - the correlation of regional adrenal metabolism with structure.[44] It therefore serves as a bridge between the laboratory determination of adrenal function and anatomic imaging procedures such as CT and ultrasound. Adrenal imaging with radionuclides fills an important role in distinguishing carcinoma from adenoma and in establishing the presence or absence of autonomous (non-suppressible) function.[2]

Presently used radiopharmaceuticals for adrenal imaging suffer from a number of deficiencies; e.g., the need for multiple imaging examinations and pharmacologic manipulation, interference from medication such as diuretics and anti-hypertensives, higher-than-optimal radiation dose, and the need for close cooperation from the patient and the referring physician.[44] Dexamethasone suppression is necessary to increase the sensitivity of adrenal imaging in abnormal aldosterone biosynthesis. Following suppression, either unilateral or bilateral adrenal visualization within 3 to 5 days (depending on dose) is consistent with adrenal disease and is 90% accurate.

RECENT ADVANCES IN HEPATOBILIARY IMAGING

Hepatobiliary radionuclide imaging is well suited for determining the patency of the cystic duct and the common bile duct, as well as the effectiveness of drainage of bile through biliary-enteric bypasses.[2] Studies with substituted aminodiacetic acids (IDA) seem to have a bright future. From 2 to 8 mCi (depending on liver function) of technetium-99m HIDA, PIPIDA, DISIDA, or another IDA is injected into the fasting patient. Images are taken for up to one hour in normal patients, but jaundiced patients require delayed imaging at up to 24 hours. The indications and accuracy of these agents are still under investigation, but they may be uniquely helpful in patients with jaundice and biliary dilatation to detect flow of bile into the gastrointestinal tract.[45]

A primary hepatocellular carcinoma presented as a focal defect on technetium sulfur colloid scan and was well visualized on scintiangiography and a gallium scan. A biliary scan also demonstrated uptake.[46] The IDA scanning agents therefore may help to differentiate primary hepatomas from hemangiomas or gallium-avid metastatic tumors. Further study of biliary agents for evaluating different histologic grades of hepatoma, hepatic adenoma, or cholangiocarcinoma is indicated, and they may also be useful in assessing functional radiation injury to the liver.

Out of 3600 patients evaluated for metastatic disease with technetium sulfur colloid scans, 40 had equivocal scans because of an apparent solitary defect on the inferior margin of the right lobe. Using technetium-labeled biliary agents, the gallbladder was clearly identified as occupying the discrete defect in 31 of the 40 patients. In 8 patients the gallbladder did not correspond to the defect and all of these were found to have metastases on laparoscopy. One patient whose gallbladder did not visualize at all was found to have cancer of the gallbladder.[47]

RECENT ADVANCES IN RENAL IMAGING

Renal scintigraphy is recognized as an accurate method for distinguishing renal tumor, cyst, abscess, or infarct from normal variants in renal morphology.[48] Normal variants take up radioactive renal tracers while true mass lesions appear as "cold" areas. For renal imaging technetium-99m glucoheptonate in a dose of 15 mCi is injected, and 2-second serial images of the renal area showing blood flow are obtained followed by static views at 10 minute intervals for 60 minutes.

The sensitivity of glucoheptonate in renal mass lesions is high, about 96%, with a specificity of about 75%.[49] Forty patients were evaluated also with arteriography. Nineteen had mass lesions and the scan was abnormal in 17, for a relative sensitivity of 89%.[48] There were 12 cysts, 2 carcinomas, 2 infarcts, and 1 abscess. Peripelvic lesions are difficult to evaluate with radionuclides because of defects caused by fat and other hilar structures. These lesions are best studied by CT. False masses due to fetal lobulation and hypertrophied columns of Bertin are best resolved by technetium glucoheptonate scans.[49]

RECENT ADVANCES IN DETECTION OF GASTROINTESTINAL BLEEDING

Gastrointestinal bleeding from neoplastic disease most commonly arises distal to the ligament of Treitz and must be differentiated from diverticular disease, angiodysplasia, and inflammatory bowel disease.[50]   When bleeding occurs from the upper tract in patients with solid tumors, it is not usually due to the tumor itself.   More commonly, bleeding in such patients is caused by hemorrhagic gastritis, peptic ulcer, esophagitis, or varices.   In the diagnosis of lower tract bleeding, both colonoscopy and barium enema imaging are compromised in the presence of active bleeding. For this reason, radionuclide studies and angiography have been more useful in the emergency management of lower than upper gastrointestinal bleeding, where endoscopy is more definitive.   Angiography for the diagnosis and treatment of lower tract bleeding can be more precisely directed if preceded by a radionuclide study. Positive scans decrease the time necessary for the angiographer to locate the bleeding point, and a negative scan may predict that an angiogram will not be helpful. Red blood cells labeled in vivo or in vitro with technetium-99m offer the opportunity to detect intermittent bleeding over a 24 hour period; upper as well as lower tract bleeding can be detected.[51]   Red cells can be labeled in vivo by injecting stannous pyrophosphate followed by 15 to 20 mCi of technetium-99m pertechnetate.[52]   Serial imaging is carried out for 4 hours, or until the bleeding site is located.   In 18 patients studied, brisk bleeding was often seen immediately as a contrast blush. With occult bleeding, longer and delayed imaging was necessary. Ten patients with gross bleeding per rectum were studied with this technique, and seven had positive scintigrams. Three of the 7 were also found to have extravasation of contrast on arteriography. Scans correctly located the site of hemorrhage in 4 patients with bleeding diverticula.   There was a single false-negative in a slow bleeder.   There was some accumulation of gastric activity in 50% of controls; since there was no thyroid activity in these subjects, the gastric secretion may not be caused by free pertechnetate. Eighty percent of the bleeding patients were undergoing simultaneous gastric suction, which can therefore be used to minimize the problem.

RECENT ADVANCES IN DETECTION OF VENOUS THROMBOSIS

Venous thrombosis occurs commonly in cancer patients, particularly with prostatic and pancreatic primaries, and tumor recurrences in the pelvis can often be confused with (or promote) lower extremity venous thrombi.

Nuclear medicine techniques have been useful in evaluating the need for prophylactic therapy in patients who have experienced or are at risk of developing deep venous thrombosis, and in monitoring therapeutic regimens.[53] Three distinct monitoring methods have been used: fibrinogen uptake tests, radionuclide venography, and thrombus scintigraphy. The disadvantages of the fibrinogen uptake test are that it takes days to complete, it is limited to evaluating the extremities, the radiopharmaceutical is expensive, and one usually does not obtain direct images with I-125 labeled fibrinogen.

Radionuclide venography visualizes flow patterns as with radiopaque venography studies, but without pain and the risk of sensitivity reactions to contrast media (Figure 5). However, failure to demonstrate particle entrapment of macro-aggregated albumin (MAA) on delayed imaging is not a reliable indicator of the absence of thrombi in patients receiving heparin, because of false negatives from interference with surface charge on the thrombus.[54]

The clinical situation should govern the approach to the diagnosis of thrombophlebitis. Patients with suspected pulmonary emboli should have lower extremity technetium-99m MAA venography and a lung scan. In patients at high risk of thrombophlebitis who are on low-dose heparin therapy, an iodine-125 fibrinogen study is optimal. Where available, iodine-123 fibrinogen may be used for venography and followed 6 to 24 hours later with imaging. Iodine-123 radiolabeled fibrinogen scintigraphy is of limited availability because of production problems, but it can be of value for differential diagnosis and determination of the extent of disease and therapeutic response, particularly in the pelvis and groin.

Other authors report that indium-111 labelled platelets are promising agents. Platelets are isolated by differential centrifugation and are labeled with indium-111 oxine and then washed. Twenty patients suspected of thromboembolism were studied, and increased uptake was seen in the lower extremities of 12 patients.[54] Of 7 patients with confirmed deep venous thrombosis, 6 had abnormal images for a sensitivity of 86%.

RECENT ADVANCES IN LYMPHOSCINTIGRAPHY

Technetium-99m antimony sulfide colloid with a particle size of 4-12 millicrons is rapidly removed by lymphatic flow after interstitial injection. For imaging of retroperitoneal lymph nodes 2.5 mCi of this tracer is injected into the web of the first and second toe and gamma camera images performed 1-2 hours later after the patient has walked for an hour. In patients with obstruction to lymphatic drainage from metastatic involvement, an increase in tracer appears in a medial band of lymphatics in the thigh, called the "flare" sign.[55] It is possible that the imaging of abdominal lymph nodes may be improved with tomographic devices.

SUMMARY AND CONCLUSION

As can be judged from this review of recently published studies, nuclear medicine has a wide and varied role to play in the diagnosis, staging and follow-up of abdomino-pelvic malignancies. Although nuclear medicine can rarely be considered the primary diagnostic modality, there are many instances where the unique ability of radionuclides to achieve high contrast and evaluate functional status make them an invaluable adjunct or screening tool. Further improvements in instrumentation and radiopharmaceuticals should assure a place for nuclear medicine in the management of patients with abdomino-pelvic malignancies in the future.

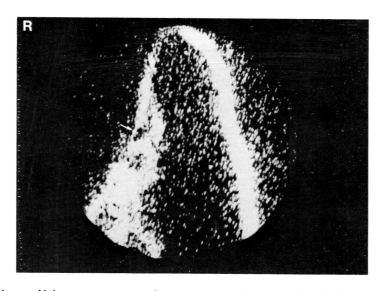

Figure 5. Radionuclide venogram in venous thrombosis; 66-year-old man with adenocarcinoma of lung, post-surgical resection of right upper lobe and multiple courses of chemotherapy for bone metastases. Patient presented with hard, cord-like veins in right groin. Venous flow studies confirmed interruption of flow in right ilio-femoral vein (arrow), and collateral flow pattern secondary to venous thrombosis. Treatment was symptomatic.

REFERENCES

1. Kaufman L: Nuclear Medicine: Physical Principles, Margulis AR, Burhenne J (eds.); Alimentary Tract Radiology vol 3 Abdominal Imaging, C.W. Mosby Co., St. Louis, 1979, p. 22.

2. Grossman ZD, Thomas FD: Position of Nuclear Imaging in the Age of Transmission Computed Tomography and Ultrasound, Freeman LM, Weissman HS (eds.); Nuclear Medicine Annual 1980. Raven Press, New York, 1980. pp. 367-391.

3. Kaufman L: Nuclear Medicine: Instrumentation, Alimentary Tract Radiology, vol 3 Abdominal Imaging, C.W. Mosby Co., St. Louis, 1979, pp. 48-53.

4. Murphy PH, DePuey G, Sonnemaker RE, Burdine JA: Emission Computed Tomography: A Current Status Report, Freeman LM, Weissman HS (eds.); Nuclear Medicine Annual 1980. Raven Press, New York, 1980, pp. 83-125.

5. Ter-Pogossian M: Relative Merit Instrumentation, Alimentary Tract Radiology, vol 3 Abdominal Imaging, C.W. Mosby Co., St. Louis, 1979. pp. 63-65.

6. Jaffe CC: Cognitive Dissonance: The Meaning of Discordant Imaging Results, JAMA 242:1741-1742, 1979.

7. Potsaid MS: Diagnostic Imaging in Perspective, JAMA 243:2412-2417, 1980

8. Fineberg HV, Wittenberg J, Ferrucci JT: Cost-effectiveness: Instrumentation, Alimentary Tract Radiology, vol 3 Abdominal Imaging, C.W. Mosby Co., St. Louis, 1979. pp. 68-71.

9. Wittenberg J, Fineberg HV: Evaluating Efficacy, Am. J. of Roentgenol. 134:1277-1279, 1980.

10. Turner DA: An Intuitive Approach to Receiver Operating Characteristic Curve Analysis, J. Nucl. Med. 19:213-220, 1978.

11. Turner DA: Observer Variability: What to do Until Perfect Diagnostic Tests are Invented, J. Nucl Med 19:435-437, 1978.

12. McNeil BJ, Pauker SG: The Patients Role in Assessing the Value of Diagnostic Tests, Radiology 132:605-610, 1979.

13. Pauker SG, Kassirer JP: Clinical Application of Decision Analysis: A Detailed Illustration, Sem. in Nucl Med 8:324-335, 1978.

14. Pauker SG, Kassirer JP: The Threshold Approach to Clinical Decision Making, New England J Med 302:1109-1118, 1980.

15. Ronai PM: Hepatobiliary Radiopharmaceuticals: Defining Their Clinical Role Will be a Galling Experience. J. Nucl Med 18:488-489, 1977.

16. Sullivan D, Gottschalk A: Nuclear Medicine: Liver and Biliary Tract, Alimentary Tract Radiology, vol 3 Abdominal Imaging, C.W. Mosby Co., St. Louis, 1979, pp. 203.

17. McAfee JG, Grossman ZD, Wistow BW, Bryan BT, Cohen W: Relative Merits: Liver and Biliary Tract, Alimentary Tract Radiology, vol 3 Abdominal Imaging, C.W. Mosby Co., St. Louis, 1979, pp. 243-245.

18. Freitas JE, Dworkin HJ: Optimizing the Detection of Hepatic Metastases, J Nucl Med 20:264-265, 1979.

19A. Snow JH Jr, Goldstein HM, Wallace S: Comparison of Scintigraphy, Sonography, and Computed Tomography in the Evaluation of Hepatic Neoplasms, Am. J. Roentgenol 132:915-918, 1979.

19B. Doiron, M.J., Bernardino, M.E. A Comparison of Non-Invasive Imaging Modalities in the Melanoma Patient. Cancer 47:2581-2584, 1981.

20. Aburano T, Tonami N, Hisada K: Radioimmunoassay for Carcinoembryonic Antigen as an Adjunct to Liver Scan in the Detection of Liver Metastases from Digestive Tract Cancer, J. Nucl Med 20:232-235, 1979.

21. Echevarria RA, Bonnano C: Value of Routine Abdominal Nuclide Angiography as Part of Liver Scan, Clin. Nucl Med 4:66-78, 1979.

22. Tetalman MR, Kusumi R, Gaughran G, Baba N: Radionuclide Liver Spots: Indicator of Liver Disease or a Blood Flow Phenomenon, Am. J. Roentgenol 130:219-296, 1978.

23. Broderick TW, Gosink B, Menuch L, Harris R, Wilcox J: Echographic and Radionuclide Detection of Hepatoma, Radiology 135:149-151, 1980.

24. Sandler MA, Petrocelli RD, Marks D, Lopez R: Ultrasonic Features and Radionuclide Correlation in Liver Cell Adenoma and Focal Nodular Hyperplasia, Radiology 135:393-397, 1980.

25. Kaplan WD, Drum DE, Lokich JJ: The Effect of Cancer Chemotherapeutic Agents on the Liver-Spleen Scan, J. Nucl Med 21:84-87, 1980.

26. Shirkhoda A, McCartney WH, Staab EV, Mittelstaedt CA: Imaging of the Spleen: A Proposed Algorithm, Am. J. Roentgenol 135:195-198, 1980.

27. Beahrs JR, Stephens DH: Enlarged Accessory Spleens: CT Appearance in Post Splenectomy Patients, Am. J. Roentgenol 135:483-486, 1980.

28. Sober A Jr, Mintzis MM, Lew RA, Lo H, Whalen C, McKusick KA, Potsaid MS, Vialotti C, Pearson B: The Significance of Augmented Radiocolloid Uptake by the Spleen in Patients with Malignant Melanoma, J. Nucl Med 20:1232-1236, 1979.

29. Hoffer P: Status of Gallium-67 in Tumor Detection, J. Nucl Med 21:394-398, 1980.

30. Halpern S, Hagan P: Gallium-67 Citrate Imaging in Neoplastic and Inflammatory Disease; Freeman L, Weissman H (eds.) Nuclear Medicine Annual 1980.   Raven Press, New York, 1980.   pp. 219-265.

31. Longo DL, Schilsky RL, Blei L, Cono R, Johnston GS, Young RC: Gallium-67 Scanning: Limited Usefulness in Staging Patients with Non-Hodgkins Lymphoma. Am. J. Med 68:695-700, 1980.

32. Pechman R, Tetalman M, Autonmattei S, Bekerman C, Olsen J, Chiles J: Diagnostic   Significance   of   Persistent   Colonic   Gallium   Activity: Scintigraphic Patterns, Radiology 128:691-695, 1978.

33. Biello DR, Levitt RG, Melson CL: The Roles of Gallium-67 Scintigraphy, Ultrasonography, and Computed Tomography in the Detection of Abdominal Abscesses, Sem in Nucl Med 9:58-65, 1979.

34. Fawcett HD, Lautiere RL, Frankel A, McDougall IR: Differentiating Hepatic Abscess from Tumor: Combined [111] In White Blood Cells and [99m]Tc Liver Scans, Am. J. Roentgenol, 135:53-56, 1980.

35. Kahn PC, Milunsky C, Dewanjee MK, Rudders RA: The Place of [57]Co-Bleomycin Scanning in the Evaluation of Tumors. Am. J. Roentgenol 129:267-273, 1977.

36. Bekerman C, Moran EM, Hoffer PB, Hendrix RW, Gottschalk A: Scintigraphic   Evaluation   of   Lymphoma: A   Comparative   Study   of ^{67}Ga-Citrate and ^{111}In-Bleomycin, Radiology 123:687-694, 1977.

37. Hisada K, Tonami N, Mujamae T, Hiraki Y, Yamazaki T, Maeda T, Nakajo M: Clinical Evaluation of Tumor Imaging with [201]Tl. Chloride, Radiology 129:497-500, 1978.

38. Goldenberg DM, DeLand F, Kim E, Bennett S, Primus JF, Van Nagell JR, Estes N, De Simone P, Rayburn P: Use of Radiolabelled Antibodies to Carcinoembryonic Antigen for the Detection and Locatization of Diverse Cancers by External Photoscanning, New England J. Med 298:1384-1388, 1978.

39. Mach JP, Carrel S, Forni M, Ritschard J, Donath A, Alberto P: Tumor Localization of Radiolabeled Antibodies Against Carcinoembryonic Antigen in Patients with Carcinoma: A Critical Evaluation, New England J. Med 303:5-10, 1980.

40. Hubner KF, Andrews GA, Washburn L, Wieland BW, Gibbs WD, Hayes RL, Butter TA, Winebrunner JD: Tumor Localization with 1-aminocyclopetane (^{11}C) Carboxylic Acid: Preliminary Clinical Trials with Single-Photon Detection, J. Nucl Med 18:1215-1221, 1977.

41. Partain CL, Staab EV, McCartney WH: Multiple Imaging Modalities for the Study of Pancreatic Disease, Sem in Nuclear Medicine 9:36-42, 1979.

42. Gaston EL, Gaspard CL, Brooks AC, Dukes A: Multiplane Tomographic Imaging of the Pancreas, J. Nucl Med Technol 8:28-29, 1980.

43. Buonocore E, Hubner KF: Positron-Emission Computed Tomography of the Pancreas: A Preliminary Study, Radiology 133:195-201, 1979.

44. Gross MD, Thrall JH, Beierwaltes WH: The Adrenal Scan: A Current Status Report on Radiotracers, Dosimetry, and Clinical Utility: Freeman LM, Weissman HS (eds.) Nuclear Medicine Annual 1980. Raven Press, New York, 1980. pp. 127-175.

45. Seltzer SE, Jones B: Imaging the Hepatobiliary System in Acute Disease, Am. J. Roentgenol 135:407-416, 1980.

46. Utz JA, Lull RJ, Anderson JH, Lambrecht RW, Brown JM, Henry W: Hepatoma Visualization with Tc-99m Pyridoxylidene Glutamate, J. Nucl Med 21:747-749, 1980.

47. Rao BK, Pastakia B, Leiberman LM: Evaluation of Focal Defects on Technetium-^{99m} Sulfur Colloid Scans with New Hepatobiliary Agent, Radiology 136:497-499, 1980.

48. Older RA, Korobtein M, Workman J, Cleeve DM, Cleeve LK, Sullivan D, Webster GD: Accuracy of Radionuclide Imaging in Distinguishing Renal Masses from Normal Variants, Radiology 136:443-448, 1980.

49. Leonard JC, Allen EW, Goin J, Smith CW: Renal Cortical Imaging and the Detection of Renal Mass Lesions. J. Nucl Med 20:1018-1022, 1979.

50. Kahn PC: Renal Imaging with Radionuclide, Ultrasound and Computed Tomography, Sem in Nucl Med 9:43-57, 1979.

51. Alavi A, McLean GK: Radioisotopic Detection of Gastrointestinal Bleeding: An Integrated Approach With Other Diagnostic and Therapeutic Modalities; Freeman LM, Weissman HS (eds.) Nuclear Medicine Annual 1980. Raven Press, New York, 1980, pp. 177-218.

52. Winzelberg GG, McKusick KA, Strauss HW, Waltman AC, Greenfield AJ: Evaluation of Gastrointestinal Bleeding by Red Blood Cells Labeled In Vivo with Technetium-99m. J. Nucl Med 20:1080-1086, 1979.

53. Smith RK, Arterburn G: Detection and Localization of Gastrointestinal Bleeding Using Tc-99m-Pyrophosphate In Vivo Labeled Red Blood Cells, Clin Nucl Med. 5:55-60, 1980.

54. Krohn KA, Knight LC: Radiopharmaceuticals for Thrombus Detection: Selection, Preparation, and Critical Evaluatin, Sem in Nucl Med 7:219-228, 1977.

55. DeNardo SJ: Role of Nuclear Medicine in the Detection of Venous Thrombosis, Freeman LM, Weissman HS (eds.) Nuclear Medicine Annual 1980. Raven Press, New York, 1980, pp. 341-365.

56. Davis HH II, Siegel BA, Sherman LA, Heaton WA, Welch MJ: Scintigraphy with ^{111}In-labeled Autologous Platelets in Venous Thromboembolism, Radiology 136:203-207, 1980.

57. Jackson FI, Lentle BC: The Scintilymphangiographic "Flare" Sign of Lymphangitis Obstruction. Clin Nucl Med 2:211-213, 1977.

Chapter 9

Percutaneous Needle Biopsy in the Thorax

Marshall Bein, M.D.

When a persistent new abnormality is detected on chest radiographs, it is usually mandatory that a definitive diagnosis be obtained. In the patient with a smoking history and an uncalcified nodule, appropriate management may be critically influenced by a benign or a malignant diagnosis. Furthermore, the initial clinical staging and treatment of patients with primary extrathoracic neoplasms will usually be significantly affected if there are pulmonary nodules or enlarged mediastinal nodes that prove to be metastases. During the subsequent course of a malignant disorder, new chest radiographic abnormalities may indicate metastases, opportunistic infection, or drug-induced lung disease. If the lung parenchyma is thought to be involved in the staging of lymphoma, patient management may be critically altered. It may also be important to distinguish between hematogenous involvement of the lung (Stage IV), and local extension of tumor into the lung from hilar lymph nodes ("E" stage).

Several different modalities may be employed for diagnosing these intrathoracic abnormalities in malignancy. Thoracotomy and open mediastinal exploration are definitive diagnostic procedures. However, they are associated with significant morbidity and some mortality, depending upon patient risk factors. Fiberoptic bronchoscopy is a much less invasive procedure and may be useful in diffuse pulmonary disease where multiple brush or forceps biopsies may be obtained. Bronchoscopy may also be diagnostic when a lesion is visible endobronchially and can be subsequently biopsied (see Chapter 4). Percutaneous needle biopsy is also less invasive than thoracotomy and has potential advantages over bronchoscopy for small, peripheral lesions that are not visible endoscopically, or for discrete lesions of any size or location that do not impinge on the bronchial lumen.[1,2] It may also be used for evaluating mediastinal lesions.

Percutaneous needle studies may be performed by cutting needle or by aspiration techniques. Complications are less with the latter.[3] The following discussion will focus upon percutaneous aspiration biopsy of the lung parenchyma and the mediastinum, and the results of several published reviews will be summarized.[4-6]

Aspiration biopsies may be performed with a variety of needles, the choice of which is usually dictated by operator familiarity and by the quality of histopathologic or cytopathologic assistance. Several types of aspiration needles have been modified to obtain tissue for histologic evaluation, and these are recommended for institutions with limited cytopathologic expertise.

Aspiration biopsy may be performed on an inpatient or outpatient, depending upon the risk factors for complications in the individual patient. The lesion is first localized in frontal and lateral radiographic projections, and with the image amplifier. Following local anesthesia of the skin and chest wall, the needle is passed above a rib margin to avoid intercostal vessels and nerves, using the shortest and most direct available approach to the lesion. It is then advanced into the lesion under fluoroscopic guidance, and confirmation of the needle position within the lesion is obtained ideally by fluoroscopy in both the frontal and lateral projections. Aspiration for cytology and/or histopathology is then performed and the material given directly to a qualified individual for appropriate handling. Post-biopsy radiographs are obtained immediately to monitor for possible complications.

The most common complication of percutaneous biopsy in the chest is pneumothorax, which may be small and is observed in approximately 10-40% of patients. The number requiring a chest tube varies from 1-14%, however. The rate of postbiopsy pneumothorax increases with the following factors: (1) increased patient age; (2) increased depth of the lesion within the lung; (3) increased outer diameter of the biopsy needle used (below 18-gauge); (4) the presence and severity of emphysema; (5) multiplicity of needle punctures; (6) decreased nodule size (below 2.5 cm in diameter); and (7) less experience in the person performing the biopsy. Postbiopsy hemoptysis occurs in 2-19% of patients and is almost always small and self-limited. Implantation or spread of tumor cells and postbiopsy infections are not significant concerns, and mortality of this procedure approaches zero.

The accuracy of diagnosis in percutaneous aspiration biopsy is variable and is critically related to the skill of the cytopathologist or histopathologist. True positive diagnoses for malignancy range between 72% and 99%, depending upon the number of aspiration biopsies obtained per nodule. A falsely positive diagnosis of malignancy may occur in up to 4% of cases. A precise benign diagnosis can be made in 55-87%. The overall accuracy of percutaneous needle aspiration in the chest ranges between 82% and 96%.

Indications for aspiration biopsy include the following: (1) suspected lung cancer in an inoperable patient; (2) single or multiple nodules in a patient with a known extrathoracic malignancy; (3) probable Pancoast tumor; (4) a cryptic nodule in a marginal surgical candidate; (5) a localized and persistent pneumonic infiltrate; and, occasionally, (6) an undiagnosed nodule in an operable patient. With respect to the latter group, it has been recommended by some that aspiration biopsy be performed preoperatively for the diagnosis of malignancy, or to obtain a precise histologic diagnosis even when a malignancy is known (e.g., small cell cancer of the lung). In practice, however, the operable patient is still often brought to thoracotomy without a preoperative needle biopsy. On the other hand, if the accuracy of a well-performed (and interpreted) percutaneous aspiration biopsy can now approach 95% or better, a negative biopsy might appropriately indicate radiographic follow-up rather than thoracotomy and an argument might be advanced for the "routine" use of percutaneous biopsy in otherwise operable patients. Spirited discussion of the indications for percutaneous biopsy in this group of patients will undoubtedly continue.[7]

Contraindications to percutaneous biopsy include an uncooperative patient, an uncontrolled cough, pulmonary arterial hypertension, a hemorrhagic diathesis, bullous emphysema, a suspected vascular lesion, or a prior contralateral pneumonectomy.

Radiologically directed percutaneous aspiration biopsy of the mediastinum has been shown to be safe and accurate. While not employed as frequently as parenchymal lung biopsy, it may be used more often in the future as its ease of performance becomes more widely realized. The indications include: (1) suspected lung cancer with possible mediastinal metastases; (2) a known extrathoracic malignancy with suspected mediastinal metastases; (3) suspected recurrence of previously-diagnosed mediastinal disease; and (4) confirmation of a suspected benign mediastinal abnormality such as a cyst. Cytopathologic techniques alone may not be optimal for the initial diagnosis of lymphoma, thymoma or a germ cell neoplasm.

Several other considerations relative to the use of percutaneous biopsy in the chest may be added. Computed tomography (CT), with its transaxial image display, has been useful in the biopsy of anterior mediastinal masses by delineating precisely the separation between mass and great vessels, thereby minimizing the risk of inadvertent needle passage through the mass into vascular structures (Figure 1). While most previous attempts at percutaneous mediastinal biopsy have been confined to anterior and posterior masses and have avoided the middle mediastinum because of the great vessels, the biopsy of large right paratracheal masses may be performed from a posterior approach with fluoroscopic guidance (Figure 2). The great vessels are easily avoided, since these masses are posterior to the superior vena cava, right innominate vein, and innominate artery, and lateral to the trachea. It may also be possible to biopsy smaller right paratracheal lesions with CT guidance.

In summary, percutaneous needle aspiration biopsy of the lung parenchyma and the mediastinum has developed as an accurate technique with acceptable complications. Its judicious application, especially in those situations where it may reasonably be expected to obviate more expensive and dangerous surgical procedures, should be encouraged. The efficacy of the needle approach will be further enhanced with additional collaborative experience involving radiologists and pathologists.

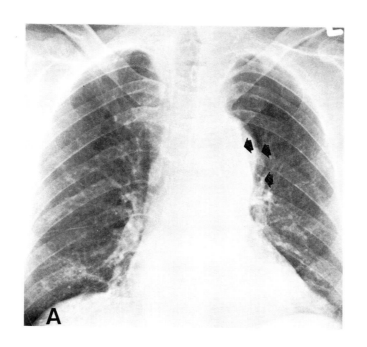

FIGURE 1

Posteroanterior chest radiograph in a patient with recent nephrectomy for hypernephroma demonstrates left-sided mediastinal lymphadenopathy (arrows in (a)). On the lateral projection, there is increased density in the retrosternal air space (arrows in (b)). Computed tomography (CT) clearly delineates left anterior mediastinal lymphadenectomy adjacent to the aortic arch (arrows in (c)). Biopsy with CT guidance using an anterior approach and a 22-gauge Chiba needle (open arrow) confirmed the suspicion of metastatic hypernephroma. The percutaneous biopsy obviated a mediastinal exploration.

Key for Figure C: S = superior vena cava; A = aortic arch; T = trachea.

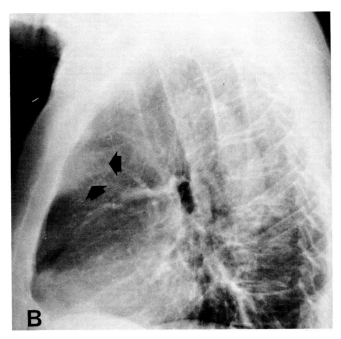

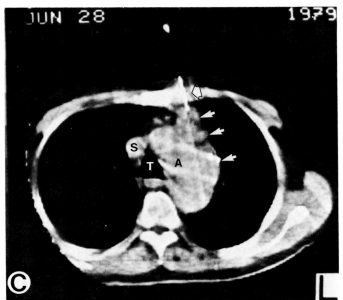

Figure 1, continued.

234

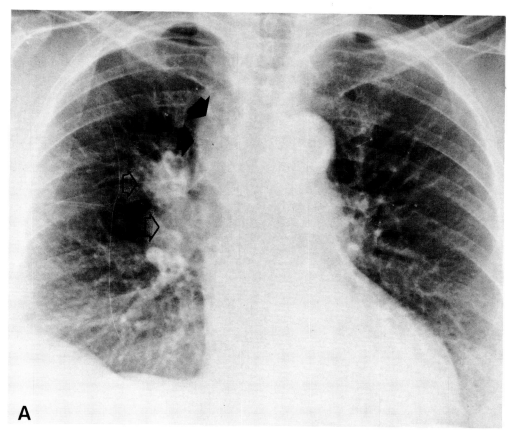

A

FIGURE 2

Another patient with previous nephrectomy for hypernephroma developed right paratracheal (arrows) and right hilar (open arrows) lymphadenopathy (a, b). CT (c) demonstrated enlarged paratracheal nodes (arrows) but no anterior mediastinal lymphadenopathy. Biopsy of the right paratracheal nodes (arrows in (d)) was performed with fluoroscopic guidance using a posterior approach and a 22-gauge Chiba needle. Metastatic hypernephroma was confirmed.

Key for Figure C: S = superior vena cava; A = aortic arch; DA = descending aorta; T = trachea.

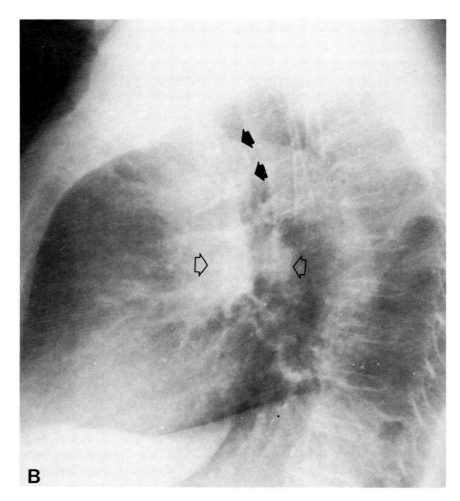

Figure 2, continued.

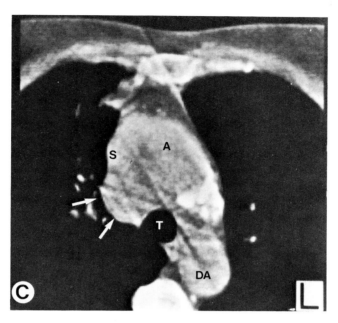

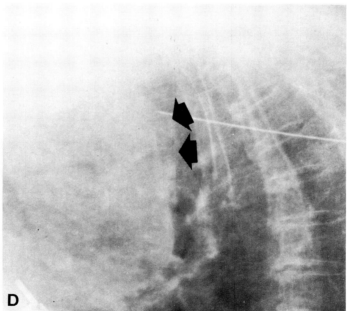

Figure 2, continued.

BIBLIOGRAPHY

1. Carter, D.   Biopsies of the lung.   In <u>Pulmonary System.   Practical Approaches to Pulmonary Diagnosis.</u> Siegelman, S.S., Stitik, F.P., Summer, W.R., eds. New York: Grune and Stratton, 1979:141-159.

2. Mark, J.D.B., Marglin, S.I., Castellino, R.A. The role of bronchoscopy and needle aspiration in the diagnosis of peripheral lung masses. <u>J. Thorac. Cardiovasc. Surg.</u> 1978; 76:266-268.

3. Herman, P.G., Hessel, S.J.   The diagnostic accuracy and complications of closed lung biopsies. <u>Radiology</u> 1977; 125:11-14.

4. House, A.J.S.   Biopsy techniques in the investigation of diseases of the lung, mediastinum and chest wall. <u>Radiol. Clin. N. Amer.</u> 1979; 17:393-412.

5. Sagel, S.S., Forrest, J.V. Fluoroscopically-assisted lung biopsy technique. In <u>Special Procedures in Chest Radiology.</u> Sagel, S.S., ed. Philadelphia: W.B. Saunders Company, 1976; 22-68.

6. Stitik, F.P.   Percutaneous lung biopsy.   In <u>Pulmonary System. Practical Approaches to Pulmonary Diagnosis.</u> Siegelman, S.S., Stitik, F.P., Summer, W.R., eds. New York: Grune and Stratton, 1979:181-219.

7. Kagan, A.R., Steckel, R.J., Braun, R.   Asymptomatic peripheral lung nodule. <u>AJR</u> 1980; 135:417-422.

Chapter 10

Thin Needle Aspiration Biopsy in the Abdomen and Pelvis (and Related Radiologic Procedures)

Zoran L. Barbaric, M.D.

INTRODUCTION

Needle aspiration biopsy can be an invaluable aid for obtaining a primary diagnosis of cancer in the abdomen, and/or in confirming metastatic spread. An example of the former is the needle biopsy confirmation of pancreatic cancer in a patient presenting with cholestatic jaundice; an example of the latter application is needle biopsy confirmation of a liver metastasis in a person with a known colon primary. Needle biopsy cannot be used when it is necessary to rule out malignancy. Even in these situations, however, it can sometimes be helpful, as when fluid is obtained unexpectedly from the biopsy needle with a renal cyst or a pancreatic pseudocyst that was thought originally to be a solid mass. Occasionally, frank pus may be aspirated (from an abscess), rather than the expected malignant cell sample. When endoscopic visualization of the primary is possible and no mass is palpable externally (as in a gastric carcinoma), an endoscopic biopsy is preferable to an attempted percutaneous needle aspiration. However, most malignancies in the pelvis and the abdomen are not amenable to endoscopic diagnosis, except for peritoneoscopy (laparoscopy) which requires specialized expertise and is attended by some morbidity. Since abdominal spread from ovarian primaries may still be quite treatable, laparotomy should be done directly following the establishment of malignant cytology (from ascitic fluid) when this diagnosis is suspected; needle biopsy of a pelvic or peritoneal mass will not adequately confirm the diagnosis.

Most primary and secondary malignant tumors within the abdomen or pelvis are, in fact, easy to diagnose using standard clinical and laboratory methods. A combination of history, physical examination, laboratory tests and simple radiographs will, in most instances, be sufficient to arrive at the proper clinical diagnosis. When the diagnosis must be verified histologically prior to deciding on appropriate management, specimens may be acquired either by exfoliative cytology or by the use of a biopsy procedure. Locally persistent or recurring tumors, for which the patient has already undergone one or more surgical interventions, may present particularly perplexing problems. Iatrogenic mishaps, such as ureteral injuries resulting in strictures, small hematomas, postoperative lymphoceles, and intra-abdominal abscesses, can all mimic recurrent or persistent neoplastic disease. In many such instances, exploratory laparotomy was formerly the only means available for excluding or confirming the presence of a malignancy.

Before subjecting a patient to exploratory laparotomy today, an alternative method for obtaining histological material should be considered. Thin-needle transperitoneal aspiration biopsy of such lesions has become the method of choice in many such instances. The technique is simple and can be done on outpatients with an extremely low likelihood of morbidity. While no radiological procedure alone (including computerized axial tomography) is

240

capable of establishing a tissue diagnosis, radiologic assistance in the performance of directed needle biopsy of a suspected malignancy is crucial to the success of this diagnostic procedure.

BRIEF HISTORY OF THE TECHNIQUE

Although Ferguson described aspiration biopsy of the prostate in 1930,[1] the technique remained practically dormant for almost 30 years. Following Papanicolaou's work, Franzed re-introduced the technique, employing a more sophisticated aspirating needle.[2] Applications of needle biopsies for the thyroid and salivary glands and for peripheral lymph nodes followed quickly. In the mid-60's, percutaneous biopsy of lung nodules was popularized, followed by percutaneous biopsy of the breast. In 1968, a large series of patients were reported with ovarian carcinoma who had transperitoneal aspiration biopsies in the hope of establishing a pre-operative diagnosis.[3] This was probably the first published report of a diagnostic transperitoneal puncture of an intra-abdominal mass. Biopsies of the pancreas and stomach followed,[4] and it became apparent that an anterior transperitoneal approach to the retroperitoneum was also feasible and could be effected with a very low incidence of complications. This was true despite the fact that the peritoneal cavity and intraperitoneal organs, including often the bowel and stomach, were traversed by the needle. Biopsies of the other intra- and retroperitoneal structures soon followed. Lymph nodes which showed abnormalities on a lymphangiogram were biopsied under radiologic guidance to differentiate inflammatory changes from metastases.[5,6,7] This experience has helped to improve the diagnostic accuracy of lymphangiographic examinations. Aspiration of periureteral lesions was another logical development,[8,9] and in fact practically every intra- and retroperitoneal structure has proved susceptible now to aspiration biopsy.

DESCRIPTION OF TECHNIQUE

The patient is pre-medicated with 0.6 mg of Atropine, subcutaneously, and the abdominal wall is cleansed with Betadine. After choosing the point of needle entry, a small amount of local anesthetic is introduced. This has proved to be the most unpleasant part of the examination for many of our patients. The tip of the aspirating needle (22 gauge) is introduced into the area of interest, the needle obturator is removed, and a 20 cc syringe is attached tightly. Suction is applied either directly, or with a special syringe handle which enhances the force of aspiration. During aspiration, the tip of the needle is moved back and forth slightly in the suspected lesion for several seconds. Aspiration is then discontinued, the needle withdrawn, and the aspirate smeared and fixed immediately in 95% alcohol by a cytopathology technologist.

Usually, three aspirating attempts are made, each time in a slightly different location within the lesion. Most smears are stained immediately, and an experienced cytopathologist determines specimen adequacy. If the specimens are inadequate, repeated aspirations are made.

To maximize diagnostic accuracy, the needle must of course be placed precisely within the area of interest; depending on the size and location of the lesion to be biopsied, various imaging modalities are used to assist in needle placement. Ultrasound and, in particular, computerized axial tomography have become popular in the last few years, allowing precise placement of the tip of the needle within the desired area.[10,11,12,13,14] Computerized tomography seems to have a slight advantage over ultrasound, since the needle tip is more readily visible on the display monitor using the former method. Placement of various skin markers or grids may further facilitate precise needle placement.[15,16] Fluoroscopy probably remains the most common imaging method employed. It is frequently augmented by the intravenous, intra-arterial, pyeloureteral (retrograde or antegrade), cholangiographic, or intralymphatic administration of contrast material.[4-9,17,18]

PRACTICAL APPLICATIONS OF NEEDLE BIOPSY

A. Liver: In many instances where histologic confirmation of metastatic malignancy in the liver is desired, thin-needle aspiration biopsy is the method of choice. This is particularly true if a known mass lesion is relatively small or is located deep within the liver parenchyma. With the help of ultrasound or CT, it is relatively easy to position the tip of the percutaneous needle precisely in the desired area of the liver.

B. Pancreas: Large pancreatic masses suspected of being carcinomas may be judged unresectable solely on the basis of clinical and radiologic criteria. However, there frequently is a need to confirm the diagnosis histologically, so that palliative treatment can be attempted. Needle biopsy is frequently indicated in these situations. Pancreatic pseudocysts and inflammatory masses may sometimes mimic pancreatic carcinomas, and their management of course is quite different.

C. Common Bile Duct: Obstructions of the common bile duct by carcinomas, benign strictures, or active inflammatory processes may commonly result in jaundice. In recent years many of these patients have had their biliary tracts decompressed with percutaneous (transhepatic) placement of a draining catheter above the level of obstruction. An antegrade cholangiogram done by instillation of contrast material through the catheter will identify the proximal extent of an obstructing lesion and may also suggest the cause. However, it is often impossible to arrive at an exact diagnosis by ductal opacification alone. Knowing where the point of the obstruction is, a thin aspirating needle can be inserted under fluoroscopic control into the area of interest and a specimen acquired for histologic diagnosis. Depending upon clinical circumstances, if the aspirate is positive for malignant cells one may then choose to place a percutaneous stent across the area of stenosis. As an option, the stent can be completely internalized, allowing for continuous drainage of bile into the second part of the duodenum.

D. Upper Urinary Tract Obstruction: A large autopsy series has shown ureteral metastases to be present in 4.3% of patients dying with disseminated cancer. In some forms of cancer, the single most common cause of death is bilateral ureteral obstruction. This is particularly true for prostatic and cervical carcinomas, where up to 37% of autopsied patients were reported to have died of this cause.[19] Most patients with metastatic deposits in or around the ureter do not exhibit hematuria, and radiologically metastatic obstruction is often indistinguishable from a nonmalignant stricture. Benign inflammatory, radiation-induced or post-operative ureteral strictures following cancer treatment are less common than malignant obstructions but are found in 1-2% of patients dying with cancer. These patients could benefit from aggressive surgical management to preserve renal function. Obviously, a correct diagnosis of the cause of ureteral obstruction is an important one to make becuase of the different treatments indicated, and a directed needle biopsy at the point of obstruction may be determinative.

E. Lymph Nodes: On lymphangiographic study, it is frequently impossible to distinguish a focal metastatic process within the lymph node from inflammatory or fibro-fatty node replacement, particularly with carcinomas or testes tumors. Aspiration biopsy of questionable nodes under fluoroscopic control has greatly improved the diagnostic accuracy of the lymphangiogram. However, aspiration biopsy of questionable retroperitoneal lymph nodes in lymphomas has not proved as successful. The tissue consistency of certain lymphomas may make them more difficult to aspirate successfully.

F. Other Retroperitoneal Masses: Retroperitoneal metastases from any primary carcinoma can be diagnosed using thin-needle aspiration, provided the lesion can be localized by clinical or radiologic means. In our experience this has been helpful for metastatic carcinomas of the appendix, rectum, bladder, prostate, cervix, breast, and others. In all cases, management of the patient was influenced by histologic verification of a disseminated process.

DIAGNOSTIC ACCURACY

In a number of reported series, thin-needle aspiration biopsy has yielded true positive results for malignancy in 80 to 100% of cases. False positive findings do not occur. True negative biopsy results are reported in approximately 60%, and false negatives in about 40%. It is obvious, therefore, that a negative needle biopsy may not contra-indicate further study in a particular patient (including exploratory surgery); however, the high yield of true positive results for confirmation of malignancy makes the technique extremely attractive. Since the study can be done on an outpatient basis with negligible morbidity (see below), it should be highly competitive with alternative procedures such as laparoscopy or exploratory surgery.

COMPLICATIONS

A fear of potential complications still precludes more liberal use of this biopsy technique in some medical centers. What is remarkable is the lack of major complications despite the fact that the peritoneal cavity and visceral organs are often transversed by the biopsy needle. Biopsy in a patient with a frank bleeding diathesis obviously is to be avoided. Peritonitis or a major hemorrhage have not been reported, and if these occur they must be very infrequent.   Smith, et al have pointed out that the caliber of the aspirating needle is smaller than commonly used suture needles.[20]   Mild vasovagal reactions are fairly frequent, and for this reason we advise pre-treatment with Atropine.[21]   We are aware of one (unreported) rectus sheath hematoma.   In our own series, antegrade placement of a nephroureterostomy catheter in one patient apparently introduced an infection into the renal collecting system which subsequently cleared.

Possible dissemination of malignancy by the biopsy procedure, either through local spillage of malignant cells, seeding along the needle tract, or hematogenous dissemination, has received considerable attention.   Few instances have actually been reported, and these occurrences must be extremely rare.[22,23,24]   In our own series we have never observed subsequent evidence of tumor seeding along the needle tract.

Continued application of transperitoneal, retroperitoneal and subperitoneal needle biopsies for confirmation of suspected abdominal and pelvic malignancies promises to have an increasing impact on the management of these patients in the future.

References

1. Ferguson, R.S.:   "Cytology of Prostate Specimens Obtained by Peri neal Aspiration Biopsy." Am. J. Surg. 9:507-511, 1930.

2. Franzen, S., Giertz, G., Zajicek: "Cytological Diagnosis of Prostatic Tumors by Transrectal Aspiration Biopsy: A Preliminary Report."   Urol. 32:193-196, 1960.

3. Kjelklgren, O., Angstrom, T., Bergman, F., Wiklund, D.E.:   "Fine   Needle Aspiration Biopsy in Diagnosis and Classification of Ovarian Càrcinoma." Cancer 28:967-977. 1960.

4. Oscarson, J., Stromby, N., Sundgren, R.:   "Selective Angiography   in Fine-Needle Aspiration Cytodiagnosis of Gastric and Pancreatic Tumors." Acta Radiolog. Diag. 12:737-743, 1972.

5. Gothlin, J.H.: "Post Lymphangiographic Percutaneous Fine-Needle Biopsy of Lymph Nodes Guided by Fluoroscopy." Radiology 120: 205-207, 1976.

6. Zornoza, J., Wallace, S., Goldstein, H.M.:   "Transperitoneal   Percutaneous Retroperitoneal Lymph Node Aspiration Biopsy." Radiology 122:111-115, 1977.

7. Zornoza, J., Johsson, K., Wallace, S., Lukeman, J.M.:   "Fine-Needle Aspiration Biopsy of Retroperitoneal Lymph Nodes and Abdominal Masses." Radiology 125:87-88, 1977.

8. Gothlin, J.M., Barbaric, Z.L.:   "Fluoroscopy-Guided   Percutaneous Transperitoneal Needle Biopsy of Renal and Periureteral Masses." Urol. 11:300-302, 1978.

9. Freiman, D.B., Ring, E.J., leaga, J.A., et al: "Thin Needle Biopsy in the Diagnosis of Ureteral Obstruction With Malignancy." Cancer 42:714-716, 1978.

10. Holm, H.H., Pedersen, J.F., Kristensen, J.K., et al: "Ultrasoni caily Guided Percutaneous Puncture." Radiol. Clin. North Am. 13:493-503, 1975.

11. Haaga, J.R., Alfidi, R.J.:   "Precise Biopsy Localization by Computed Tomography." Radiology 118:603-607, 1976.

12. Haaga, J.R., Reich, N.E., Havrilla, T.R., Alfidi, R.J.:   "Interventional CT Scanning." Radiol. Clin. North Am. 15:449-456, 1977.

13. Hancke, S., Pederson, J.F.: "Percutaneous Puncture of Pancreatic Cysts Guided by Ultrasound." Surg. Gynec-Obst. 140:361-364, 1975.

14. Hancke, S., Holm, H.M., Koch, F.: "Ultrasonically Guided Percutaneous Fine Needle Biopsy of the Pancreas." Surg. Gynec-Obst. 140:361-364, 1975.

15. Ferucci, J.T., Wittenberg, J.: "CT Biopsy of Abdominal Tumors: Aids for Lesion Localization." Radiology 128:739-744, 1978.

16. Jacques, P.F., Staab, E., Richey, W., et al: "CT Assisted Pelvic   and Abdominal Aspiration Biopsies in Gynecological Malignancy."   Radiology 128:651-655, 1978.

17. Ho, C.S., McLaughlin, M.J., McHattie, J.D., Tad, C.C.: "Percutaneous Fine Needle Aspiration Biopsy of the Pancreas Following Endoscopic Retrograde Colangiopancreatography." Radiology 125:351-353, 1977.

18. McIntosh, P.K., Thompson, K.R., Barbaric, Z.L.: "Percutaneous Trans peritoneal Lymph Node Biopsy as a Means of Improving Lymphographic Diagnosis." Radiology 131:647-649, 1979.

19. Sotto, L.S.J., Graham, J.B., Pickeren, J.W.: "Post Mortem Findings in Cancer of the Cervix: Analysis of 108 Autopsies in the Past 5 Years." Am. J. Obstet. Gynecol. 80:791-812, 1960.

20. Smith, E.H., Bartrum, R.J., Chang, Y.C.: "Percutaneous Aspiration Biopsy of the Pancreas Under Ultrasonic Guidance." N. Engl. J. Med. 292:825-828, 1975.

21. Bigongiari, L.R.: "Vagal Pseudohemorrhage After Percutaneous Biopsy." Invest. Radiol. 15:350-352, 1980.

22. von Scheeb, T., Arner, O., Skousted, G., Wingstad, N.: "Renal Adenocarcinoma: Is There Risk of Spreading Tumor Cells in Diag nostic Puncture?" Scand. J. Urol. 1:270-276, 1967.

23. Labardini, M.M., Nismith, R.M.: "Perineal Extension of Adenocarci noma of the Prostate Gland After Punch Biopsy." J. Urol. 97: 891-898, 1967.

24. Sinner, W.N., Zajicek, J.: "Implantation Metastasis After Percutane ous Transthoracic Needle Biopsy." Acta Radiol. Diag. 17:473-476, 1976.

Chapter 11

Radiologic Techniques in
Breast Cancer Screening and Diagnosis

Richard H. Gold, M.D.

It is a paradox that while the breast is the female organ most accessible to palpation, half of all breast cancers go undetected until they have already undergone regional or disseminated metastasis. Mammary carcinomas that are accidentally discovered by patients are commonly in the range of 3.5 cm in diameter. Tumors of this size are accompanied by axillary lymph node metastases in 65% of cases and are associated with five-year survival rates of only 50%. Smaller carcinomas are less frequently accompanied by axillary lymph node metastases, and in the absence of node metastases a five-year survival rate greater than 80% may be attained. Because breast cancer is generally detected "by accident", it is often locally advanced (with microscopic dissemination to distant sites) and remains the leading cause of cancer deaths in American women.

Physicians may be able to palpate a centrally located or deep breast mass as small as 1 cm in diameter, but mammography (using either film or xeroradiographic images), can disclose the presence of even smaller carcinomas - lesions that are not yet symptomatic or palpable - which are truly localized and hence potentially curable. Indeed, the primary role of x-ray mammography is the detection of breast cancer before it has grown large enough to become palpable. Mammography is the only imaging modality which now permits the detection of some cancers when they are still "minimal" - i.e., minimally invasive carcinomas whose diameter is no greater than 0.5 cm (Figure 1), or even carcinomas in situ. The importance of early detection and treatment is underlined by the fact that minimal breast cancer is associated with a 20-year survival as high as 93%.[1]

History of Mammography

An historical overview may be helpful to place mammography in perspective as a cancer detection tool. Salomon,[2] as early as 1913, used x-rays to study his surgical mastectomy specimens, but Warren (in 1930)[3] became the first to report on the clinical use of mammography. Thereafter, poor technical quality coupled with difficulties in image reproducibility led to a decline in the use of mammography. A new era began in 1956 when Egan,[4] after exhaustive trials using various x-ray techniques, developed a simple approach which gave improved image detail and was easily reproduced by others.[5]

In 1967, Gros[6] introduced molybdenum (in place of tungsten) as a more suitable material for x-ray tube targets in mammography. This resulted in improvement in image detail, but with one serious disadvantage: compared to the Egan technique, radiation exposures to the breast surface were doubled - from approximately 4 R to 8 R. Fortunately, the problem of increased dose with the molybdenum target was overcome in 1973 with the development of an imaging system incorporating a single-emulsion film and a high-definition intensifying screen, all contained with an air-evacuated polyethylene envelope. Surface exposure was reduced to one-eighth of that previously required (from approximately 8 R to 1 R per image), without degrading image quality. Beginning in 1975, several improved versions of the reduced-dose, film-screen system became available, many of which required less than one-half the exposure (500 mR) of the original version. Similarly, many manufacturers of x-ray equipment have marketed improved molybdenum target units dedicated to mammography.

Xeroradiography (xeromammography), an electrostatic technique which provides edge enhancement in x-ray-generated images, became widely available in 1972.[8,9] The radiation exposure required by this technique was similar to that originally required by the Egan film technique. However, through a combination of added filtration and internal modifications of the xeromammographic system, it has been possible to reduce the surface exposure considerably (from 3 R to less than 1 R per image).[10] It is possible further to reduce the dose by approximately 30%, by performing xeromammography in the negative mode (where soft tissues and pathologic structures appear white and the background blue instead of vice versa).

Benefits of Mammography for Screening

In the past decade mammography has undergone a striking improvement in image detail along with a corresponding decrease in radiation exposure. Improved image quality is obvious when mammograms of the 1960s, such as those performed under the auspices of the Health Insurance Plan (HIP) of New York, are compared to those of the 1970s' Breast Cancer Detection Demonstration Project (BCDDP).[11] The importance of this improvement is implied by comparing the results of the two projects. Both of these studies used a combination of physical examination and mammography. Mammography alone was responsible for the biopsy recommendation in 46.0% of the cancers in the BCDDP study, compared with 33.3% in the older HIP study. When limited to the age group under 50 years, mammography alone was responsible for the biopsy recommendation in 45.3% of the cancers detected in the BCDDP study, but in only 19.4% of those detected in the HIP study. In the later BCDDP investigation the significant contribution by mammography to case detection, especially in the detection of very early breast cancer, occurred in all age groups. Women under 50 years of age as well as 50 years of age and older had similar experiences.

As promising as these results seem, legitimate criticisms have been leveled against them, for the efficacy of mammography in a screening program has yet to be validated in women under the age of 50 years. This lack of validation stems from several factors: First, it is possible that mortality was not lowered in the age group under 50 years among casecontrolled HIP screenees, because very few cancers 1 cm or less in diameter were discovered among these screenees; on the other hand, approximately one-third of the cancers detected among the BCDDP screenees were less than 1 cm (as stated, a possible explanation for the HIP failure to detect more small cancers was the poorer image detail in the older HIP mammography technique, as compared to more current BCDDP mammography techniques). Furthermore, image detail is of particular importance in mammography with younger women, whose breasts normally contain less fat to serve as a contrasting background upon which one can see a cancer. Second, the BCDDP was not a case-controlled study. BCDDP screenees lacked a suitable control group against which breast cancer mortality might be measured. It is not possible, therefore, to accept uncritically the proposition that the high proportion of early stage breast cancers detected in BCDDP screenees is evidence of benefit, for it is not known when and at what stage of disease those cases would ordinarily have been detected without formal screening. Finally, and of extreme importance, there is a lack of knowledge about the natural history of patients classified in the BCDDP as "noninfiltrating cancers", some of whom conceivably might never have developed clinical disease.

As shown in the BCDDP study, mammography is capable of detecting breast cancer in a preclinical state, before the appearance of a palpable mass. Over an eight-year period after diagnosis in the HIP screening program, breast cancer paients who were positive only on mammography had a case fatality rate of 14%, compared to 32% for patients positive only on physical examination and 41% for those positive by both modalities. Excluding mammography would have reduced the benefit of screening by an estimated one-third.[12] Although the impact of these HIP results was confined to women 50 years of age and older, it is possible that with the newer mammography equipment younger women would have benefited. Clearly, with the striking technical advances and lower doses that are now possible in mammography, randomized control trials under the age of 50 years, with long-term follow-up as advocated by the Beahrs Group[11] and by Thier[13], are defensible. This will be the only way to resolve questions concerning: (a) the magnitude of benefit achieved in screening with mammography and physical examination under the age of 50 years; (b) the magnitude of the benefit attributable to mammography alone, in this age group; (c) the effect when screening is scheduled less frequently than annually; and (d) the effect on survival, if any, when in situ carcinomas are detected.

Risks of Mammography for Screening

The report of Upton and his NCI Working Group on the Risks Associated with Mammography in Mass Screening for the Detection of Breast Cancer[14] noted that epidemiologic studies had revealed an excess of breast cancer in three groups: (1) American women treated with x-ray radiation of the breast for postpartum mastitis; (2) American and Canadian women subjected to multiple fluoroscopic examinations of the chest during artificial pneumothorax treatment of pulmonary tuberculosis; and (3) Japanese women surviving atomic bomb irradiation.

In two of these three groups, women who were fluoroscoped and Japanese bomb survivors, the risks of irradiation decreased with age. The risk appeared to be greatest in young women, and a considerably lower risk was observed in women over 35 years. In the postpartum mastitis study there was no difference in risk according to age, but few women in that study were over 40 years. While the relationship between dose and "response" (number of cancers) was assumed to be linear, at the lowest calculated dose levels (0 to 9 rads) there was no observed difference in the number of breast cancers between women who were not exposed to radiation and those who were exposed. Thus, it would seem that women who are at the greatest risk of developing breast cancer, those over 40 years, have the least risk of developing it as a result of radiation to the breast, and, in fact, in two of the three studies evaluated by Upton little or no risk was observed.

According to Upton, a single examination performed with a mammographic technique that involves an average dose to the breast of less than 1 rad should be expected to increase a woman's subsequent risk of breast cancer by much less than 1% of the natural risk (which is 7% at age 35), and by a progressively smaller percentage with increasing age at examination. To put it another way, risk at 35 years would increase from 7% to 7.07%.

It is now possible for a radiologist to perform a complete, highquality mammographic examination using considerably less than 500 millirads (0.5 R) to the mid-breast. The BCDDP provided information on the lowest dose to the breast then attainable through mammography that was still consistent with maintenance of high diagnostic quality. In June, 1977, according to the BCDDP data gathered by the Regional Centers for Radiologic Physics and compiled by the American Association of Physicists in Medicine, the average mid-breast dose in a complete film examination was 0.067 rad (67 millirads) and in a complete xeromammographic examination 0.61 rad. Assuming that the risk analysis of Upton and his group is the best currently available, a total dose of 1 rad to the mid-breast would allow 13 annual mammographic examinations before the patient's breast cancer risk was increased from the "natural" risk level of 7% to a risk level of 8%. A dose of 0.5 rad to the mid-breast during each examination would permit 26 annual mammograms to be performed before the 7% risk was increased to 8%; and a dose of 1/3 rad to the breast would permit 39 annual mammograms to occur before the risk was increased to 8%. At the University of California, Los Angeles (UCLA), using film-screen technique with a Phillips "mammo Diagnost" x-ray unit, the mid-breast dose is 100 millirads (0.100 R) for a complete two-view examination. At this dose level, more than 100 annual mammographic examinations should be possible before the risk is increased by 1%!

Xeromammography and film-screen mammography, while excellent methods for cancer detection, each have drawbacks as well as advantages. Relative soft-tissue densities are sometimes evaluated more reliably with film-screen images, while calcifications are sometimes seen better in xeromammographic images. Film-screen mammography tends to evaluate fatty or fibro-fatty breasts more reliably than xeromammography, while the latter tends to image dense, dysplastic breasts better than the former.

At UCLA, both film-screen and xeromammographic techniques are available and have been used fo tailor individual mammographic examinations to obtain the greatest information with the lowest possible doses of radiation. With women under 35 years who have strong indications for mammography (usually meaning signs or symptoms which raise a possibility of breast cancer), two film-screen images of each breast are obtained. With some women between 35 and 49 years, depending upon the film images obtained, a single negative-mode, highly filtered xeromammogram (150 millirads to mid-breast) may be added. For some women 50 years and over, a single positive-mode, highly filtered xeromammogram (200 millirads to the mid-breast) may be used to complement the filmscreen images. A correlative physical examination of the breasts by the mammographer or by a nurse under his/her supervision is routinely performed with each mammographic examination, to aid the mammographic interpretation.

In summary, with current techniques early (nonpalpable) breast cancer can be detected through mammography with x-ray exposures that are below the levels at which any cancers have been identified in any of the published studies of radiation hazard. Referring physicians and their patients will nevertheless do well to question the radiologist regarding his/her dose: most radiologists are extremely aware of the sensitive nature of this problem and are quite willing to provide the requested information.

An essential requirement of any technique for cancer detection is that it provide the greatest benefit with the least risk. When performed and interpreted by experienced, well-trained personnel using highly specialized and carefully-monitored equipment, mammography in combination with physical examination can satisfy this requirement. Careful and continued monitoring is essential! Bicehouse[15] examined the surface exposures delivered by mammography units in 70 medical facilities in eastern Pennsylvania and found that some facilities were delivering excessive radiation, while others were employing too little radiation to permit adequate image detail. Since that time, the Bureau of Radiological Health of the Food and Drug Administration has developed a mammography quality assurance program to minimize patient exposures and to improve image quality. This joint FederalState program, called BENT (Breast Exposure: Nationwide Trends), currently operates in most of the 50 states and the District of Columbia, serving over 3,500 mammography units.[16] The BENT program operates in four phases: groundwork, evaluation, follow-up survey, and re-evaluation. Facilities are mailed a dosimetry card for each mammographic unit. The card is exposed to x-rays as if it were a breast and returned to the State-based agency for analysis; the mammography facility subsequently receives a report on its exposure level. High or unusually low exposures lead to follow-up visits by State physics personnel who recommend specific improvements in mammographic technique. Finally, the effects of implementing these recommendations are assessed by subsequent mailing of dosimetry cards several months later. The Bureau of Radiological Health in cooperation with members of the Committee on Mammography Equipment of the American College of Radiology, is now evaluating mammography physics phantoms for the purpose of developing better methods for image quality control.

Education programs in mammography have yielded improved technical and interpretive ability and a renewed awareness by radiologists of its potential risks and benefits. In 1975 the National Cancer Institute supported a new training program at seven U.S. institutions in a threeyear effort to re-orient radiologists and their technologists to more advanced mammographic techniques and improved interpretation for the detection of early breast cancer. At these demonstration teaching institutions, highly filtered xeromammography, reduced-dose film-screen mammography, physical examination, and thermography were taught through on-the-job training as well as by didactic teaching and audiovisual materials supplied by the American College of Radiology. Anatomic, physiologic, and pathologic correlations were stressed as well as the need (and reasons) for dose reduction. Epidemiology, pre-operative needle localization of clinically occult but suspicious lesions, and specimen radiography were fundamental components of these week-long, continuous training programs.

For the past two decades, the American College of Radiology has also supported and planned annual week-long multidisciplinary conferences and workshops aimed at the earlier detection and treatment of breast cancer. Similarly, a large number of skilled mammographers and technologists have continued to present local postgraduate refresher courses and workshops in mammography. While these initiatives have stimulated the training of radiology residents in mammography, an equally important stimulus was the decision of the American Board of Radiology to include questions specifically relating to mammography in both the written and oral certifying examinations.

Indications for X-Ray Mammography

What can now be considered a reasonable overall approach to the performance of mammography? Are there groups of women at higher risk for the development of breast cancer, and is it reasonable to examine these women earlier and with greater regularity than the average woman? Some risk factors correlate highly with the development of breast cancer: for example, a patient with a previous history of breast cancer has an increased risk for a second cancer of five-to-seven times; if a patient's mother had breast cancer, there is a 2-to-3-times greater risk than average, and if the mother had bilateral premenopausal breast cancer, the increased risk is nine-fold. Furthermore, evidence indicates that risk factors are additive: the greater the number of risk factors, the greater the chance of breast cancer.

Given our present knowledge of benefits and potential risks, the following is a reasonable approach:

(1) Mammography should be performed at any age when clinical findings indicate a suspicion of cancer. On the other hand it should not be performed in women under the age of 35 except when there are specific, strong clinical indications. The incidence of carcinoma in this age group is quite low.

(2) A single baseline mammogram should be performed in the age period of 35 to 40 years, for several reasons: a small but significant number of early cancers will be detected; a single study will provide the essential baseline for assessing subtle changes in subsequent mammograms that may indicate cancer; and there is increasing evidence that the radiologic breast patterns can be used to a certain extent as indicators of higher or lower risk categories.

(3) Periodic mammography with low-level radiation factors may be performed in women between the ages of 35 and 49 years, but the periodicity of such examinations should be linked to an individual analysis of relative risk factors. For asymptomatic women 50 years of age and older, annual or at least periodic mammography is statistically justified to screen for breast cancer.

Mammography is important not only for examining palpable breast lesions before they can be evaluated by the pathologist, but also for evaluating both breasts pre-operatively for mammographic signs of clinically occult cancer. Should ominous findings be detected in an area other than the area to be biopsied, a biopsy specimen of the radiographically suspicious area also should be obtained.

Just as mammography should not be expected to replace a good physical examination, physical examination of the breast does not replace mammography. A negative mammogram or a negative physical examination should never deter the biopsy of a suspicious lesion that has been detected by either method. Mammography cannot be relied upon invariably to differentiate benign from malignant disease. The capability of mammography to reveal a carcinoma or an alteration in breast architecture that might signify an underlying carcinoma is largely dependent upon the presence of sufficient fat in the breast to serve as a contrasting radiolucent background. Mammography may indicate an obvious carcinoma that is only a few millimeters in diameter in a breast in which all glandular tissues have been replaced by fat (Figure 1). However, in breasts that contain predominantly radiopaque tissues instead of fat (such as those of young, nulliparous, pregnant or lactating women, and in breasts manifesting severe mammary dysplasia), even a large carcinoma may be obscured by the dense tissue surrounding it. Thus mammography should be considered to be of limited value in severe dysplasia, pregnancy, or lactation.

Preoperative Needle Localization and Specimen Radiography

All suspicious clusters of calcifications recognized on mammography should be biopsied, with the expectation that in some cases they will be found to result not from malignancy but from benign disease (usually sclerosing adenosis). Similarly, any alteration of breast architecture that could signify a malignant desmoplastic reaction requires a biopsy, although benign disorders such as sclerosing adenosis and fat necrosis may manifest an identical fibrous connective tissue response to that of cancer.

To reduce the size of the biopsy specimen and to improve the accuracy of localization of suspicious findings, percutaneous transfixion of the lesion with a narrow-gauge needle may be performed just prior to surgery (Figure 2A). As an alternative to leaving the needle in place, after confirmatory mammograms show the needle to be in close proximity to the lesion a drop of methylene blue may be injected pre-operatively and the needle then withdrawn; the dye then acts as a surgical landmark.

Pre-operative needle localization does not alter the need for a postoperative specimen radiograph to confirm that the lesion was actually included in the excised biopsy specimen (Figure 2B). If the radiograph of the surgical specimen fails to reproduce the suspicious mammographic findings, excision of additional tissue, followed again by radiography, is required until the findings are corroborated. However, since the processing of xeromammograms and film-screen mammograms takes 90 seconds or less, the performance of additional specimen radiography should not unduly prolong the operation.

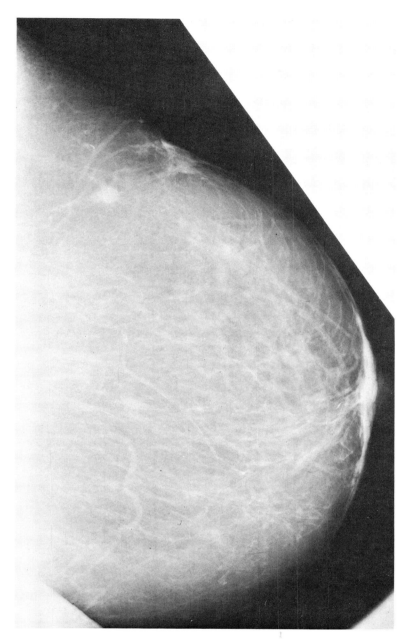

Figure 1. Five-mm. carcinoma in the upper hemisphere of the breast. On histologic examination only minimal invasion was detected, permitting the lesion to be classified as a "minimal" carcinoma. The cancer is welloutlined by surrounding fat. However, were this to have been a dysplastic, dense breast, there is a strong likelihood that the carcinoma would have gone undetected because of the lack of a contrasting (radiolucent) background.

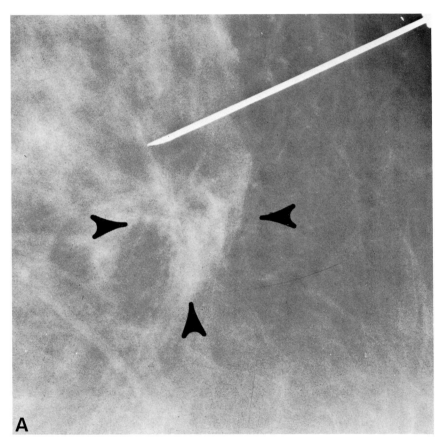

Figure 2. One-centimeter scirrhous carcinoma: (A) to reduce the size of the biopsy specimen and to improve the accuracy of localizing the suspicious findings, percutaneous transfixion of the lesion with a narrowgauge needle has been performed just prior to surgery; (B) a radiograph of the excised biopsy specimen confirms that the lesion is within the specimen.

Figure 2, continued.

For the detection, excision, and evaluation of nonpalpable breast cancer, the surgeon, mammographer, and pathologist muork together closely as a team. Only permanent histologic sections should be relied upon for the diagnosis of lesions less than 0.5 cm in diameter. Following confirmation of the lesion on a specimen radiograph, the specimen should be cut into serial slices 3 to 4 mm in thickness, the slices laid out and numbered with radiopaque markers, and radiographs made of them. The mammographer then identifies for the pathologist the radiographically suspicious region(s) within a given tissue slicethat is likely to provide the most productive area for permanent histologic sections. If the permanent sections reveal that a lesion is indeed malignant, additional treatment may be undertaken after further consultation with the patient and with added confidence in the diagnosis.

The Mammographic Examination

The mammographic examination includes mediolateral and cephalocaudal views of both breasts. Since these views are at right angles to each other, they permit the mammographer to make a three-dimensional assessment which allows suspicious lesions to be localized not only by their breast quadrant but also by their "clock face" location and relative depth. The mediolateral view may include the axilla. A special view of the axilla itself is not obtained routinely, because it results in more radiation exposure than the other views and seldom provides information about the axillary nodes that is not readily obtainable through palpation. Lymph node metastases arising from mammary carcinoma rarely exhibit characteristic malignant-type calcifications. Furthermore, the apparent size of axillary lymph nodes as displayed radiographically, is a poor measure of metastatic involvement. Small nodes may harbor metastases while large ones may be free of tumor. Some film-screen mammographers use an oblique view as a supplement to, or in place of, the mediolateral view. The oblique view often permits visualization of more of the posterior portion of the breast than the mediolateral view.

Basic Mammographic Features of Benign and Malignant Disease

Breast cancer is normally distributed in patterns that appear bilaterally symmetric on mammograms. Asymmetry of the breast patterns may result from mammary dysplasia or a prior surgical excision or, most importantly, deposition of fibrous connective tissue in response to a carcinoma (Figure 3). Cooper's ligaments are normal tooth-like projections of the peripheral skin to the superficial layer of the superficial fascia. Carcinomas may evoke fibrosis in their vicinity, causing the Cooper's ligaments to shorten, a condition that is the basis for the skin retraction often associated with an underlying malignancy. Similarly, elaboration of fibrous tissue in response to a carcinoma may thicken the walls of ducts within the breast, increasing their prominence on mammograms, and eventually causing them to shorten and to result in nipple retraction.

A cluster of tiny, finely stippled, angular, lacy or branching calcifications is characteristic, albeit not pathognomonic of malignancy (Figure 4). Unfortunately, cancers exhibit these mammographic calcifications in no more than half the cases. Moreover, some benign disorders such as fat necrosis, apocrine metaplasia and sclerosing adenosis (Figure 3B) may occasionally

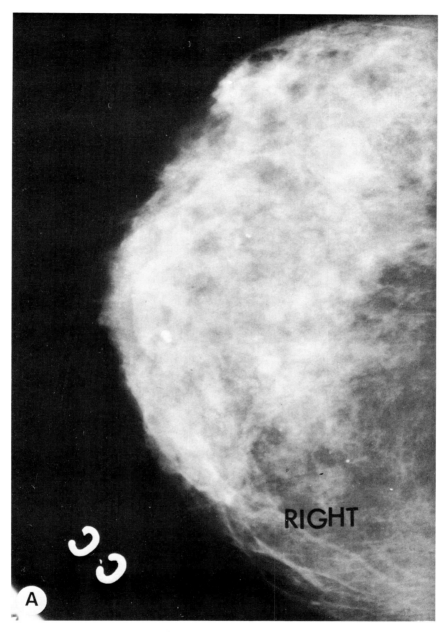

Figure 3. Nonpalpable carcinoma of the left breast in an asymptomatic woman: (A) diffuse nodularity in the right breast signifies mammary dysplasia, but no sign of malignancy is seen; (B) in the left breast, an area of duct prominence and fibrillary, fibrous tissue proliferation (encircled by small arrowheads) results from a carcinoma; a 5 mm cluster of microcalcifications (large arrowhead), while suspicious for carcinoma, was actually in a focus of sclerosing adenosis.

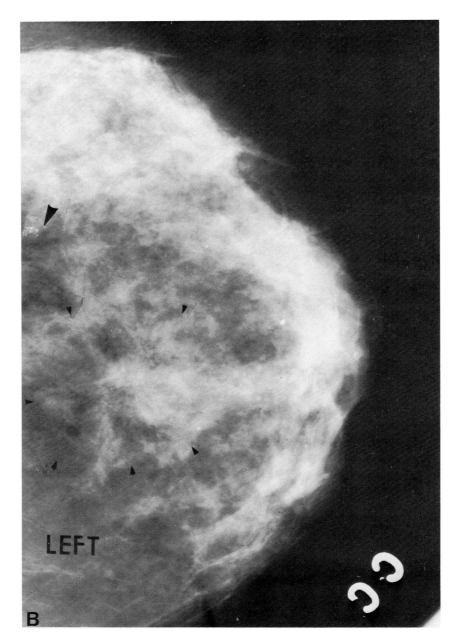

Figure 3, continued.

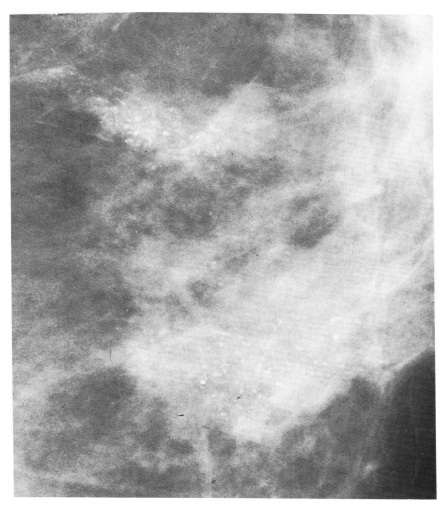

Figure 4. Multicentric carcinoma as signified by two clusters of numerous, tiny, finely stippled, angular and branching microcalcifications. The upper lesion measured 1.5 cm in greatest diameter, and the lower 2.0 cm.

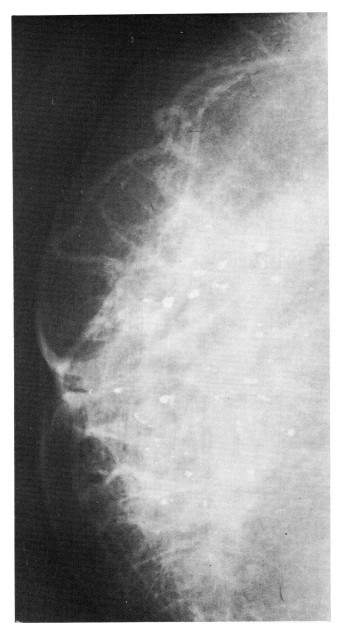

Figure 5.   Scattered, ring-shaped calcifications reflecting benign secretory disease.

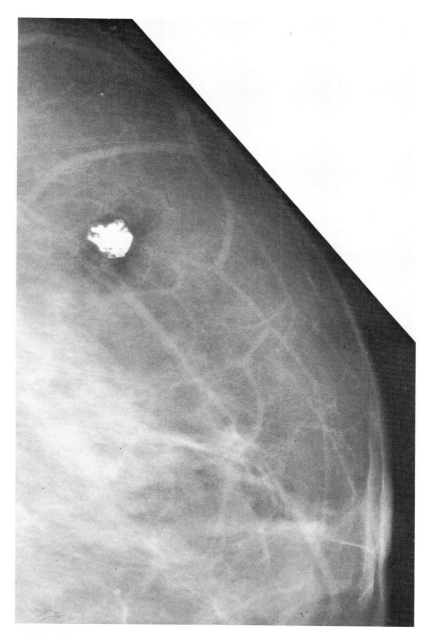

Figure 6. Calcifying fibroadenoma: here the characteristically large, amorphous calcification has completely replaced the fibroadenoma.

manifest identical calcifications. The calcifications in these benign disorders, however, are usually rounder in shape and tend to be fewer in number and more scattered in distribution than the more numerous and irregularly shaped calcifications associated with carcinomas. Intraductal papillomas may contain a rosette pattern of several small calcifications that sometimes mimics those of malignancy. Scattered, ring-shaped, or coarse linear calcifications are characteristic of benign secretory disease (Figure 5). Fibroadenomas, the most common solid benign tumor of the breast, may hyalinize and form large, amorphous calcifications that may eventually replace the mass (Figure 6). Calcified arteries appear mammographically as broken parallel lines of calcium in the breast.

"Early cancer" is defined as cancer of the breast that is asymptomatic, too small to be palpable, and without metastases. The mammographic features of such lesions include one or more of the following: a circumscribed cluster

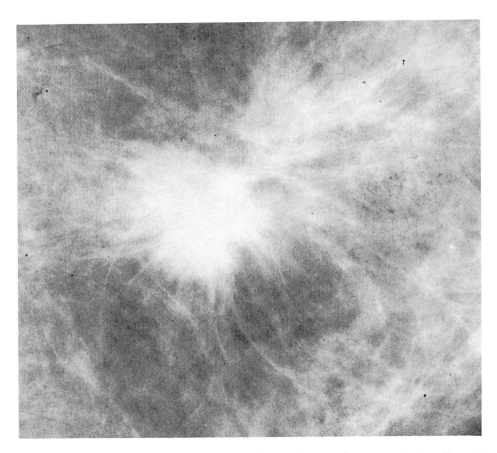

Figure 7. Scirrhous carcinoma measuring 2 cm in greatest diameter, and characterized by an irregular border consisting of spicules of fibrous connective tissue and cords of tumor cells aggressively infiltrating the surrounding breast tissue.

of stippled microcalcifications (as described above), a segmental prominence of one or more ducts, and a localized distortion of the breast architecture (Figure 3B). The latter two features reflect a desmoplastic reaction. Indeed, if the cancer is truly early or minimal, any or all of these signs are usually noted <u>in the absence of mammographic evidence of a mass.</u>

Breast carcinoma tends at the beginning to grow slowly and sometimes remains intraductal for years, but it eventually invades the ductal basement membrane. The vast majority of these are designated infiltrating ductal carcinomas, but they are also described as <u>scirrhous carcinomas</u> because of the prominent desmoplastic reaction that they incite, which results in a characteristic rock-hard induration. The key mammographic feature which distinguishes a locally-advanced carcinoma from most benign breast masses is its irregular margin, reflecting spicules of fibrous connective tissue and cords of tumor cells that aggressively infiltrate the surrounding tissue (Figures 7 and 8). Less aggressive carcinomas may appear more circumscribed and may

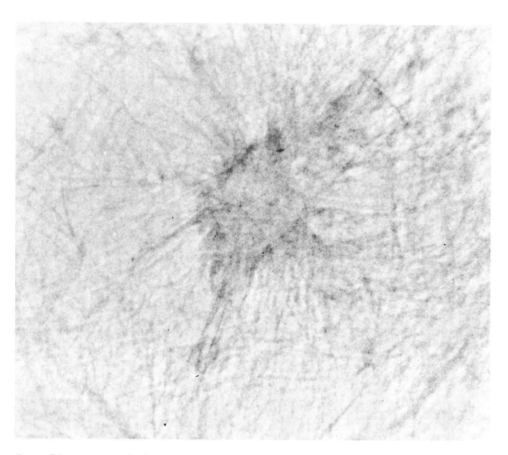

<u>Figure 8.</u> Close-up of 2 cm carcinoma from a xeromammogram: this is the same lesion shown on the film study in Figure 7, and illustrates well the characteristic spiculated border of a scirrhous carcinoma.

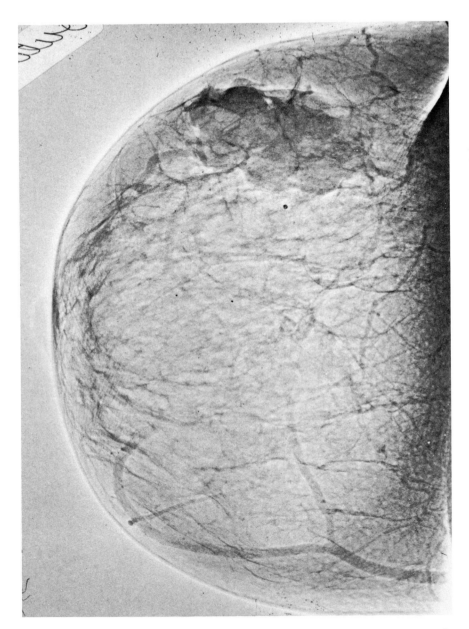

Figure 9. Papillary carcinoma shown on a xeromammogram: the lesion is characterized by an irregular and indistinct margin, but without spiculation. This is an example of a less aggressive, well-circumscribed carcinoma which has a more favorable prognosis than scirrhous carcinoma.

resemble benign lesions, both clinically and mammographically. Examples of these well-circumscribed carcinomas include <u>papillary carcinomas</u> (Figure 9), <u>medullary carcinoma</u>, and <u>colloid (mucinous) carcinomas</u>. These less aggressve (and less frequent) lesions have a more favorable prognosis than scirrhous carci-nomas. While the majority of breast carcinomas are infiltrative, benign masses such as <u>cysts</u> (Figure 10) and <u>fibroadenomas</u> (Figure 11) appear sharply circumscribed on the mammograms.

Comedocarcinoma of the breast frequently results in a characteristic branching pattern of calcifications (Figure 12). This tumor forms plugs of desquamated cells within the ducts. When these cells become necrotic they may calcify, accounting for the branching pattern as the calcifications follow the duct ramifications. In many cases comedocarcinoma may extend throughout much of the duct system and still remain entirely intraductal (noninvasive) and

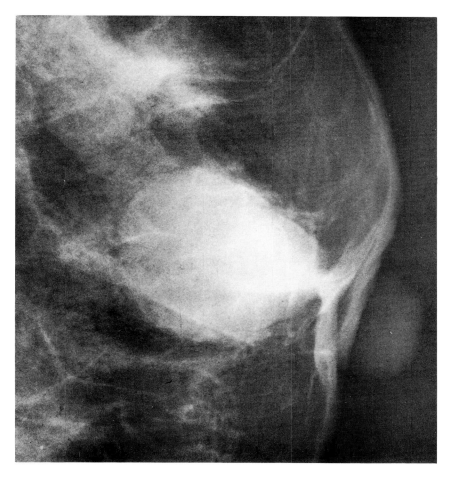

<u>Figure 10</u>. Cyst measuring 2 cm in greatest diameter and characterized by a smooth, sharp border.

frequently   nonpalpable;   accordingly,   the   importance   of   mammographic
recognition of the characteristic calcifications cannot be over-emphasized.

Lobular carcinoma is a less common type and is difficult to detect
mammographically.   It is usually found in dysplastic breasts and tends not to
form a distinct mass.   When calcifications are associated with a lobular
carcinoma, they tend to occur in smaller numbers and are more scattered in
distribution than the usual calcifications of scirrhous carcinoma.

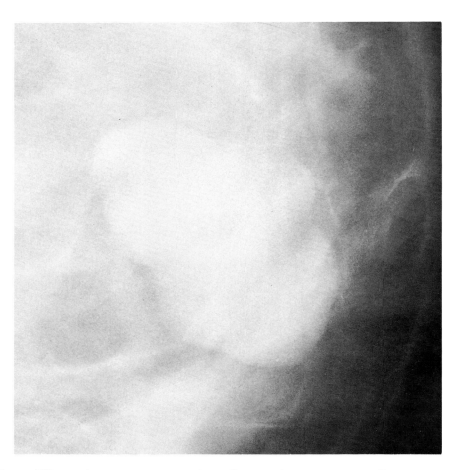

Figure 11.   Fibroadenoma, measuring 3 cm in greatest diameter and characterized by a smooth margin and a lobulated shape.

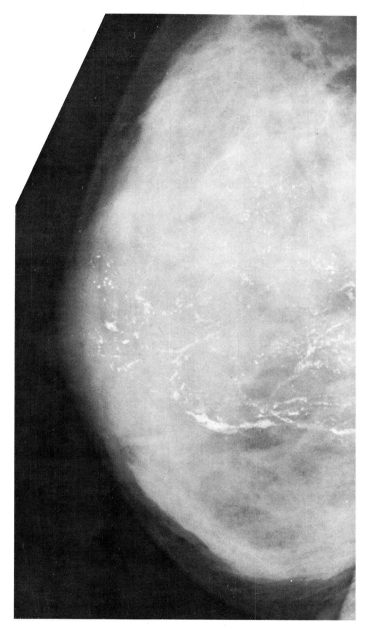

Figure 12. Comedocarcinoma characterized by branching, punctate micro-calcifications extending throughout much of the duct system. The patient was only 28 years old; the lesion, while extensive, was not palpable and on histologic examination was shown to be completely intraductal (noninvasive).

Parenchymal Patterns as Risk Markers for Breast Cancer

According to Wolfe,[17] mammographic patterns can be used to predict which women are most likely to develop breast cancer and which are least likely. Wolfe's four patterns, in order of increasing risk, are as follows: N1, lowest risk - breast parenchyma composed entirely of fat with (at most) small amounts of dysplastic tissue and no visible ducts; P1, low risk - parenchyma is primarily fat with prominent ducts in the anterior portion of the breast which occupy up to one-fourth of the breast volume or (alternatively, this pattern may be relected by a thin band of ducts extending only into one quadrant); P2, high risk -prominent ducts occupying more than one-fourth of the breast volume; and DY, highest risk - severe dysplasia, which in its most severe form appears homogenous and may obscure an underlying prominent duct pattern. A fifth pattern, QDY (Question DY), is useful in the classification of women with an apparent "DY pattern" who are under the age of 40, because of a tendency for this pattern to revert to a lower risk pattern at about that age.

Stated more generally, N1 and P1 together may be considered as lowrisk patterns, whereas P2 and DY together may be considered as high-risk patterns. At the extremes Wolfe noted a 37-times greater incidence of breast cancer n the highest risk group (DY) as in the lowest risk group (N1). Others have confirmed Wolfe's results qualitatively, but have found a much lesser risk differential between the DY and N1 groups.

The Wolfe classification appears to have two applications: first, a woman in the highest-risk group should probably be watched more carefully for the development of breast cancer, with a regimen that includes instructions in breast self-examination, periodic physical examination and mammography with appropriate indication. The second application concerns screening for breast cancer, where parenchymal patterns may eventually be coupled with other risk factors to permit the concentration of mammographic screening on a smaller segment of the population, thus improving the benefit-to-risk ratio.

The mammographic appearance of parenchymal breast patterns can also be correlated with histology. N1 breasts show normal stroma, ducts, and lobules. P1 breasts have mild-to-moderate periductal and perilobular fibrosis, with some atypical lobules and low-grade lesions. P2 breasts are similar to P1 breasts, but with more fibrosis and more atypical lobules. DY breasts have even more atypical lobules and extensive, confluent fibrosis. The highest grades of precancerous epithelial abnormality are also found in the P2 and DY categories, seldom in P1 and very rarely in N1. In short, mammographic patterns and histologic risk grading reveal an overall close correlation.

Computer-Assisted Tomographic (CAT) Mammography

In CAT scanning a narrow x-ray beam rotates about the anatomical part being examined to produce a cross-sectional image with the assistance of a computer. The intravenous administration of radiopaque contrast medium may increase the quantity of information available.

Although the results of preliminary investigations on the detection of breast cancer and precancerous lesions by CAT scanning have been promising, two current drawbacks are the risk of intravenous injections of iodinated contrast material and the high cost of a scanner dedicated to breast diagnosis. The results of preliminary investigations[18] have revealed preferential uptake of iodine and, hence, significant contrast enhancement in CAT scans for carcinoma (Figure 13), fibroadenoma, and atypical duct hyperplasia. Only minimal contrast enhancement seems to occur in other benign (predominantly fibrotic and cystic) lesions.

Thermography

The future of thermography as a screening modality for detecting early breast cancer is clouded. Thermography was positive in only 43% of the cases of cancer detected during the first two years of the BCDDP.[11] Moreover, if thermography had been used in conjunction with physical examination but without mammography, 37.1% of the cancers less than 1 cm in diameter would have gone undetected in the first annual screen and 44% in the second annual screen. Thus, most false negatives with thermography, seem to occur in cancers that are subclinical and therefore most amenable to therapy. At present, thermography is most valuable as an adjunct to mammography and physical examination; it should never be used as the sole modality in a screening program.

A number of investigators have shown that the sensitivity of breast thermograms is directly related to cancer size and that a direct correlation also exists between aggressive cellular characteristics, shorter tumor doubling times, and the degree of thermographic positivity. Conceivably then, the degree of positivity could prove to be a useful semiquantitative means of assessing prognosis.

Microfocal Spot Magnification Mammography for the Assessment of Calcifications

Conventional mammography with either film-screen or xeroradiographic recording systems has two major limitations in the evaluation of isolated clusters of breast calcifications. First, it does not detect all of the microcalcifications that are present histologically. Second, conventional mammography is often unable to differentiate benign from malignant calcifications (see above); this results in equivocal interpretations, that may in turn lead to many biopsies of benign lesions and/or to deferred biopsies for what may later prove to be carcinomas. Magnification mammography using a microfocal spot x-ray tube can address this problem by producing sharper, more detailed images of microcalcifications in the breast.[19]

Laboratory investigations have shown that 1.5 X magnification mammograms are superior in quality to the best conventional mammographic images because of increased resolution and reduced image mottling.[20] Clinical evaluations have also been encouraging, indicating that improved image quality leads to increased accuracy of diagnostic interpretation. At the present time, microfocal spot magnification mammography is ready to be used as an adjunct to conventional mammography and may permit a substantial reduction in the number of biopsies for benign breast lesions. Unfortunately, magnification

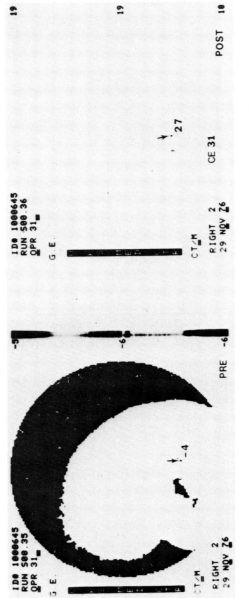

Figure 13. Minimal carcinoma of the breast detected by computed tomography. Pre-contrast injection scan on the left: no sign of cancer. Post-contrast injection scan on the right: there is a tiny area with considerable contrast enhancement (a change of 31 CT units, or a 6.2% increase in density), indicating cancer (Courtesy C.H. Joseph Chang, M.D., and the American Journal of Roentgenology.

mammography requires an increased radiation exposure in comparison to conventional screen-film mammography. This limitation has prevented magnification mammography from taking the place of non-magnified images for routine mammographic examinations. Methods to diminish the radiation exposure are now being investigated. One of these[21] is the use of a fast, double-emulsion film/double-screen combination together with a microfocal spot x-ray tube having a rotating anode and a high-heat load capacity (in place of the single-emulsion film/single-screen combination and stationary anode microfocal spot x-ray tube currently in use). Although the imaging properties of a fast film-screen system are generally less than optimal, overall image quality has been considerably enhanced as a result of magnification.

References

1. Frazier, T.G., Copeland, E.M., Gallager, H.S., Paulus, D.D. Jr., White, E.C.: Prognosis and treatment in minimal breast cancer. Am J Surg 133:697-701, 1977.

2. Salomon, A.: Beitrage zur pathologie und klinik des mammakarzinoms. Arch f Klin Chir 101:573-668, 1913.

3. Warren, S.L.: Roentgenologic study of the breast. Am J Roentgenol 24:113-124, 1930.

4. Egan, R.L.: Experience with mammography in a tumor institution. Evaluation of 1,000 studies. Radiology 75:894-900, 1960.

5. Clark, R.C., Copeland, M.M., Egan, R.L., Gallager, H.S., Geller, H., Lindsay, J.P., Robbins, L.C., White, E.C.: Reproducibility of the technic of mammography (Egan) for cancer of the breast. Am J Surg 109:127-133, 1965.

6. Gros, C.M.: Methodologie. Symposium sur le sein. J de Radiologie d'Electrol 48:638-655, 1967.

7. Ostrum, B.J., Becker, W., Isard, H.J.: Low-dose mammography. Radiology 109:323-326, 1973.

8. Wolfe, J.N.: Xerography of the breast. Radiology 91:231-240, 1968.

9. Martin, J.E.: Xeromammography - an improved diagnostic method: review of 250 biopsied cases. Am J Roentgenol 117:90-96, 1973.

10. Van de Riet, W.G., Wolfe, J.N.: Dose reduction in xeroradiography of the breast. Am J Roentgenol 128:821-823, 1977.

11. Beahrs, O.H., Shapiro, S., Smart, C., et al: Report of the working group to review the National Cancer Institute - American Cancer Society Breast Cancer Detection Demonstration Projects. J Natl Cancer Inst 62:640-709, 1979.

12. Shapiro, S.: Evidence on screening for breast cancer from a randomized trial. Cancer 39:2772-2782, 1977.

13. Thier, S.D.: Breast cancer screening: a view from outside the controversy. New Eng J Med 297:1063-1065, 1977.

14. Upton, A.C.: Report of NCI Ad Hoc Working Group on the risks associated with mammography in mass screening for the detection of breast cancer. J Natl Cancer Inst 59:481-493, 1977.

15. Bicehouse, H.J.:   Survey of mammographic exposure levels and tech
    nique used in Eastern Pennsylvania.   In Proceedings of the Seventh
    Annual National Cancer Conference on iation Control.   Hyannis,
    Massachusetts, April 27-May 2, DHEW Publication 76-8026, 1975.

16. Jans, R.G., Butler, P.F., McCrohan, J.L. Jr., Thompson, W.E.:   The
    status of film-screen mammography.   Results of the BENT Study.
    Radiology 132:197-200, 1979.

17. Wolfe, J.N.:   Risk for breast cancer development determined by
    mammographic parenchymal pattern. Cancer 37:2486-2492, 1976.

18. Chang, C.H.J., Sibala, J.L., Fritz, S.L., Dwyer, S.J. III,   Templeton,
    A.W.: Specific value of computed tomographic breast   scanner (CT/M)
    in diagnosis of breast diseases. Radiology 132:   647-652, 1979.

19. Sickles, E.A.: Further experience with microfocal spot magnifica   tion
    mammography in the assessment of clustered breast microcalci   fications.
    Radiology 137:9-14, 1980.

20. Haus, A.G., Paulus, D.D., Dodd, G.D., Cowart, R.W., Bencomo, J.:
    Magnification mammography: evaluation of screen-film and xero
    radiographic techniques. Radiology 223-226, 1979.

21. Arnold, B.A., Eisenberg, H., Bjarngard, B.E.:   Magnification mammo
    graphy: a low-dose technique. Radiology 131:743-749, 1979.

Chapter 12

Automated Ultrasound Mammography
of the Whole Breast

Richard H. Gold, M.D.

Ultrasound mammography, in its present state of development, has not yet been shown to be as reliable as x-ray mammography for the detection of subclinical cancer. Nevertheless, because it is noninvasive and requires no ionizing radiation there is continuing impetus toward its further improvement. Ultrasound, at diagnostic power levels, has to date produced no known ill effects in humans and therefore may be performed repeatedly on patients regardless of their age.

Features of the Ideal Scanning System

Several companies are currently marketing automated systems dedicated to ultrasound scanning of the whole breast. These systems have one or two transducers immersed in a water bath, in which the breast is suspended (Figure 1). Each of these systems attempts to incorporate the following features: adequate resolution for detection of small lesions; high sensitivity to small differences in tissue textures; controllable image enhancement; high-speed operation to facilitate rapid examinations; a means of display that permits rapid evaluation of images; and patient privacy and comfort. An ideal design would also permit three views of any suspicious area in the breast to help ensure diagnostic accuracy: longitudinal and transverse B scans (planes perpendicular to the chest wall) as well as "C scans" (planes parallel to the chest wall).

Diagnostic Criteria

Ultrasonic reflection images reveal differences in the acoustic impedance of the tissues and are displayed by means of a calibrated grey scale. Five major criteria of ultrasonic diagnosis are used: (1) delineation (or nondelineation) of a mass; (2) presence or absence of internal echoes; (3) regularity of the contour of the mass; (4) character of the far wall of a lesion; and (5) extent of through-transmission of sound deep to the lesion. A combination of these criteria, rather than any single one leads to the sonographic diagnosis.[1,2,3] For example, the outline of a scirrhous carcinoma is characteristically irregular, with tiny internal echoes and striking attenuation of the echo beam by the tumor (Figures 2 and 3). Both the images of fibroadenoma (Figure 4) and of medullary carcinoma (Figure 5) have slightly irregular borders and few internal echoes. Cysts (Figure 6) have smooth borders and no internal echoes, and are associated with strong echoes beyond their posterior margins.

Advantages

Ultrasound mammography is useful: (1) to distinguish between cystic and solid palpable masses, especially in dysplastic nodular breasts that are difficult to evaluate clinically and by x-ray mammography; and (2) in conjunction with x-ray mammography, to increase diagnostic accuracy for the detection of

278

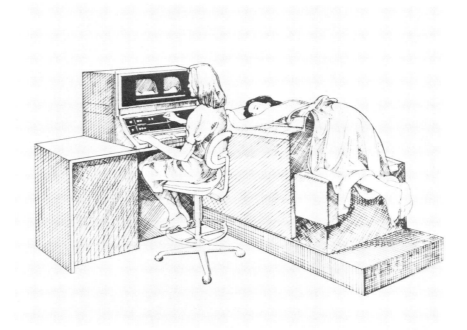

Figure 1. Diagnostic ultrasound system designed specifically for examination of the breast. The apparatus is a high-resolution, real-time water-path scanner. The breast is suspended in a water bath. The operator sits at a console which features various image-enhancement and data-manipulation features, as well as provisions for display of patient and instrument status data (courtesy of Technicare Corporation).

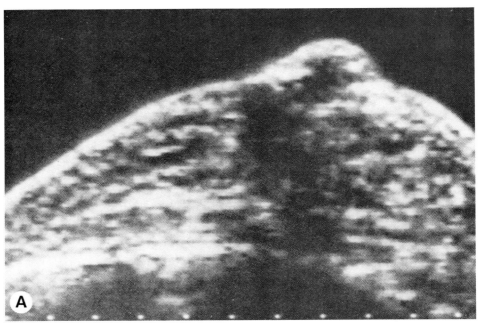

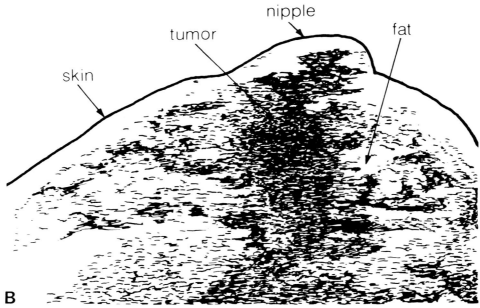

Figure 2. Infiltrating duct carcinoma. A. Ultrasound scan. The outline of this scirrhous carcinoma is typically irregular, with tiny internal echoes and striking attenuation of the echo beam by the tumor. B. Drawing of the same breast section pointing out relevant normal and abnormal features. C. Gross pathological section. D. Histopathological whole breast section (courtesy of Technicare Corporation).

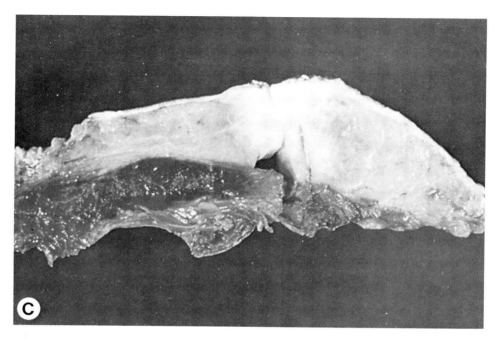

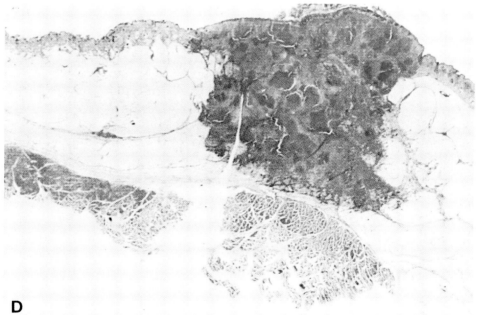

Figure 2, continued.

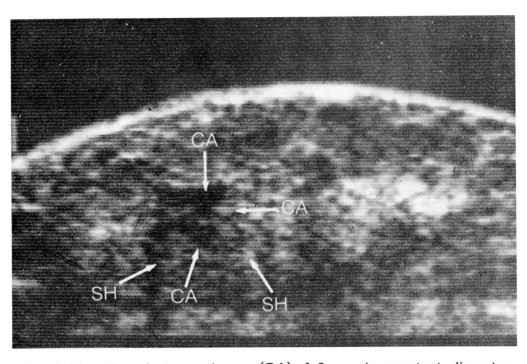

Figure 3. Infiltrating duct carcinoma (CA), 1.2 cm. in greatest diameter. The border of the lesion is irregular. The shadowing (SH) behind the lesion is a characteristic feature (courtesy of Technicare Corporation).

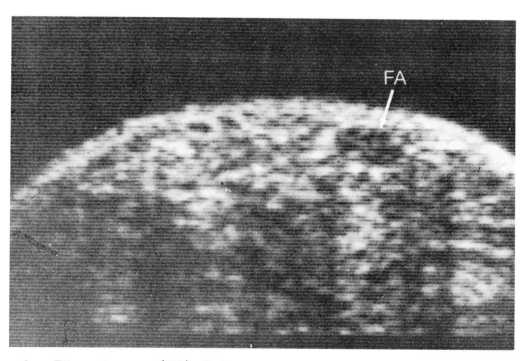

Figure 4. Fibroadenoma (FA), 1.2 cm. in greatest diameter, characterized by a smooth border and few internal echoes (courtesy of Technicare Corporation),

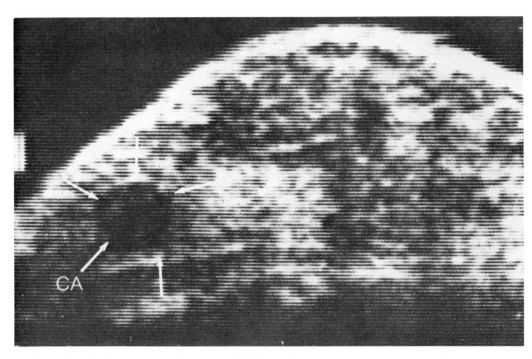

Figure 5. Medullary carcinoma (CA), 1.5 cm. in greatest diameter. Since these cancers are generally well-circumscribed with low-level internal echoes, they mimic fibroadenomas (courtesy of Technicare Corporation).

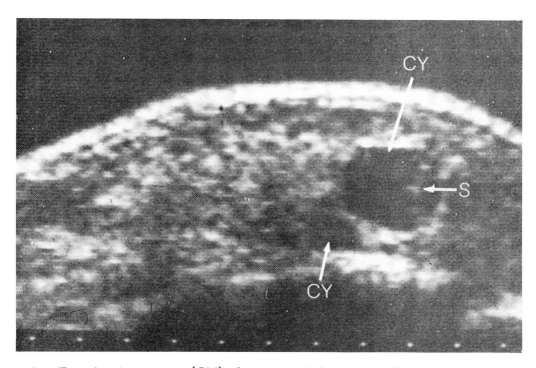

Figure 6. Two benign cysts (CY), 1 cm. and 2 cm. in diameter, the largest of which is septated (S). Cysts have smooth borders and, unless septated, have no internal echoes and are associated with strong echoes beyond their posterior margins (courtesy of Technicare Corporation).

cancer. In a breast that is dense and dysplastic, ultrasound may be capable of disclosing an uncalcified or minimally calcified carcinoma better than x-ray mammography, because the low-level echo content of the cancer stands out from the strong echo pattern of the surrounding fibrous tissue. However, in a fatty breast the carcinoma is usually more easily detected by x-ray mammography.

Limitations

Clinical evaluations of symptomatic patients with several prototype units have shown promising results[3,4,5] but it has not yet been proven that these units are as reliable as x-ray mammography in detecting subclinical cancer (Figure 7). Two important limitations associated with ultrasound breast diagnosis are nipple attenuation and difficulties in imaging microcalcifications.[5] Masses located deep to the nipple may not be detected because the nipple attenuates the sound beam, resulting in an acoustic shadow. At least one system employs a mechanized compression device which alleviates this problem.[3] In its present state of development, ultrasound is not as capable of imaging microcalcifications as x-ray mammography. Nevertheless, there may be a place for the combined use of x-ray mammography and ultrasound mammograhy, since x-ray mammography tends to give the best results in breasts that are relatively fatty, while ultrasound mammography may prove to be the more reliable technique in breasts that are relatively dense.

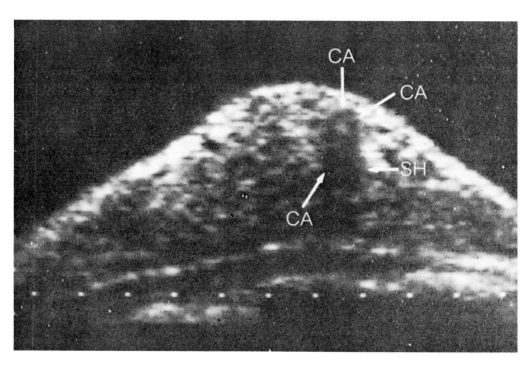

Figure 7. Infiltrating duct carcinoma (CA), 1 cm. in diameter. This lesion was clinically occult and remained undetected by x-ray mammography. The extensive shadowing (SH) posterior to the lesion is characteristic (courtesy of Technicare Corporation).

References

1. Teixidor, H.S. and Kazam, E.: Combined mammographic-sonographic evaluation of breast masses. <u>AJR</u> 128:409-417, 1977.

2. Kobayashi, T.: Gray-scale echography for breast cancer. <u>Radiology</u>
122:207-214, 1977.

3. Cole-Beuglet, C.M., Goldberg, B.B., Patchefsky, A.S., Rubin, C.S., Schneck,
C.D., Soriano, R.Z.: <u>Atlas of Breast Ultrasound.</u> Correlation of:
Anatomy, Pathology, Mammography, Ultrasonography. Somerset, New Jersey,
Technicare Corporation, 1980.

4. Maturo, V.G., Zuzmer, N.R., Gilson, A.J., Smoak, W.M., Janowitz, W.R.,
Bear, B.E., Goddard, J., Dick, D.E.: Ultrasound of the whole breast
utilizing a dedicated automated breast scanner. <u>Radiology</u> 137:457-463,
1980.

5. Harper, P., Kelly-Fry, E.: Ultrasound visualization of the breast in
symptomatic patients. <u>Radiology</u> 137:465-469, 1980.

Chapter 13

Diagnosis of Metastatic Cancer
with an Unknown Primary Site

A. Robert Kagan, M.D.
Richard J. Steckel, M.D.

Diagnostic persistence in working up metastatic cancer with an unknown primary site may be wasteful and unnecessary.[1] However, disseminated tumors for which effective treatment is now available include laryngopharyngeal carcinomas metastatic to lymph nodes in the upper two-thirds of the neck, certain germinal cell malignancies, hormone-dependent carcinomas originating in the breast, prostate, or endometrium, and some thyroid carcinomas and malignancies of neural crest origin. Finding the primary tumor might be useful in these patients. Several malignant tumors in infants and young children can also be treated effectively even when they are disseminated, but their site of origin can usually be identified with relative ease using a combination of histologic and clinical findings. With metastatic nodes in the upper cervical chain containing epidermoid or poorly differentiated carcinoma, a primary site of origin in the pharynx, larynx, or nasopharynx can usually be identified through a meticulous ENT examination.

Of 7,000 new cancer patients seen at the UCLA Hospital between 1968 and 1974, 255 were coded as having an unknown primary site.[1] Two hundred thirty-one of these 255 patients have expired, and autopsy results were available in 34. In 20 out of these 34 patients the primary site COULD NOT BE FOUND EVEN AT AUTOPSY. None of the remaining malignancies would have been treatable, even if they had been characterized before death. This review showed that, despite the persistent desire of some physicians to discover the primary site of a metastatic tumor, discovery of the primary rarely benefits the patient.

In this retrospective study, 255 unknown primaries out of 7,000 new cancer patients (or 3.6%) was a minimum estimate, since many of the cases were recoded by the physician or the UCLA Registry from an "unknown primary" to a "known primary" by what might be characterized as a "best-guess" method. At another large Los Angeles hospital registry (the Sunset Hospital of the Southern California Permanente Medical Group), the tumor registrar may eventually recode unknown primaries but does not erase the initial "unknown" coding from the registry record. During 1979, a total of 834 new patients with cancer were registered at the Sunset Hospital. Sixty-five patients were coded as "unknown primary" on the initial tissue or cytologic diagnosis, representing 7% of the total new cancer patients seen that year. The tumor registrar subsequently recorded 40 of these 65 into a "known" primary site, based on her interpretation of the doctor's progress notes, leaving only 3% of the patients coded persistently as "primary unknown."

In the Sunset Hospital series there were 15 patients with an initial liver biopsy of cancer, primary site undetermined. Nine biopsies were adenocarcinoma, 2 were poorly differentiated carcinoma, 2 were "malignant tumor" (type unspecified), and 1 each was interpreted as choriocarcinoma and squamous cell carcinoma. Of these, a primary site subsequently was inferred in seven patients: two colonic cancers were diagnosed by barium enema, two pancreatic and one gallbladder cancer were suggested by transhepatic cholangiograms, and one hepatoma was diagnosed by serum alphafeto-protein determination (which was 500-times normal). Another stomach primary was diagnosed at autopsy. The remaining nine patients presenting with liver metastases had extensive abdominal carcinomatosis in addition to liver involvement, and it was felt that the primary could have arisen anywhere. Unfortunately, no single diagnostic study in <u>any</u> of these patients precluded an eventual exploratory laparatomy. The large amount of tumor present in the abdomen often made surgery extremely difficult. In addition, the type of bypass procedure that was chosen in some of the patients was minimally influenced by the prior diagnostic workup, which often included abdominal ultrasound, computed tomography, barium enema, upper gastrointestinal series, small bowel series, itravenous pyelogram, liver scan, bone scan, and/or mammography. While the use of pancreatic and hepatic angiography to diagnose a rare metastatic islet cell tumor is relatively specific, angiography may be indicated only when the initial percutaneous liver biopsy suggests a tumor of endocrine origin.

There were 19 patients in the Sunset Hospital series presenting initially with malignant pleural effusion or ascites. Of 7 patients with positive abdominal cytologies, 6 were interpreted a adenocarcinoma and one as "nonspecific malignant cells." Of 12 patients with malignant cells in their pleural fluid, 7 were adenocarcinoma, 1 probable oat cell, 1 lymphoma, 1 carcinoma and 2 "malignant cells, unspecified." Subsequent diagnostic imaging studies failed to define the primary in any of the patients with ascites (a primary in the ovary was identified <u>later</u> in 2, the stomach in one, and in the colon in one). In the 12 patients with positive pleural cytology the primary remained unknown in 6, whereas a lung primary was eventually diagnosed in 3, a kidney primary in 1 (by a renal arteriogram), and probable breast and endometrium primaries in 1 each (inferred by <u>previous histories</u> of carcinomas at these sites). Often the chest roentgenogram revealed the presence of one or more pulmonary masses following a thoracentesis. The three "unknown primary" patients with malignant pleural effusions who were eventually coded as having primary lung cancer, either had chest radiographs strongly suggesting lung cancer or a positive bronchoscopy. The patient with "probable oat cell cancer" on pleural cytology had no mediastinal or lung mass, and hence was coded as a persistent unknown primary by the Registry.

In summary, for the malignant ascites patients, except for one positive barium enema, no radiologic examination was informative in locating the primary tumor site, and no imaging study precluded a subsequent exploratory laparotomy. Similarly, in the patients with malignant pleural effusions, most diagnostic imaging studies proved not to be helpful. Bronchoscopy and chest radiographs should be sufficient to diagnose a lung primary, which in the vast majority of patients will not alter therapy or prognosis. It is unlikely that intrathoracic lymphoma or oat cell carcinoma can be diagnosed by ordering additional diagnostic imaging studies.

There were 10 patients in the Sunset Hospital series with metastatic cancer which presented initially in lymph nodes; 7 in the neck and 3 in the mediastinum. Four were squamous cell carcinomas, 3 carcinomas of unspecified type, 1 lymphoepithelioma, 1 large cell carcinoma, and 1 adenocarcinoma. In six of these 10 patients the primary was never determined, and in four the lung was eventually judged the primary site (based on bronchoscopy, chest radiographs, mediastinoscopy and/or thoracotomy). Radiographic studies of the paranasal sinuses, multiple imaging examinations, radiographic bone surveys, and radionuclide scans of various types were not helpful. The patient with metastatic lymphoepithelioma was irradiated empirically to the neck and nasopharynx, after negative panendoscopy and nasopharyngeal biopsy.

Four other patients who presented with unknown primaries required a diagnostic brain biopsy, with two revealing metastatic adenocarcinoma, 1 an apparent oat cell, and 1 carcinoma. In only one of these patients was the apparent primary subsequently established: a hilar mass on the chest roentgenogram.

Four patients presented initially with metastases to the soft tissues. In one a xerogram eventually defined a breast primary; in another a chest roentgenogram led to bronchoscopy, which in turn was positive for lung cancer, and in two no primary site was ever found.

One patient required an emergency laminectomy for metastatic carcinoma, and the primary was never found. In another, a solitary lung nodule proved to be a leiomyosarcoma, and no primary could be demonstrated subsequently in the intestinal tract, bladder or uterus. Another solitary lung nodule was diagnosed as adenocarcinoma of nonbronchogenic origin, and the primary site remained unknown following (among other studies) a bone survey, thyroid scan, liver scan, barium enema, upper gastrointestinal seies, bronchoscopy, and computerized tomograms of the chest and abdomen.

Rectal biopsies of stenotic lesions in two patients revealed squamous carcinoma in one and adenocarcinoma in the other. In the former, chest roentgenograms showed multiple nodules, and therefore an abdomino-perineal resection was not done; in the latter, the managing physicians felt the adenocarcinoma could have originated either in the bowel or the ovary.

Four patients presented first with metastatic carcinoma in the omentum. Barium enema subsequently demonstrated a primary in the splenic flexure of the colon in one, and a primary site could not be established at the time of exploratory laparotomy in the other 3.

Two patients presented with adenocarcinomas metastatic to bone. Diagnostic studies including prostate biopsies, computed tomograms, upper gastrointestinal series, intravenous pyelograms, barium enemas, etc., were all negative, and no primary sites could be established.

One patient had an undifferentiated metastasis in the orbit and another presented with squamous cell carcinoma in a parotid lymph node; no primary could be found in either patient.

An overall summary of these findings in these 65 patients with unknown primaries is in order. Only 19 of the 65 patients had their primary tumor site diagnosed eventually through additional diagnostic studies (Table I). In the patients with tumors metastatic to liver or omentum, and/or with malignant ascites, the only diagostic procedure that was helpful (and then rarely) was a barium enema. The results of a preoperative barium enema may also warn the surgeon occasionally to order the bowel prepared for a palliative bypass procedure or colostomy (4 patients in this series). If biopsy of a liver metastasis suggests a tumor of endocrine origin (islet cell), a subsequent visceral arteriogram may prove diagnostic, but nonfunctioning endocrine malignancies are rare.

With metastatic cancer presenting in cervical lymph nodes, or as a malignant pleural effusion, diagnostic chest roentgenograms should be all that are necessary. Occasionally, chest tomography will help if the plain films are equivocal. If these relatively. simple radiologic examinations do not help, more imaging studies will not solve the problem. Endoscopy and possible directed biopsy of the posterior tongue, tonsil, nasopharynx, larynx or hypopharynx might prove to be much more useful.

Further diagnostic imaging studies (beyond chest radiographs) in a patient who presents initially with brain metastases will not be rewarding. Demonstrating an occult hypernephroma, for instance, will not alter the survival of a patient with widespread metastases. Xerograms to establish a breast primary will be helpful if the presenting lesion is a metastatic axillary node, and may even contribute to a treatment decision in the face of more distant metastases if hormonal therapy is a consideration. The presence of an ovarian primary in association with peritoneal carcinomatosis can only be proved by an operative procedure, and even at laparotomy proof can sometimes be difficult. As with the earlier series of unknown primaries reported from UCLA[1], 90% of the patients from the Southern California Permanente series are now dead. In spite of the often dogged persistence of the oncologist in trying to establish a primary tumor site, little was gained in length or in quality of survival. While chest roentgenograms, barium enemas, or visceral angiograms may occasionally be helpful in selected patients, no diagnostic imaging study is productive enough to be used "routinely."

The Sunset Hospital tumor registrar eventually recoded 40 of the original 65 patients presenting with unknown primaries as having an "identified" primary site, but on review we recoded 15 of these 40 again as unknown primaries. There was a tendency to overcode the pancreas and the lung as putative "primary sites" in the presence of widespread metastatic disease, a tendency that has been noted by others.[2,3] Therefore, in this series 40 of 845 new cancer patients had persistently unknown sites of origin (5%).

It should be emphasized that the clinician may not be entirely to blame for the overuse of diagnostic studies (and the underuse of clinical judgment) in patients with unknown primaries. The pathologist's report often suggests that the clinician consider lung, stomach, colon and/or kidney as primary sites, rather than stating simply that metastatic carcinoma is present and that the tumor origin is occult. Covering one's ignorance by listing a variety of differential possibilities does no one a service, least of all the patient. In an excellent report, Fermont reviews 139 patients with malignant cervical adenopathy and no obvious clinical primary, with a crude survival at 5 years

TABLE I

FINAL DIAGNOSIS OF PATIENTS PRESENTING WITH METASTATIC CARCINOMA

Source of initial diagnosis of metastatic tumor	Number of patients presenting with "unknown primaries"	Final diagnosis remained "unknown primary"#	Helpful diagnostic studies (Preoperatively)
Liver	15	9	transhepatic cholangiogram (3) barium enema (2) alphafeto-protein (1)
Abdominal Fluid	7	3	barium enema (1)
Pleural Fluid	12	6	renal arteriogram (1) chest radiographs (3)
Lymph Nodes	10	6	chest radiographs (4)
Brain	4	3	chest radiographs (1)
Soft Tissues	4	2	chest radiographs (1) xerogram of breast (1)
Laminectomy	1	1	none
Lung Nodule	2	2	none
Rectum	2	1	none*
Omentum	4	3	barium enema (1)
Bone	2	2	none
Orbit	1	1	none
Parotid	1	1	none
TOTAL	68	40	19

*Positive chest examination (for showing metastases) prevented an abdomino-perineal resection, however.

#According to hospital Tumor Registry (see text).

294

of 5%.[4]   In 5 of these patients the site of the tumor primary was found during the patient's lifetime, and eight more were found at postmortem examination.   Panendoscopy is suggested by the author in all patients presenting with malignant cervical adenopathy, but he adds that it is also important to rule out primaries in the thyroid, breast, kidneys and prostate. How far should one go to rule out all of these primary sites?   One intravenous urogram was positive in our 65 patients with unknown primaries, and even in this single patient the therapeutic approach and the outcome were not changed.   One xerogram of the breast did alter management, but thyroid scans were of no help and prostate biopsies were not useful in our series.

Common sense and clinical judgment are more important than a battery of diagnostic tests in patients presenting with metastatic tumors and unknown primaries.   The reluctance of the physician to tell a patient that he does not know the primary site and that knowing will probably not alter the patient's clinical course, remains a persistent impediment to humane and rational management.

REFERENCES

1. Steckel, Richard J., and Kagan, A. Robert: Diagnostic Persistence in Working Up Metastatic Cancer with an Unknown Primary Site. Radiology 134(2):367-369, 1980.

2. Cassiere, S. Germain, McLain, David A., Emory, W. Brooks, and Hatch, Hurst B.: Metastatic Carcinoma of the Pancreas Simulating Primary Bronchogenic Carcinoma. Cancer 46:2319-2321, 1980.

3. Cechner, Ronald L., Chamberlain, William, Carter, John R., Milojkovic-Mirceta, and Nash, Nancy P.: Misdiagnosis of Bronchogenic Carcinoma: The Role of Cigarette Smoking, Surveillance Bias, and Other Factors. Cancer 46:190-199, 1980.

4. Fermont, D.C.: Malignant Cervical Lymphadenopathy Due to an Unknown Primary. Clinical Radiology 31:355-358, 1980.

Chapter 14

Interventional Radiologic Techniques

Frederick S. Keller, M.D.
Josef Rösch, M.D.

INTRODUCTION:

In recent years, interventional radiologic therapy has become a rapidly growing adjunct to diagnostic - particularly cardiovascular - radiology. Especially designed tools, mainly vascular catheters, and new techniques are now used for the percutaneous treatment of lesions that could previously be treated only by surgery. These procedures are performed in the radiology department under local anesthesia and with minimal stress and risk. Early ambulation and decreased cost are some of the other advantages of interventional radiologic therapy. In addition, the avoidance of a major surgical procedure with accompanying pain and morbidity in patients with terminal malignant disease can be an obvious benefit. Interventional percutaneous therapeutic techniques can be used selectively to deliver chemotherapeutic agents to the primary tumor or metastases, to infarct malignant tumors by transcatheter embolization of their arterial supply, to drain bile ducts obstructed by biliary or pancreatic cancers or by lymph node metastases in the porta hepatis, and to relieve urinary obstructions caused by pelvic malignancies.

LIVER:

The selective infusion of chemotherapeutic drugs via percutaneously introduced hepatic arterial catheters was one of the earliest interventional radiology applications used in many institutions for patients with hepatic metastases or unresectable primary liver tumors.[1] The advantages of this approach over intravenous administration of certain cytotoxic agents include the potential for increasing the local tumor dose while simultaneously decreasing systemic side effects (Figure 1A, B). The infusion of radioactive particles directly into vessels which supply either primary or secondary hepatic neoplasms, to deliver high-dose local radiation, is another interventional radiologic therapy technique for hepatic malignancies.[2,3]

When more than one major vessel supplies arterial blood to the liver (as occurs in 15-20% of the population), separate chemotherapeutic infusions into each of the feeding vessels must be done if an effort is made to treat the entire liver. However, at one large cancer institution the radiologists have occluded one of two major arteries supplying blood to the liver and have noted that collateral vessels rapidly develop from the remaining hepatic artery and perfuse those areas of the liver previously supplied by the occluded hepatic branch. Therefore, in patients with a dual hepatic arterial supply one of the feeding arteries is occluded and the chemotherapy infusion catheter placed in the other. With this method, the entire liver can be infused at one session.[4]

298

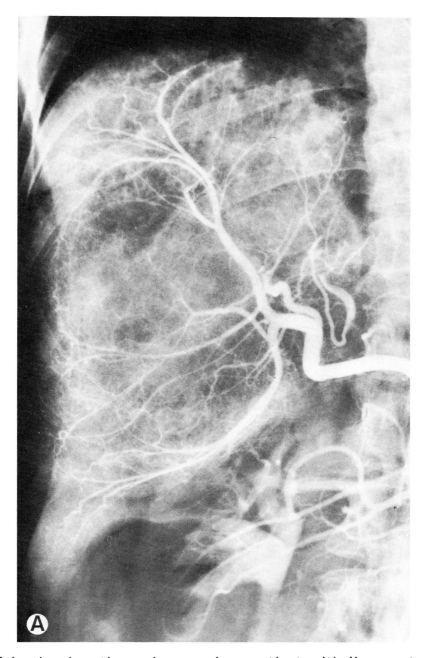

Figure 1. Selective hepatic angiograms in a patient with liver metastases from colon carcinoma, before (A) and after (B) a course of intra-arterial 5FU: there are large metastatic deposits spreading and displacing branches of the hepatic artery (A). In the post-infusion angiogram (B) the intrahepatic arteries are not displaced and the liver has decreased in size.

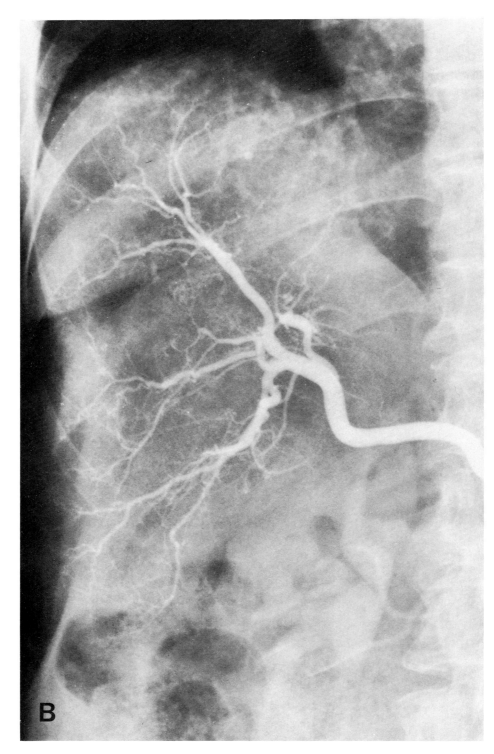

Figure 1, continued.

Transcatheter tumor embolization is another modality used in radiologic therapy of liver malignancies. The normal liver receives 75-80% of its blood flow from the portal vein and only 20-25% from the hepatic artery. However, both primary and metastatic liver tumors receive all of their blood supply from the hepatic artery. Because of this dual blood supply, some interventional radiologists have been able successfully to embolize the arterial branches feeding the tumor or even the main hepatic artery without causing liver ischemia or necrosis.[5] However, before attempting to occlude the hepatic artery, patency of the portal vein must be confirmed beforehand.

One interventional radiologic procedure which is being used with increasing frequency is percutaneous biliary drainage for the relief of obstructive jaundice caused by malignant disease.[6-8] The drainage procedure is usually preceded by a percutaneous transhepatic cholangiogram (PTC) to define the level of the obstructing lesion and anatomy of the ductal system. After obtaining diagnostic information from the PTC, a suitable duct is selected and punctured percutaneously under fluoroscopic guidance with a sheathed needle. With the aid of various types of guidewires, an angiographic catheter can then be manipulated through the ductal system to the site of obstruction. The catheter may be left in place and the proximal biliary system decompressed by external drainage (Figure 2A). Frequently, however, it is possible to advance the guidewire and catheter (either at the time of initial decompression or a few days later) past the obstructing lesion and into the duodenum. With catheter sideholes both above and below the site of obstruction, the external end of the catheter may be capped and internal drainage of bile from the liver to the duodenum occurs (Figure 2B).[6-13] Internal biliary drainage is preferable to external drainage since the inconvenience of an external drainage bag is eliminated and, more important, there is no loss of bile salts with resulting digestive abnormalities and electrolyte imbalances. Successful external drainage can be achieved in 92-100% of patients with obstructive jaundice, while internal drainage can be accomplished in 75-90% of patients.

Although percutaneous biliary drainage does not increase the mean survival time in these individuals, it does afford relief from intractable pruritis and precludes the need for surgery with its accompanying pain, morbidity, and even mortality. Occasionally, in patients with biliary-enteric anastomoses who have developed anastomotic strictures, transhepatic dilatation of the stricture can be accomplished with an angiographic balloon catheter (Figure 3).[14]

Major complications of percutaneous biliary drainage are few and are primarily related to catheter dislodgement, rarely to peritoneal bile leaks or to hemoperitoneum. Several cases of hemobilia following percutaneous biliary drainage have been reported.[15] For those patients with external biliary drainage, serum electrolytes must be monitored periodically to prevent imbalances from loss of bile salts and fluids.

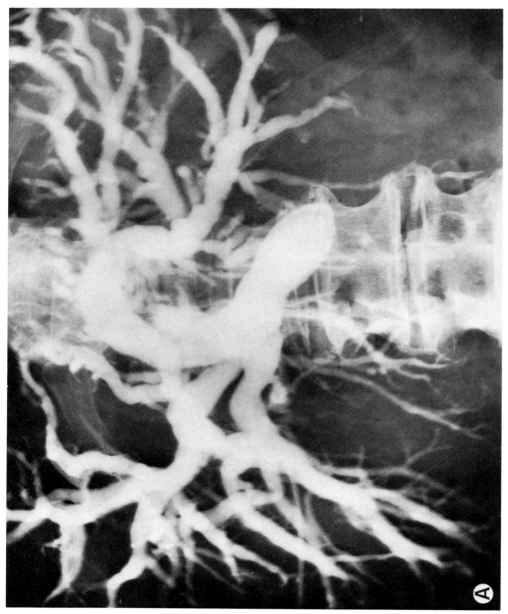

Figure 2. External biliary drainage in a patient with pancreatic carcinoma: (A) a drainage catheter has been inserted percutaneously by the transhepatic approach. The common bile duct is occluded by the tumor at the level of the pancreas. (B, following page) Five days later the catheter has been advanced through the obstructing lesion so that its tip lies in the duodenum. With catheter side-holes located above and below the obstruction, internal biliary drainage is achieved.

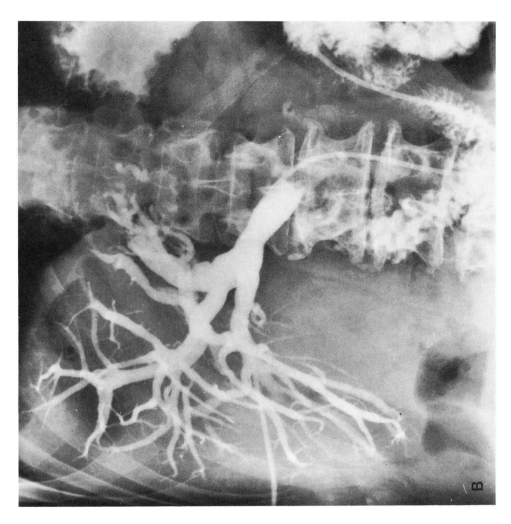

Figure 2, continued.

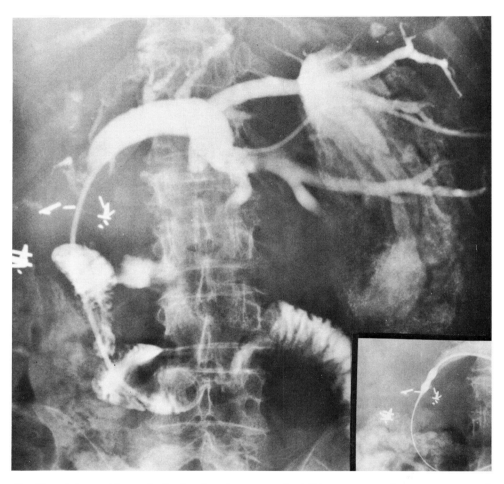

Figure 3. Transhepatic choledochoplasty of biliary-enteric anastamosis after right hepatic lobectomy for cholangiocarcinoma: the biliary drainage catheter entered from the left lobe, and the anastomotic stricture was dilated with an angiographic balloon dilating catheter (insert).

KIDNEY:

The kidney, like the liver, is a parenchymal organ well suited for several forms of interventional radiologic therapy. For patients with malignant renal tumors, therapeutic infarction by vaso-occlusion is the most frequent form of interventional radiologic treatment (Figure 4A-B). Percutaneous transvascular renal infarction has been used pre-operatively with extremely vascular tumors to reduce blood loss during surgery. In addition, some urologic surgeons have reported that dissection of the kidney is facilitated after renal embolization, because edema makes the peri-renal tissue planes more distinct. Another potential advantage of pre-operative infarction is that it might permit initial ligation of the renal vein without the risk of tumor engorgement.[16,17]

Usually, however, renal tumor infarction is performed for palliation, as with patients with large inoperable tumors or patients who have resectable cancers but are not acceptable surgical candidates because of other underlying medical problems. Embolization may be particularly effective in helping to control local symptoms and signs such as pain and severe tumor-induced hematuria.[17] Furthermore, there has been evidence that tumor infarction sometimes prolongs survival. In several cases reduction of size of the primary tumor or complete disappearance of tumor metastases has been documented after embolization, possibly through immunologic mechanisms.[17,18] Renal tumor infarction may also be used for other malignancies that have metastasized to the kidney and are causing hematuria or severe pain (Figure 5A-B).

After successful vaso-occlusion of renal tumors, especially large ones, the patient usually develops a characteristic symptom complex known as the "post-infarction syndrome." This consists of severe pain, three or four days in duration and usually requiring narcotic analgesics, fever, leukocytosis, and serum LDH elevation. Mild-to-moderate gastrointestinal symptoms are common and frequently respond to temporary restriction of oral intake and intravenous fluids. Occasionally, however, fairly profound paralytic ileus may occur, necessitating insertion of a nasogastric tube for several days.

Potential complications of renal tumor infarction include post-infarction renal abscesses, occurring when bacteriurium and/or pyelonephritis were present at the time of embolization. Renal failure from the administration of too much contrast medium can complicate an otherwise successful procedure. This complication usually occurs as a result of performing the diagnostic and the interventional angiographic procedures at the same sitting. The occasionally-reported complication of peripheral ischemia, caused by reflux of embolized material back into the aorta, can be avoided by carefully controlled embolization techniques.

Relief of urinary tract obstruction from malignant disease by the use of percutaneous nephrostomy is another form of interventional radiologic therapy.[17,19] It can be used as a temporary measure prior to definitive surgery to permit the kidney to recover from obstruction pre-operatively, or as a permanent, long-term diversion for the upper urinary tracts in patients

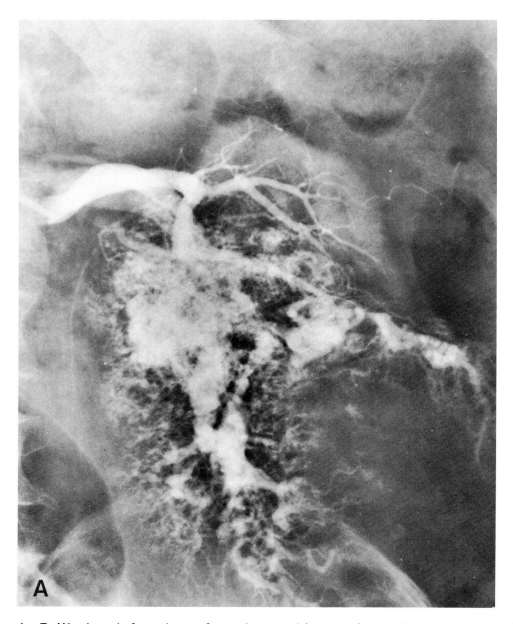

Figure 4. Palliative infarction of an inoperable renal carcinoma: control left renal angiogram (A) demonstrates a large hypervascular malignant tumor extending beyond the margins of the left kidney. There is early shunting of contrast to the left renal vein. The post-embolization left renal angiogram (B) demonstrates occlusion of the left renal artery (Gianturco coil spring occluder is marked by the white arrow).

Figure 4, continued.

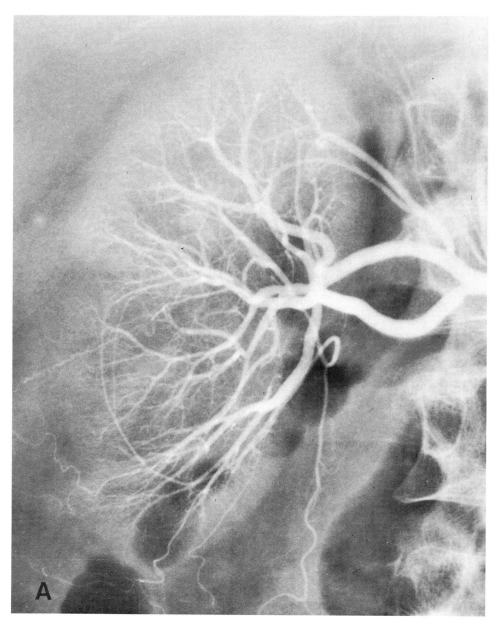

Figure 5. Palliative infarction of right kidney for pain and hematuria caused by metastasis from a squamous cell lung primary: the control right renal angiogram (A) demonstrates stretching and tumor encasement of intrarenal arteries in the inferolateral portion of the kidney. Post-embolization plain abdominal film (B) reveals intravascular renal arterial casts which are composed of embolized acrylic material. The patient's pain and hematuria were controlled by the embolization.

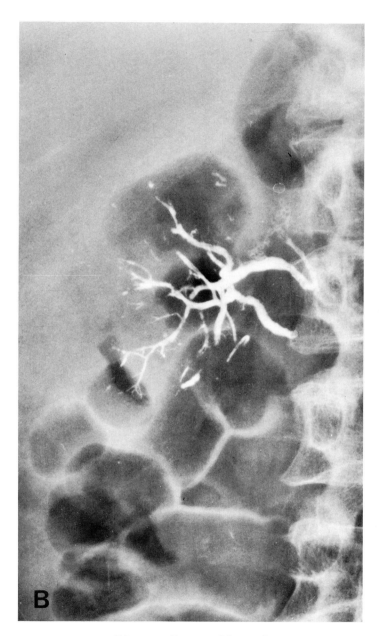

Figure 5, continued.

with unresectable tumors. Permanent occlusion of the ureter, combined with a percutaneous nephrostomy in patients with ureteral fistulae, eliminates the chronic discomfort and inconvenience of constant urine leakage.

Percutaneous nephrostomy is performed under fluoroscopic guidance after the urinary collecting systems have been opacified with intravenous contrast material. For those patients with non-visualizing pelvi-calyceal systems, ultrasonography may provide adequate guidance for the initial puncture. In patients with obstruction at the uretero-pelvic junction, the tip of the nephrostomy catheter is deliberately coiled within the dilated pelvis (Figure 6A-B). With more distal obstructions, the nephrostomy catheter may be threaded more distally so that its tip is well within the ureter. Often it is possible to pass the nephrostomy catheter beyond the site of obstruction and into the bladder. With catheter side holes placed above as well as below the obstructing lesion, the external end of the catheter may be capped and urine allowed to drain internally from the collecting system to the bladder, thus eliminating the need for external drainage bags.[20]

PELVIS:

Interventional radiologic techniques have also been used successfully for the palliation of unresectable tumors within the pelvis. Arterial embolization of primary and secondary tumors involving the pelvic bones may alleviate severe pain associated with these neoplasms (Figure 7A-B). In addition to the relief of pain, regression in size of osseous lesions with calcification of their margins indicating some degree of healing, has often been noted following embolization.[21]

A primary indication for arterial embolization in pelvic bone tumors has been the failure of previous therapy including surgery, radiation, and chemotherapy to relieve pain. The main blood supply to these tumors usually comes from branches of the internal iliac artery. Additional arterial supply frequently originates from the lower lumbar, middle sacral, external pudendal, and circumflex iliac branches. For the best therapeutic results, the maximum possible number of feeding arteries should be embolized. The exact mechanism by which tumor embolization relieves bone pain is not known; however, it has been postulated that vascular occlusion initially decreases the size of the tumor and retards its progression. As a result, there is less expansion or stretching of the periosteum which contains the sensitive nerve endings responsible for pain.

In addition to the palliation of severe bone pain, transcatheter arterial embolization has been employed successfully to control vaginal hemorrhage from advanced gynecologic cancers, hematuria from bladder and prostatic neoplasms, and lower gastrointestinal hemorrhage from involvement of the sigmoid colon or rectum by pelvic malignancies.[22-24] Surgical management of hemorrhage in these cases may be technically unfeasible because of extensive tumor encasement or radiation-induced tissue fibrosis. Furthermore, these patients are often severely debiliated and poor surgical risks. In most reported cases the vaginal, bladder, or rectal hemorrhage was successfully and permanently controlled by arterial embolization. However, in occasional cases bleeding

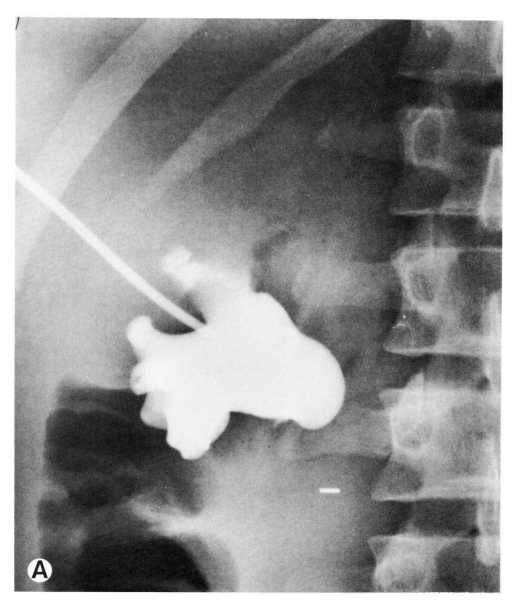

Figure 6. Percutaneous nephrostomy in a young patient with right ureteropelvic obstruction caused by lymph node metastases from a testicular carcinoma: the nephrostogram (A) shows a slightly dilated right renal collecting system with no flow of contrast material into the right ureter. After aspiration of contrast via the nephrostomy catheter, its coiled position in the right renal pelvis can be appreciated (B).

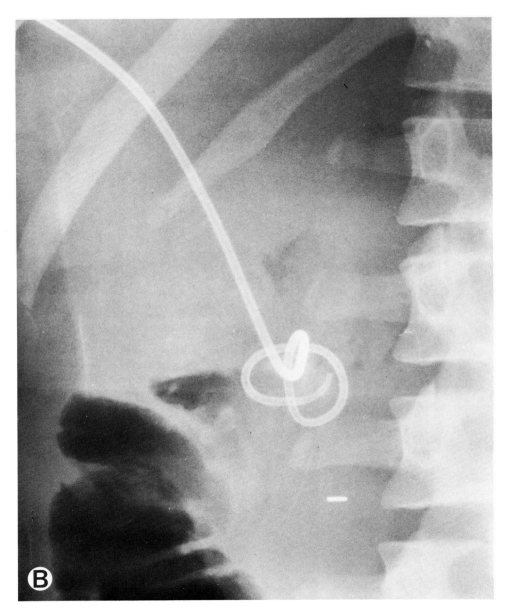

Figure 6, continued.

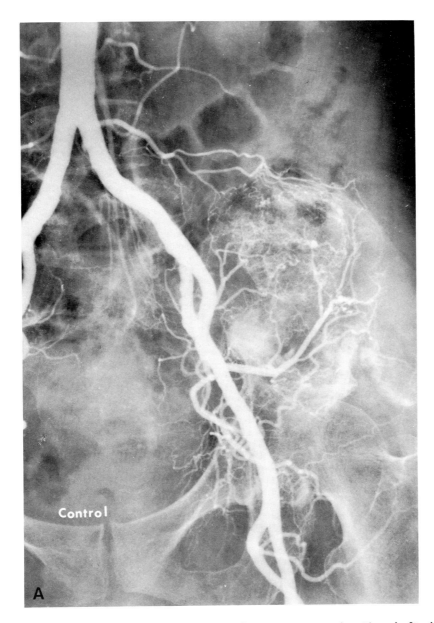

Figure 7A-B Palliative embolization of a fibrosarcoma in the left iliac bone: the control pelvic angiogram demonstrates a hypervascular malignant tumor involving the left iliac wing. It is fed by branches of the left internal iliac and fourth lumbar arteries. After transcatheter embolization of the feeding arteries with acrylic material, the pelvic angiogram reveals essentially no blood supply to the tumor. The small white arrowheads mark the radiopaque acrylic embolic material.

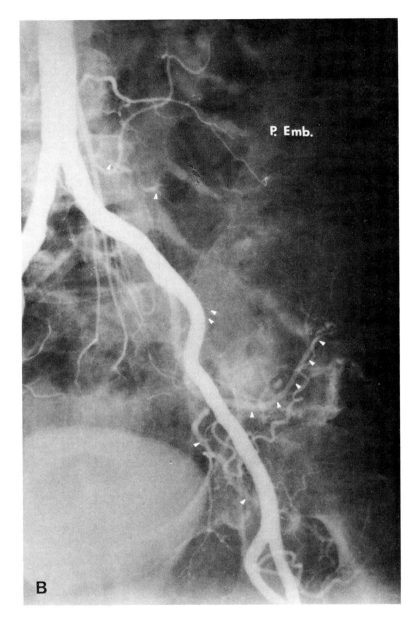

Figure 7, continued.

314

recurred, usually after several months, requiring a second and sometimes even a third embolization.

MISCELLANEOUS:

Hospitalized patients with malignancies are of course subject to all the potential complications seen in patients severely ill with non-malignant disease. Interventional radiologic techniques can sometimes contribute dramatically to the treatment of these complications. Upper gastrointestinal hemorrhage from stress ulcers or post-surgical bleeding can frequently be controlled, either by transcatheter infusion of vasoconstrictors or by embolization, thereby avoiding emergency surgery in an already compromised patient.[25] Iatrogenic complications such as sheared segments of central venous catheters which have embolized to the heart or the pulmonary arteries also occur, and these catheter fragments can become a nidus for infection or may eventually even perforate the myocardium causing cardiac tamponade. Successful percutaneous retrieval of these intravascular foreign bodies can be accomplished in a high percentage of cases by an experienced radiologist using interventional vascular techniques.[26]

REFERENCES

1. Wirtanen GW, Bernhardt LC, Mackman S, Ramirez G, Curreri AR, Ansfield FJ: Hepatic artery and celiac axis infusion for the treatment of upper abdominal malignant lesions. Ann Surg 168:137-141, 1968.

2. Simon N, Silvertone SM, Roach LC, Warner RRP, Baron MG, Rudovsky AZ: Intra-arterial irradiation of tumors, a safe procedure. AJR 92:732, 1971.

3. Lang EK: Superselective arterial catheterization as a vehicle for delivering radioactive infarct particles to tumors. Radiology 98:391, 1971.

4. Chuang VP, Wallace S: Hepatic arterial redistribution for intraarterial infusion of hepatic neoplasms. Radiology 135:295-299, 1980.

5. Roche A, Franco A, Dhumeaux D, Bismuth H, Doyon D: Emergency hepatic arterial embolization for secondary hypercalcemia in hepatocellular carcinoma. Radiology 133:315-316, 1979.

6. Hoevels J, Lunderquist A, Ohse I: Percutaneous transhepatic intubation of bile ducts for combined internal-external drainage in preoperative and palliative treatment of obstructive jaundice. Gastrointest Radiol 3:23-31, 1978.

7. Nakayama T, Ikeda A, Okuda K: Percutaneous transhepatic drainage of the biliary tract. Gastroenterology 74:554-559, 1978.

8. Ring EJ, Oleaga JA, Freiman DB, et al.: Therapeutic applications of catheter cholangiography. Radiology 128:333-338, 1978.

9. Pereiras RV, Rheingold OJ, Hutson D, et al.: Relief of malignant obstructive jaundice by percutaneous insertion of a permanent prosthesis in the biliary tree. Ann Intern Med 89:589-593, 1978.

10. Ariyama J, Shirakabe H, Shimaguchi S, Schmidt L: Transhepatic biliary drainage for obstructive jaundice. Rofo 131:610-615, 1979.

11. Ferrucci JT, Mueller PR, Harbin WP: Percutaneous transhepatic biliary drainage: Technique, results and applications. Radiology 135:1-13, 1980.

12. Harbin WP, Ferrucci JT Jr: Nonoperative management of malignant biliary obstruction: A radiologic alternative. AJR 135:103-107, 1980.

13. Burcharth F, Jensen LI, Olesen K: Endoprosthesis for internal drainage of the biliary tract: Technique and results in 48 cases. Gastroenterology 77:133-137, 1979.

14. Teplick SK, Goldstein RC, Richardson PA, Haskin PH, Wilson AR, Corvasce JM, Ring EJ, Wolferth CC: Percutaneous transhepatic choledochoplasty and dilatation of choledochoenterostomy strictures. JAMA 244:1240-1242, 1980.

15. Hoevels J, Nilsson U: Intrahepatic vascular lesions following nonsurgical percutaneous transhepatic bile duct intubation. Gastrointest Radiol 5:127-135, 1980.

16. Arkell DG, Cotter KP, Fitz-Patrick JD, Shaw RE: Pre-operative arterial embolization in renal carcinoma. Br J Urol 50:469, 1978.

17. Rosch J, Keller FS, Dotter CT: Therapeutic angiography in renal disease. Chapter in Angiography, Editor, Abrams HC, Edition III. Little Brown and Company, Boston (in press).

18. Swanson DA, Wallace S, Johnson DE: The role of embolization and nephrectomy in the treatment of metastatic renal carcinoma. Urol Clin North Am 7:719-730, 1980.

19. Perinetti E, Catalona WJ, Manley CB, Geise G, Fair WR: Percutaneous nephrostomy: Indications, complications and clinical usefulness. J Urol 120:156-58, 1978.

20. Bigongiari LR, Lee KR, Moffat RE, Mebust WK, Foret J, Weigel J: Percutaneous ureteral stent placement for stricture management and internal urinary drainage. AJR 133:865-868, 1979.

21. Wallace S, Granmayeh M, DeSantos LA, Murray JA, Romsdahl MM, Bracken RB, Jonsson K: Arterial occlusion of pelvic bone tumors. Cancer 43:322-328, 1979.

22. Giuliani L, Carmignani G, Belgrano E, Zambelli S, Puppo P, Cichero A: Total pelvic arterial embolization in case of massive vesical and vaginal bleeding by pelvis carcinomatosis. Eur Urol 5:205-207, 1979.

23. Carmignani G, Belgrano E, Puppo P, Cichero A, Giuliani L: Transcatheter embolization of the hypogastric arteries in cases of bladder hemorrhage from advanced pelvic cancers: Followup in 9 cases. J Urol 124:196-200, 1980.

24. Higgins CB, Bookstein JJ, Davis GB, Galloway DC, Barr JW: Therapeutic embolization for intractable chronic bleeding. Radiology 122:473-478, 1977.

25. Goldstein HM, Medellin H, Ben-Menachem Y, Wallace S: Transcatheter arterial embolization in the management of bleeding in the cancer patient. Radiology 115:603-608, 1975.

26. Dotter CT, Keller FS, Rosch J: The transluminal catheter removal of foreign bodies from the cardiovascular system. Chapter in: Angiography Editor, Abrams HL, Edition III, Little Brown and Company, Boston (in press).

Conclusion

A. Robert Kagan, M.D.
Richard J. Steckel, M.D.

Each physician "superspecialist," by design, looks at the patient from his or her own perspective. The endoscopist determines which instrument to use in which orifice, the more relaxed radiologist which non-invasive study to use, and the more aggressive radiologist which invasive test. Diagnosis may depend on 3 cells (the cytopathologist) or on a highly-selected area in the middle of a tissue section (the electron-microscopist). Between the overuse of diagnostic procedures and an unwarranted casualness concerning cancer diagnosis, lies a middle ground which is best for the patient; however, in practice the radiologist may be flooded by requests for procedures from concerned clinicians who want to be sure that they "not miss anything." This may be illustrated in the workup of metastatic cancer from an unknown primary site (Chapter 13).

For example, in the otherwise asymptomatic patient presenting with obstructive jaundice, what information does the surgeon actually require pre-operatively? One surgeon may want to know only that the chest x-ray is negative and confirm (if possible) that the patient has a dilated biliary tree, before performing an exploration. His aim at surgery is to determine if a resection is indicated, or possibly to determine if liver metastases are present or bypass a ductal obstruction. If the pancreas, common bile duct, and gallbladder appear normal, he may use a choledochoendoscope to inspect the major hepatic ducts. Another surgeon might demand to know pre-operatively exactly where the bile duct obstruction is located, the size and location of an obstructing mass, and the condition of the liver and the anatomy of its principal vascular supply.

To confirm an initial diagnosis of cancer we usually recommend obtaining tissue for permanent sections, rather than relying solely on aspiration cytology. The error rate will be less. However, each patient requires special consideration. If a 4 cm breast mass feels like cancer and looks like cancer on the mammogram, aspiration cytology may be sufficient.

There is no doubt that pathologists receive more useful diagnostic information from a cutting needle biopsy than from cytologic aspirations. "Borderline" or equivocal results are more common with the latter, as are false negatives. Some cancers require open biopsy if precise histologic classification is desired, such as bone and soft tissue tumors, lymphomas, and sclerosing carcinomas of the biliary tree and pancreas (to name a few). Endoscopic biopsy of a mass obstructing a bronchus is often diagnostic, while an endoscopic biopsy of a gastric ulcer often cannot be relied upon to distinguish a lymphoma from a poorly-differentiated carcinoma.

If a patient has a prior diagnosis of cancer, then diagnostic radiographic findings and/or an aspiration or endoscopic biopsy are usually adequate to establish the presence of metastatic disease. For example, in a patient with ascites and a history of ovarian cancer, a positive abdominal cytology or laparoscopic biopsy are sufficient evidence of peritoneal spread after chemotherapy or radiation. Needle aspiration of an enlarged regional lymph

320

node in a patient with a known pelvic cancer or a head and neck cancer can be diagnostic of regional metastatic disease. A positive bone scan showing multiple lesions in a symptomatic patient with cancer of the breast or prostate is also relatively reliable. Thus, in the patient with an already-diagnosed aggressive malignancy and a short recurrence interval, diagnosis or exclusion of metastatic disease can sometimes be accepted without redundant laboratory or operative procedures. An exception to this may be Hodgkin's disease, since establishing or ruling out Stage III disease (with a clinically normal spleen and a normal lymphogram) is essential and often cannot be accomplished without a laparotomy. On the other hand, in non-Hodgkin's lymphoma, which tends to disseminate early, the staging laparotomy has usually not been helpful in altering treatment decisions. In the staging of lung cancer, a gallium scan may detect mediastinal adenopathy if the primary tumor is gallium-positive. However, to determine the potential resectability of a paramediastinal primary in the lung a clear plane of resection between the tumor and the mediastinum may best be demonstrated pre-operatively by a high-quality CT scan.

The "superspecialized" radiologist today may sometimes only appreciate his or her own area of interest and, occasionally, time, expense and effort are wasted when this fact is ignored. For example, the neuroradiologist, neurosurgeon and neurologist may appreciate a posterior fossa lesion on CT scan in a patient with a prior history of lung cancer. Because there is no peri-focal edema seen, a primary brain tumor may be considered. On reviewing the record, however, the patient had required a pneumonectomy for a large, centrally-located lung tumor 18 months earlier. The lung cancer was poorly-differentiated and hilar adenopathy was present. Clearly, the brain lesion was a metastasis and an additional contrast-enhanced scan, angiogram, EEG, etc., were unnecessary. If the original primary tumor had been a 1 cm peripheral lesion in the lung or a Stage I carcinoma of the breast, a more detailed workup of the new lesion might have been indicated.

A common error in choosing diagnostic studies is the absence of a defined therapeutic goal. This is illustrated by the patient who initially presents with an enlarged neck node containing metastatic tumor. Of major importance is the location of the node and its histology. Nodes confined to the lower half of the neck usually are metastatic from below the clavicle: only a chest x-ray may be required in the asymptomatic patient who presents in this way. Usually, the histology of the metastatic tumor will be characteristic if the primary is in the thyroid. Multiple enlarged nodes in the posterior cervical chains are often lymphomatous or are metastatic from the nasopharynx. If metastatic squamous cell carcinoma is found in an anterior cervical chain and involves primarily the upper cervical nodes, panendoscopy of the upper airways with directed biopsies will be more productive than a host of laboratory studies.

Patterns of cancer spread are often predictable and may be related to the initial stage (and/or grade) of the primary tumor. A patient with low back pain and a history of prior abdominal-perineal resection for Stage B$_2$ or C adenocarcinoma of the rectum may be referred initially to a neurologist or an orthopedist, before the likelihood of recurrent cancer is appreciated. Similarly, in an older patient with acute back pain and without a diagnosed malignancy, a bone scan, skeletal survey, tomograms, myelogram, IVP and barium enema may be ordered before a complete pelvic exam is done in the female, or a rectal in the male, to identify a primary malignant tumor. Since local soft tissue recurrences of rectal carcinomas usually occur in the presacral space a pelvic CT scan should be the initial study when recurrence is suspected.

To encourage better communication, the request for a radiologic consultation should indicate at least whether the study is for:

1. Initial diagnosis   _____

    Regional staging   _____

    Investigating distant metastasis   _____

and 2. Whether the radiologic findings
        could preclude or influence
        surgery, radiotherapy, or
        chemotherapy   _____

To reiterate, tissue should usually be obtained to confirm a suspected diagnosis. Radiologic or laboratory procedures, or cytology alone are often not adequate for definitive diagnosis and staging. Finally, the information obtained becomes of practical use only when the laboratory, imaging and clinical findings together "make sense", and can be correlated with the known biologic behavior of a primary tumor.

Appendix

Illustrative "Decision-Trees" for Diagnosing and Staging Cancer

Richard J. Steckel and A. Robert Kagan

"Management algorithms" or decision-trees are currently in vogue in clinical medicine. Conceivably they might serve several purposes: (1) as teaching aids and as guidelines for clinical management for physicians-in-training, and sometimes for allied health personnel ("physician extenders", nurse specialists, etc.); (2) as protocol guides for clinical investigations; (3) as audit mechanisms for health planners, governmental agencies and private insurers. In this multi-authored volume which is concerned with recent advances in cancer diagnosis, it seemed reasonable to the editors initially to develop decision-trees for all major malignancies and common cancer-related diagnostic problems, by achieving some kind of editorial consensus among our contributing authors. This proved to be a very "tall task," and of course in practice it was not achievable. In making the attempt, however, we have learned something we should have known about the "better half" of human nature, and some very important lessons not only for the clinical care of patients who have cancer but for other diseases as well.

In the first place, among a panel of expert contributors from diverse disciplines, there can be no absolute consensus on an acceptable pattern of clinical care, including the "most appropriate" diagnostic work-up (decision-tree) for a particular form of cancer. "Majority rule" among professional experts may in fact not be in the patient's best interest, and the persuasiveness of a vocal advocate for a given diagnostic study may not be either. In everyday clinical situations involving patients, the editors have learned that there is no "right way" to diagnose cancer and to stage the disease. Some excellent decision-trees were submitted to us by individual contributors to this book. When circulated to the contributors of other chapters who are experts in different diagnostic modalities, there was a healthy "give-and-take" but no consensus as to the best decision-tree for a given malignancy or clinical situation. Reluctantly (but with inescapable logic) we have come to the conclusion that there can be no "prescription" for the most appropriate diagnostic and staging strategy in a specific patient, which can then be applied to all other patients who can be similarly characterized. There is too much variability between patients, between physicians, and between institutions to achieve that!

Accordingly, we have exercised "editorial prerogative" by tailoring several illustrative decision-trees to represent the views of the Editors while we acknowledge gratefully a large number of suggestions from our contributing authors. We have done this with two caveats in mind: (1) we definitely think it advisable for each oncologist and diagnostician to develop his/her own deductive approach for diagnosing and staging specific malignancies, an approach which can then be tailored to the needs of each individual patient; (2) as a direct corollary, the Editors take sole responsibility for the recommendations which are made in the illustrative decision-trees which follow; they do not represent the views of any one contributor, nor do they represent a "consensus" of our contributing authors for the reasons given. We earnestly recommend that each of you develop flexible diagnostic guidelines for different clinical situations, and that you make your own views well known to the professional colleagues and the patients with whom you interact. We have learned, and we hope you agree, that the patient will be the ultimate beneficiary of an open "marketplace of ideas" in which informed physicians from diverse disciplines actively participate. Given the varying diagnostic and therapeutic disciplines which must be brought to bear upon each cancer patient and the unforeseen differences that obtain between patients, it is clear that one "decision-tree" for a given clinical presentation will never suffice!

The following illustrative decision trees have been included here:

1. Hodgkin's Disease: Diagnosis and Staging
2. Non-Hodgkin's Lymphoma
3. Imaging Techniques in Breast Cancer Diagnosis and Staging
4. Radiologic Evaluation of Renal Mass
5. Radiologic Evaluation of Suspected Space-Occupying Lesion(s)
        in the Liver
6. Painless Jaundice
7. Workup for Suspected Pancreatic Cancer
8. Persistent Obstructive Pneumonia or Atelectasis on Chest X-Rays
        (Tumor Suspected)
9. Solitary Pulmonary Nodule (or Lung Mass) on Plain Radiographs:
        Tumor Suspected

- The Editors

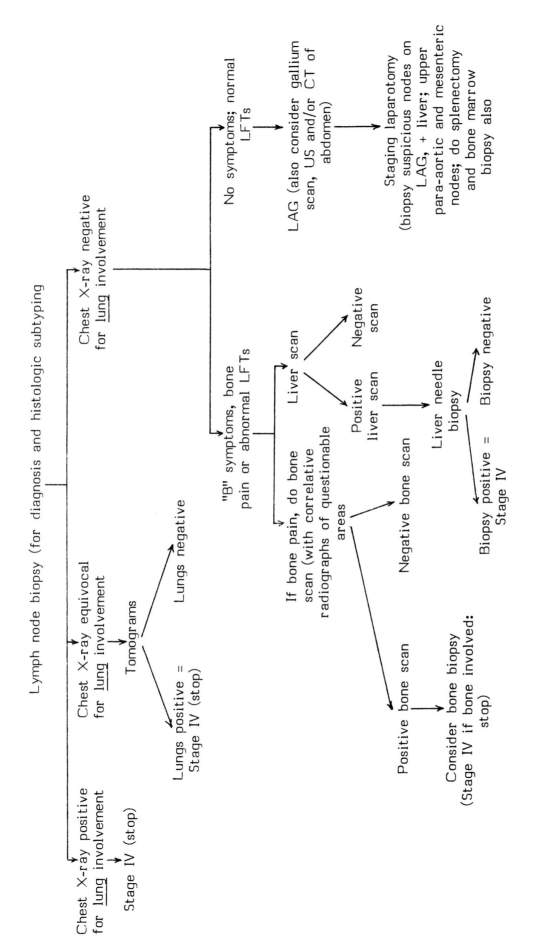

Hodgkin's Disease: Diagnosis and Staging

Therapeutic goals for staging:
Stages I, II, IIIA are treated by radiation
Stages IIIB and IV receive chemotherapy at most centers (supplemental radiotherapy may be indicated)
(Laparotomy not required if need for chemotherapy has been established)

KEY: LAG = Lymphangiogram
      LFTs = Liver Function Tests
      US   = Ultrasound
      CT   = Computerized (body) Tomograms

326

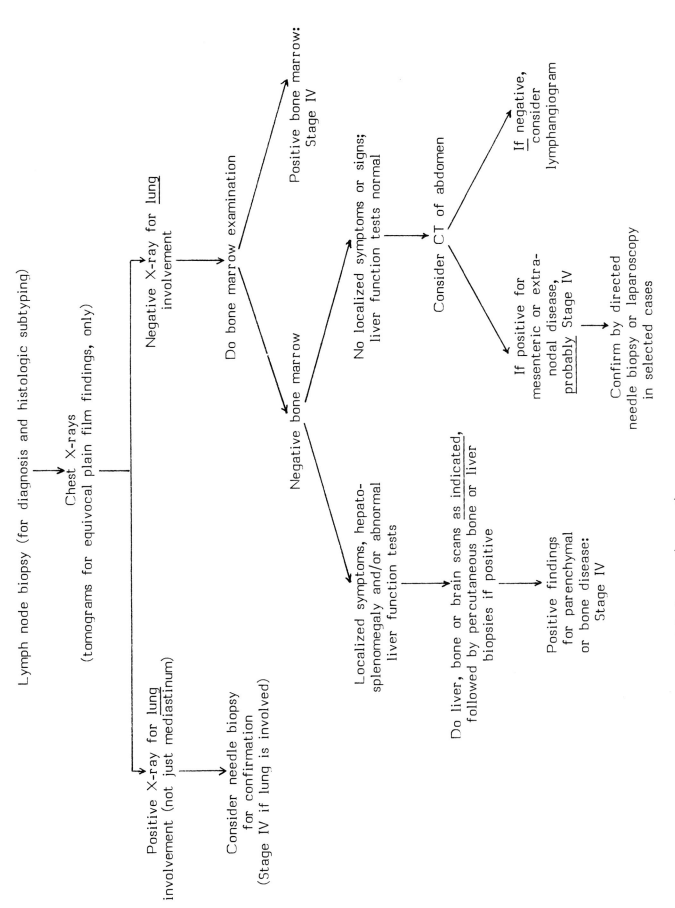

Non-Hodgkin's Lymphoma*

Lymph node biopsy (for diagnosis and histologic subtyping)

Chest X-rays
(tomograms for equivocal plain film findings, only)

Positive X-ray for lung involvement (not just mediastinum)

Consider needle biopsy for confirmation (Stage IV if lung is involved)

Negative X-ray for lung involvement

Do bone marrow examination

Positive bone marrow: Stage IV

Negative bone marrow

No localized symptoms or signs; liver function tests normal

Consider CT of abdomen

If negative, consider lymphangiogram

If positive for mesenteric or extra-nodal disease, probably Stage IV

Confirm by directed needle biopsy or laparoscopy in selected cases

Localized symptoms, hepato-splenomegaly and/or abnormal liver function tests

Do liver, bone or brain scans as indicated, followed by percutaneous bone or liver biopsies if positive

Positive findings for parenchymal or bone disease: Stage IV

*Not applicable for primary extranodal disease (unusual)

327

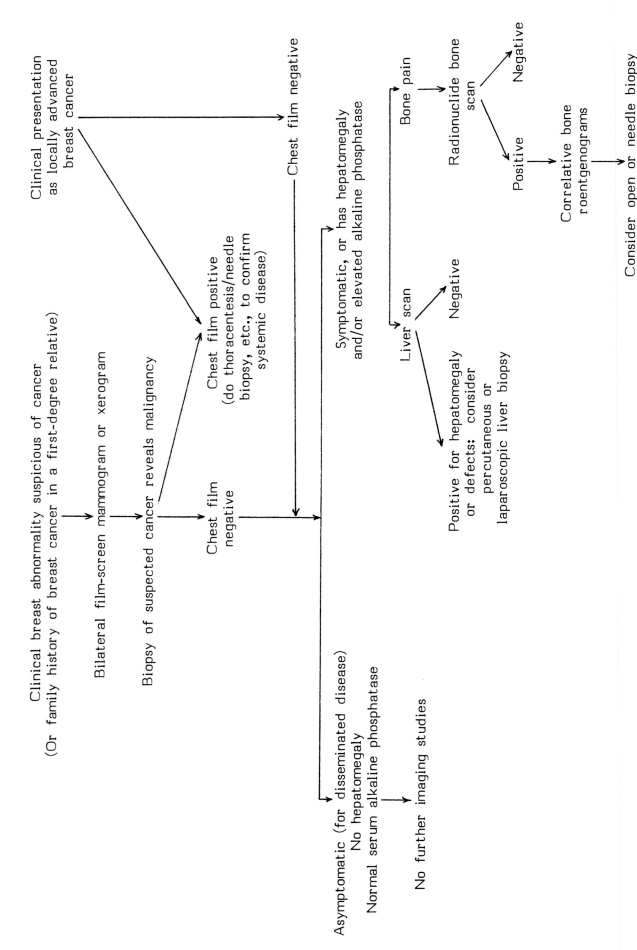

Imaging Techniques in Breast Cancer Diagnosis and Staging

Clinical presentation as locally advanced breast cancer

Clinical breast abnormality suspicious of cancer
(Or family history of breast cancer in a first-degree relative)

Bilateral film-screen mammogram or xerogram

Biopsy of suspected cancer reveals malignancy

Chest film positive
(do thoracentesis/needle biopsy, etc., to confirm systemic disease)

Chest film negative

Chest film negative

Symptomatic, or has hepatomegaly and/or elevated alkaline phosphatase

Bone pain

Radionuclide bone scan

Negative

Positive

Correlative bone roentgenograms

Consider open or needle biopsy if bone involvement is equivocal

Liver scan

Negative

Positive for hepatomegaly or defects: consider percutaneous or laparoscopic liver biopsy

Asymptomatic (for disseminated disease)
No hepatomegaly
Normal serum alkaline phosphatase

No further imaging studies

328

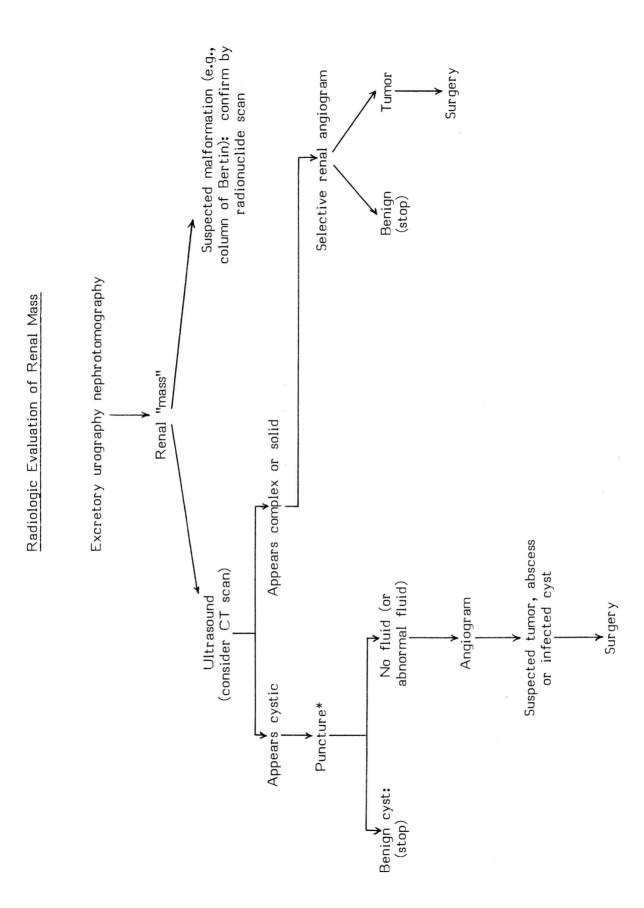

Radiologic Evaluation of Renal Mass

Excretory urography nephrotomography

Renal "mass"

Suspected malformation (e.g., column of Bertin): confirm by radionuclide scan

Ultrasound (consider CT scan)

Appears complex or solid

Selective renal angiogram

Tumor → Surgery

Benign (stop)

Appears cystic

Puncture*

No fluid (or abnormal fluid) → Angiogram → Suspected tumor, abscess or infected cyst → Surgery

Benign cyst: (stop)

*To remove fluid for analysis and introduce radiologic contrast into the cyst.

329

Radiologic Evaluation of Suspected Space-Occupying Lesion(s) in the Liver
(Clinical hepatomegaly, elevated serum alkaline phosphatase, etc.)

Liver scan (colloid)

Normal → Periodic follow-up scans, if indicated

Positive (for space-occupying lesion(s)) → Ultrasound

Ultrasound → Normal

Ultrasound → Solid or complex mass → hepatic angiogram

Ultrasound → Cystic lesion → Puncture diagnostically for fluid (or stop)

hepatic angiogram → Hemangioma: stop

hepatic angiogram → Hypervascular lesion(s) → Open biopsy (or laparoscopy for superficial lesion(s)

hepatic angiogram → Hypovascular lesion(s) → Guided needle biopsy (proceed to open biopsy, if unsuccessful)

Painless Jaundice

Ultrasound

→ Bile ducts dilated (obstructive jaundice; note that biliary calculi or pancreatic mass may also be evident on ultrasound)

→ Bile ducts normal (probable hepatocellular disease)

Radionuclide (colloid) liver scan

→ Negative for parenchymal deposits → Transhepatic cholangiography

→ Multiple rounded defects: probable liver metastases

Transhepatic cholangiography:

→ Tumor obstructing major duct(s) → Consider ERCP, CT and/or angiography to delineate local tumor extent and involvement of adjacent organs and great vessels

→ Percutaneous needle biopsy for clearly non-resectable tumors → Consider percutaneous biliary drainage or diversion procedure, if indicated

→ Surgery if resection feasible or if an operative diversion is needed

→ Common duct stone(s) or benign stricture → Surgery and/or biliary drainage

331

Workup for Suspected Pancreatic Cancer

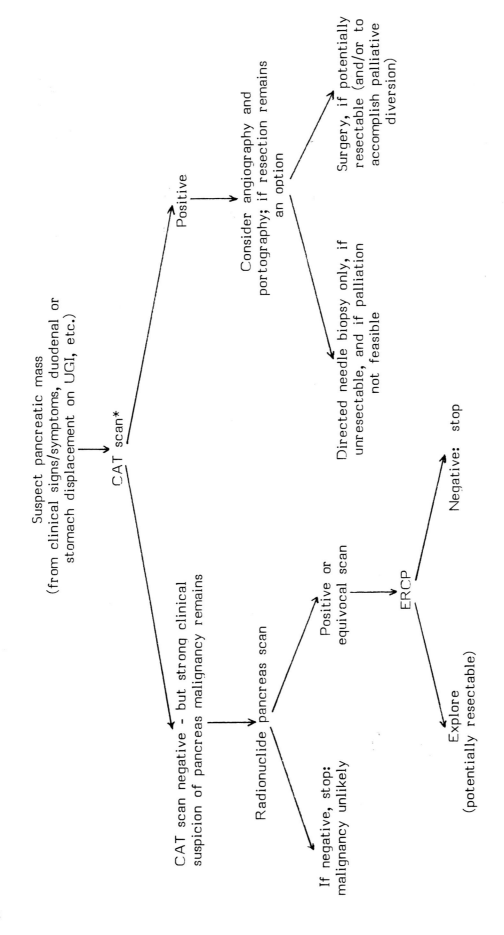

Suspect pancreatic mass
(from clinical signs/symptoms, duodenal or stomach displacement on UGI, etc.)

CAT scan*

Positive

Consider angiography and portography; if resection remains an option

Surgery, if potentially resectable (and/or to accomplish palliative diversion)

Directed needle biopsy only, if unresectable, and if palliation not feasible

CAT scan negative - but strong clinical suspicion of pancreas malignancy remains

Radionuclide pancreas scan

Positive or equivocal scan

ERCP

Negative: stop

Explore (potentially resectable)

If negative, stop: malignancy unlikely

*Ultrasound may give complementary information in cachetic patients (no retroperitoneal fat)

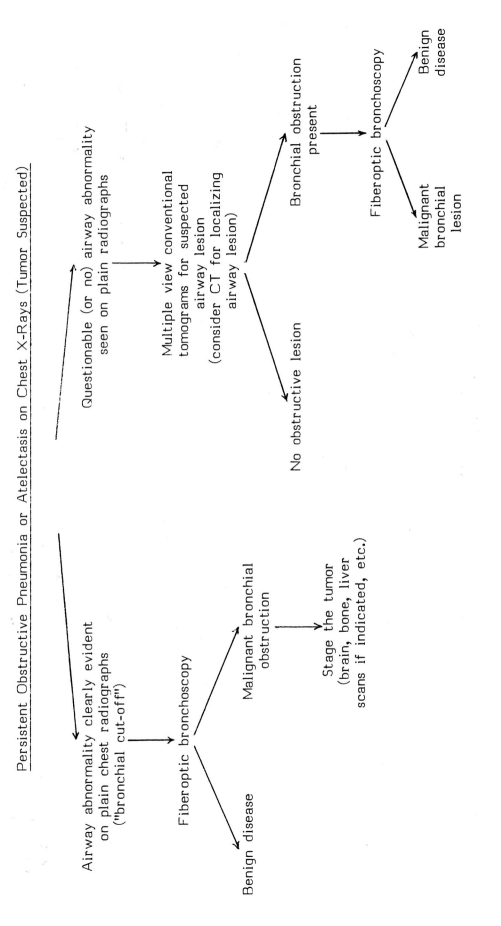

Persistent Obstructive Pneumonia or Atelectasis on Chest X-Rays (Tumor Suspected)

Airway abnormality clearly evident on plain chest radiographs ("bronchial cut-off")

Questionable (or no) airway abnormality seen on plain radiographs

Fiberoptic bronchoscopy

Multiple view conventional tomograms for suspected airway lesion (consider CT for localizing airway lesion)

Malignant bronchial obstruction

Benign disease

No obstructive lesion

Bronchial obstruction present

Stage the tumor (brain, bone, liver scans if indicated, etc.)

Fiberoptic bronchoscopy

Benign disease

Malignant bronchial lesion

Solitary Pulmonary Nodule (or Lung Mass) On Plain Radiographs: Tumor Suspected

Nodule contains "benign calcification(s): granuloma or hamartoma

No Ca++ (or small asymmetric ca++ within nodule)

Obtain old chest radiographs

Old films unavailable

Consider CT (for nodule density)

possibly malignant

probably benign

Growth observed within 2 years

No nodule growth for over 2 years

Benign

Do low kVp plain film and/or coned-down conventional tomograms

Benign-type Ca++ (benign lesion)

No ca++ (possibly malignant)

Do percutaneous aspiration biopsy

No definite diagnosis

Specific benign diagnosis

Malignant diagnosis

Determine intrathoracic extent (to determine operability, resectability)

Consider Mediastinoscopy

Consider gallium scan (for mediastinal involvement)

Multiple-view conventional tomograms (include full-lung and mediastinal tomograms)

CT (for extra-parenchymal extension)

Surgery, if disease is localized and potentially resectable

334

Index